DIABETES COMPLICATING PREGNANCY

DIABETES COMPLICATING PREGNANCY

The Joslin Clinic Method

Second Edition

Editors

Florence M. Brown, MD
John W. Hare, MD

WILEY-LISS
A JOHN WILEY & SONS, INC., PUBLICATION
New York • Chichester • Brisbane • Toronto • Singapore

Address All Inquiries to the Publisher
Wiley-Liss, Inc., 605 Third Avenue, New York, NY 10158-0012

Copyright © 1995 Wiley-Liss, Inc.

Printed in the United States of America

Under the conditions stated below the owner of copyright for this book hereby grants permission to users to make photocopy reproductions of any part or all of its contents for personal or internal organizational use, or for personal or internal use of specific clients. This consent is given on the condition that the copier pay the stated per-copy fee through the Copyright Clearance Center, Incorporated, 27 Congress Street, Salem, MA 01970, as listed in the most current issue of "Permissions to Photocopy" (Publisher's Fee List, distributed by CCC, Inc.), for copying beyond that permitted by sections 107 or 108 of the US Copyright Law. This consent does not extend to other kinds of copying, such as copying for general distribution, for advertising or promotional purposes, for creating new collective works, or for resale.

While the authors, editors, and publisher believe that drug selection and dosage and the specification and usage of equipment and devices, as set forth in this book, are in accord with current recommendations and practice at the time of publication, they accept no legal responsibility for any errors or omissions, and make no warranty, express or implied, with respect to material contained herein. In view of ongoing research, equipment modifications, changes in governmental regulations and the constant flow of information relating to drug therapy, drug reactions, and the use of equipment and devices, the reader is urged to review and evaluate the information provided in the package insert or instructions for each drug, piece of equipment, or device for, among other things, any changes in the instructions or indication of dosage or usage and for added warnings and precautions.

Library of Congress Cataloging-in-Publication Data

Diabetes complicating pregnancy : the Joslin Clinic method. — 2nd ed.
/ editors, Florence M. Brown, John W. Hare.
p. cm.
Includes bibliographical references and index.
ISBN 0-471-11031-0 (cloth : alk. paper)
1. Diabetes in pregnancy. I. Brown, Florence M., 1957– .
II. Hare, John W.
[DNLM: 1. Pregnancy in Diabetes. WQ 248 D53545 1995]
RG580.D5D519 1995
618.3—dc20
DNLM/DLC
for Library of Congress 95-8383

The text of this book is printed on acid-free paper.

To my mother Evelyn, with whom I share so many interests and passions, and her mother Anna Lerner—FMB

To the late Norbert Freinkel and to Boyd Metzger, who engendered my interest in Diabetes Complicating Pregnancy—JWH

CANTERBURY CHRIST CHURCH COLLEGE	
360411979	
Library Services UK	16/09/97
618.3DIA	£70.00

Contents

Contributors

David B. Acker, MD, Department of Obstetrics and Gynecology, Brigham and Women's Hospital, Boston, MA 02115

Vanessa A. Barss, MD, Department of Obstetrics and Gynecology, Brigham and Women's Hospital, Boston, MA 02115

Anna Maria Bertorelli, MBA, RD, Joslin Diabetes Center, One Joslin Place, Boston, MA 02215

Robert N. Blatman, MD, Vincent Memorial Obstetrics Division, Massachusetts General Hospital, Boston, MA 02114

Florence M. Brown, MD, Joslin Diabetes Center, One Joslin Place, Boston, MA 02215

John P. Cloherty, MD, Department of Neonatology, Brigham and Women's Hospital, Boston, MA 02215

Suzanne Z. Ghiloni, BSN, CDE, Joslin Diabetes Center, One Joslin Place, Boston, MA 02215

Michael F. Greene, MD, Vincent Memorial Obstetrics Division, Massachusetts General Hospital, Boston, MA 02114

John W. Hare, MD, Joslin Diabetes Center, One Joslin Place, Boston, MA 02215

Linda J. Heffner, MD, PhD, Department of Obstetrics and Gynecology, Brigham and Women's Hospital, Boston, MA 02115

Elisabeth Kay, MSW, 50 Winchester Street, Brookline MA 02146

Aviva Lee-Parritz, MD, Department of Obstetrics and Gynecology, Brigham and Women's Hospital, Boston, MA 02115

Catherine A. Mullooly, MS, Joslin Diabetes Center, One Joslin Place, Boston, MA 02215

Timothy J. Murtha, MD, Joslin Diabetes Center, One Joslin Place, Boston, MA 02215

Preface

Priscilla White first worked for Elliott Joslin as a medical student and in 1924 joined the staff of what was to become the Joslin Clinic. Dr. White had an early interest in diabetes in children and in pregnancy. Joslin had written a little about diabetic pregnancy, but Priscilla White took a life-long interest in the field and became the doyenne of diabetic pregnancy. Her first chapter on the subject, "Diabetes in Pregnancy," appeared in 1928 in the Fourth Edition of the Joslin text, *The Treatment of Diabetes Mellitus*. Her last chapter, "Pregnancy and Diabetes," appeared in the eleventh edition of *Joslin's Diabetes Mellitus*, reprinted in 1973.

For over fifty years, she devoted her career at the Joslin Clinic to the topic and almost singlehandedly elevated it to a subdiscipline of diabetes. As a result, the American Diabetes Association now has a Council on Pregnancy with a substantial number of members, all evincing an interest in what was a virtual nonentity when Dr. White began to construct this field of study.

Over time, Dr. White was assisted by many diabetologists, and she had several obstetrical colleagues as well. Throughout her half-century at the Joslin Clinic she was the leader of the pregnancy service, and therefore it was the geographic focus for diabetic obstetrical care, regardless of which Boston area hospital was being used for the deliveries. For many years the Boston-Lying-In Hospital as used for deliveries, but it has since merged twice, first to become the Boston Hospital for Women, and, more recently, to become part of the Brigham and Women's Hospital.

Priscilla White's half century of leadership of the Joslin Pregnancy Clinic ended in 1974. After that time, the modern era of obstetrical management began. In 1975 new techniques of fetal surveillance were instituted. During the latter half of the 1970s medical and neonatal management techniques also improved, and there was a clear-cut reduction in perinatal mortality to what it is today.

The successful management of these high-risk pregnancies is a result of the collegial efforts of many highly trained subspecialists. We always had been diabetologists, but now the obstetricians are perinatologists; the pediatricians are neonatologists; the nurtritionists and nurse educators are specifically identified for the pregnancy clinic; there is a fetal ultrasonographer and a perinatal social worker is part of the team. There is too much specialized knowledge for a member of a single discipline to do justice to the others and it is the recognition of the skills of many that leads to the use of all in a joint effort to complete a pregnancy with a healthy mother and infant. Unfortunately the recent trend away from specialization threatens the successful outcome of these high-risk pregnancies. More and more women with pregestational diabetes are consigned to care from a less-experienced primary care provider by their health maintenance organization (HMO). Some HMO's do not have a perinatologist on staff. Many local hospitals do not have on-site neonatal intensive care units.

We cannot overemphasize the need for a collegial effort with free communication between all those involved. As an outgrowth of Priscilla White's central role, the antenatal clinic at the Joslin Clinic meets every Tuesday morning with all participants present. We think this is one of the secrets of our success with a difficult patient population. The clinic accepts all comers, patients with stable or unstable diabetes, complicated or not, and with varying psychosocial wherewithal to manage an arduous and sometimes frightening experience. All members of the staff are in sight and hearing of one another, and any problem, small or large, can be communicated before the opportunity is lost and the situation is fogotten or imprecisely recalled.

It is the pluralistic professional interaction that we especially recommend to clinicians, although we recognize that specialists and subspecialists are not available everywhere. This book is meant to provide those faced with the challenge of managing diabetic pregnancies with a concise practical manual; it is not intended to be a repository of all that is known about the biology of diabetic pregnancy. It is a book that addresses in a straightforwad manner what the clinician needs to know.

Florence M. Brown, MD
John W. Hare, MD

SECTION I

METABOLIC CONSIDERATIONS

CHAPTER 1

Pathophysiology

John W. Hare, MD and Florence M. Brown, MD

INTRODUCTION

This chapter on the pathophysiology of the metabolism of diabetes and pregnancy draws heavily from two Banting Memorial lectures delivered to the American Diabetes Association. The first of these was by George F. Cahill, Jr. (1971) and was entitled "Physiology of Insulin in Man."[1] This excellent treatise summarizes the physiology of insulin in the nonpregnant state. The other Banting Memorial lecture was entitled "Of Pregnancy and Progeny" and was delivered by Norbert Freinkel in 1980.[2] His lecture summarizes the physiological alterations that occur during normal pregnancy as well as the alterations in physiology seen in diabetic pregnancy and elucidates how insulin secretion is perturbed.

Normal Nonpregnant Physiology

Insulin is the preeminent controller of fuel storage, release, and consumption in mammalian systems. Its levels are low during the fasted state and high in the fed state. These levels affect the availability of fuel endogenously and the storage of fuel when calories are supplied exogenously. Cahill pointed out that, in a teleologic sense, man is a mobile hunter, so that excess food, whether it is carbohydrate, protein, or fat, is all stored as fat, which is the most economical method of caloric storage. Protein is conserved to provide mobility. To meet these ends, he pointed out that there are principles, which he entitled "Rules of the Game," that humans and

Diabetes Complicating Pregnancy: The Joslin Clinic Method, Edited by Florence M. Brown, MD and John W. Hare, MD.
ISBN 0-471-11031-0 © 1995 John Wiley & Sons, Inc.

other mammals must follow, and that insulin ensures adherence to these rules. They are:

1. Plasma glucose must be maintained within narrow limits.
2. An optimal storage of glycogen must be maintained as an emergency fuel.
3. An optimal supply of protein must be maintained for use in enzymatic mechanisms of metabolism as well as for muscular mobility. Excess protein is ultimately converted to fat and the nitrogen released by the metabolism of amino acids is excreted in the urine.
4. Protein must be conserved when it is scarce and stored fat used in times of caloric need.

Human beings have a minimum glucose requirement of about 200 g per day. One hundred fifty grams are used by the central nervous system and the remaining 50 g are used by cells in the hematopoietic system and the renal medulla. All of these tissues are obligatory users of glucose. The central nervous system is capable of oxidizing glucose irreversibly to carbon dioxide but the other tissues oxidize it only to lactate. Lactate may be converted to pyruvate and reutilized, since two pyruvate molecules can be combined to form a glucose molecule. This is known as the Cori cycle and serves to preserve glucose moieties. Several hours after a meal, during what is termed the postabsorptive state, glucose needs are met from glycogen stores. If food is withheld for a longer period, a fasting state ensues and glucose is supplied by de novo synthesis from stored protein, a process termed gluconeogenesis.

If small amounts of glucose are ingested in a quantity sufficient to meet obligatory needs, sufficient insulin is secreted to limit glycemia and gluconeogenesis, thus sparing protein and limiting the amount of nitrogen that must be excreted in the urine. There is also decreased hepatic output of glucose from glycogenolysis. These mechanisms comply with rules 1, 2, and 3 above. Rule 4 (protein conservation and fat storage and use) is complied with when large amounts of glucose are ingested. Insulin is secreted in even greater amounts and there is not only a suppression of hepatic output but also a promotion of peripheral glucose uptake at higher insulin concentrations. The liver takes up only a small amount of glucose, but muscle takes up a larger amount and is able to oxidize it. Even more important, excess glucose is converted to fat and stored.

Fat is an extremely efficient form of caloric storage. Not only does each gram of fat contain nine calories as a theoretical yield, but its actual storage capacity is eight calories per gram. Thus, a large number of calories can be stored in a small amount of tissue. By comparison, use of glycogen as a fuel storage mechanism would be far less practical. While carbohydrate has a theoretical yield of four calories per gram, glycogen itself, because of its water content, actually yields only one calorie per gram. Thus, to store a large number of calories in anticipation of a time of privation would require an enormous amount of storage tissue.

INSULIN SECRETION

It is most important to understand that insulin secretion by the beta cell is central to this scheme. The beta cell must rapidly assess the glucose load that has been presented to it and make arrangements for its prompt disposal. In fact, insulin secretion occurs in less than a minute when glucose levels rise, and peripheral uptake of glucose occurs in less than 10 minutes. Thus, it can be noted that early release of insulin is essential for normal glucose tolerance. At the time of ingestion of a full meal, when insulin secretion is at its highest, fat is stored by several mechanisms. The first is glucose uptake and conversion to lipid. Second is the storage of dietary fat obtained from the meal. Third, and also important, is the slowing of lipolysis by higher insulin levels. Since an ordinary meal contains protein, it is necessary to recognize what happens during protein feeding. As protein is degraded into its constituent amino acid building blocks for entry into the circulation, insulin secretion is stimulated by these amino acids. One might expect at this point that blood sugar would fall if only protein were ingested because of the rising insulin. This does not occur, however, because glucagon, which stimulates gluconeogenesis and glycogenolysis, is also stimulated by amino acids derived from dietary protein. Thus, the blood glucose does not change. This again complies with rule 1. When carbohydrate is also in the meal, as is typically the case, the rising glucose level diminishes glucagon release. Moreover, glucose and amino acid synergistically tend to increase insulin, thus diminishing the liver's need to produce glucose when carbohydrate has been added to the meal.

PROTEIN CONSERVATION

During fasting, liver glycogen is depleted and hepatic gluconeogenesis is activated. Glucose is synthesized from amino acid building blocks released by muscle when insulin is low, as is the case during fasting. This provides glucose for the obligatory needs of the organism. During feeding, the high insulin level promotes amino acid uptake by muscle and protein synthesis to comply with rules 3 and 4, i.e., to maintain an optimal supply of protein and conserve protein for fasting. Thus, insulin is a regulator of protein metabolism and conservation. It is also of interest to note that exercise tends to inhibit the breakdown of protein; thus, it is helpful in diabetes. During fasting, the muscles compete with one another because the more active ones are less proteolytic. Thus, the muscles most used for mobility are protected and comply with teleology. Excess protein in the diet results in conversion to fat, not in increased muscle mass. The above mechanisms are semiquantitatively summarized in Table I. Also included in this table is the effect of diabetes (absence of insulin) on carbohydrate economy.

During fasting, muscle preferentially releases alanine and glutamine for gluconeogenesis. The energy for gluconeogenesis by the liver is provided by free fatty acid oxidation. When insulin is low, lipolysis is permitted to proceed at a rapid rate so that free fatty acids will be available for the liver to use as its own fuel source while converting amino acids into glucose. The oxidation of fatty acids generates ketones, which cause a mild ketoacidosis. As the pH falls a bit, the liver tends to reject glutamine as a gluconeogenic precursor, enabling the kidney to use it as a source of ammonia to titrate the ketoacids and maintain the renal role in acid–base balance. During fasting, the kidney is also capable of gluconeogenesis from glutamine so that this diversion from the liver serves a dual purpose.

Insulin has a ubiquitous effect on protein. Not only does it control its rates of synthesis and release in the muscle, it also tends to reshuffle the amino acids that are released by the muscle during fasting. This is why the muscle preferentially releases alanine and glutamine during fasting.

TABLE I. Insulin and Glucagon Levels and Hepatic Glucose Production under Various Metabolic Conditions*

Meal	Insulin level	Glucagon level	Hepatic glucose production
None	+	+	+
Small carbohydrate	++	±	0
Large carbohydrate	+++	±	0
Protein	++	++	+
Protein and carbohydrate	++++	±	0
Prolonged fast	±	++	+
Diabetes	0	++++	+++

*Adapted from Cahill GF, Jr: Physiology of insulin in man. Diabetes 20:791, 1971, with permission of the American Diabetes Association, Inc.

Therefore, the mechanism is very finely tuned and insulin is the prepotent hormone for protein metabolism. It is also of interest that insulin is required for protein synthesis during lactation.

Muscle is more sensitive than fat to low insulin levels. Its catabolic threshold occurs at a lower insulin concentration than fat. This means that a very low level of insulin will prevent the breakdown of protein and only a modestly increased level of insulin will begin to promote synthesis. The same low level of insulin that occurs during fasting and prevents protein breakdown, however, allows lipolysis to occur so that fat is provided as an alternate fuel for most of the body. The catabolic thresholds are altered by ketoacidosis, trauma, and pregnancy. Thus pregnancy, which is associated with higher insulin levels than in the nonpregnant state, also exhibits alterations in tissue sensitivity and, hence, intermediary metabolism.

During fasting, a low insulin level spares glucose by decreasing muscle uptake of glucose and decreasing glucose oxidation because the hexokinase enzyme system atrophies. This enzyme system is necessary for the entry of glucose into oxidative pathways. This is also the reason why abnormal glucose tolerance may occur during fasting. Ingested glucose is unable to be oxidized because of the atrophied hexokinase system and, thus, glucose disposal is slowed. During prolonged fasting, the central nervous system is able to use the ketones β-hydroxybutyrate and acetoacetate as fuel. This further serves to spare glucose and actually diminishes the daily obligatory need for it. Because glucose is spared, protein is spared, since amino acids are the only source of glucose during fasting.

Diabetes is the equivalent of a "superfasted" state. The lack of insulin permits the metabolic machinery to run at a faster rate and catabolism (tissue breakdown) to predominate over anabolism (tissue synthesis). All of the foregoing refers to the nonpregnant state.

PREGNANCY PHYSIOLOGY

In the pregnant state, the teleologic emphasis changes. The mother must reorder her priorities so that not only are her needs met but also those of the growing fetus. Therefore, alterations are made in normal metabolic mechanisms to protect both.

Freinkel[2] emphasized three important events that occur when the conceptus (placenta and fetus) is grafted onto the maternal organism. They are:

1. The conceptus becomes an additional site for the metabolism of maternal hormones.

2. The conceptus becomes a new site for hormone biosynthesis.
3. By its own growth, the conceptus alters maternal fuel economy.

During pregnancy, insulin secretion increases approximately twofold by the third trimester. Despite the increase in insulin secretion, it has a diminished effectiveness in the periphery for the mother. The hormonal changes responsible for this insulin resistance are increasing levels of estrogen, progesterone, and especially human placental lactogen (hPL), also known as human chorionic somatomammotropin.

hPL is a polypeptide hormone, produced by syncytiotrophoblast cells of the placenta. It is closely related to human growth hormone (hGH) and human prolactin (hPRL), sharing 87% of its 191 amino acids with hGH and 35% with hPRL.[3–5] As a result of an enlarging placenta, hPL increases linearly, reaching its maximum concentration in the maternal circulation at approximately 38 weeks gestation and then declining just prior to delivery.[6] In the mother, these increasing levels of hPL are responsible for peripheral insulin resistance, hyperinsulinemia, and carbohydrate intolerance.[7,8]

In the fasting state, when insulin levels are low, hPL enhances lipolysis[9] and, hence, the production of free fatty acids. Free fatty acids are used as an alternate fuel source for the mother, while glucose and amino acids are spared for the obligatory needs of the conceptus. The passage of glucose across the placenta (by facilitated diffusion) and amino acids (by active transport) results in maternal hypoglycemia, hypoalaninemia, and (because of enhanced lipolysis) hyperketonemia. This triad of alterations during the fasting state in pregnancy has been called "accelerated starvation" by Freinkel,[10] and is apparent after 12–16 hours of fasting.[11]

If accelerated starvation were the only newly operative mechanism during pregnancy, teleology would not be well served because the mother would be the continual loser in the metabolic tug-of-war with her offspring. Therefore, "facilitated anabolism" has also been described by Freinkel and coworkers.[12] After the oral ingestion of a 100 g glucose load in pregnant women, they noted that there was an increase in the levels of glucose as well as insulin, an increase in the levels of triglyceride, and a suppression of glucagon. This meant that there was more glucose available for the fetus, more lipid available for the mother as triglyceride, since it crosses the placenta very poorly, and less stimulus to drive maternal gluconeogenesis, glycogenolysis, and ketogenesis. There was also a small decrease in levels of hPL, which stimulates lipolysis, thus resulting in less lipolysis in the fed state in a pregnant woman. From the above, it can also be seen that there are greater oscillations in glucose and insulin levels during pregnancy when compared to the nonpregnant state. In this sense, Cahill's first rule is bent a bit. Clinically, there needs to be special attention paid to insulin treatment of the pregnant woman, because her insulin needs are different than when she is not pregnant.

Freinkel and Metzger also viewed the fetus as a natural tissue-culture experiment whose substrate availability is under placental control.[13] The available fuels are: glucose, which, although provided by facilitated diffusion, does have a saturable maximum transport; amino acids (neutral and basic), whose active transport is proportional to their concentration; and glycerol and ketones, which are provided to the fetus in proportion to maternal levels. Free fatty acids are available for utilization by the placenta, although they cross to the fetal side in only small quantities. Nonetheless, essential fatty acids are available for use by the conceptus.

Insulin is the ultimate arbiter of both the fed and fasting states during pregnancy, just as it is in the nonpregnant state, so any disturbance in insulin secretory dynamics will alter the fuel mix and alter what is available to the fetus.

INSULIN NEED

There are three levels of insulin deficit in diabetic pregnancies. The mildest of these is the woman with gestational diabetes whose only manifestation is an abnormal glucose tolerance test. The fasting state glucoses are normal, but after a glucose load or mixed meal, glucose levels are higher, indicating underutilization of glucose. If the insulin deficit is a bit more severe, the fasting plasma glucose will rise, signifying overproduction of glucose because the elevation occurs in the absence of a meal. Both of these conditions can occur in gestational diabetes, which is a relatively mild disturbance of maternal metabolism (see Chapter 2).

Insulin-dependent diabetes mellitus (IDDM), also known as Type I diabetes mellitus, occurs when there is almost total absence of insulin as a result of the autoimmune destruction of the pancreatic beta cells.[14–16] Infiltration of these beta cells by lymphocytes is termed "insulitis" and precedes the development of IDDM by years. The presence of autoantibodies to various target antigens such as insulin,[17] glutamic acid decarboxylase,[18] and islet cell cytoplasmic antigens[19] predict the development of IDDM in genetically susceptible individuals.

IDDM is a disease of polygenic inheritance. Major genetic susceptibility is conferred by the Class II histocompatibility immune response genes DR and DQ located on the short arm of chromosome 6.[20] Changes in the amino acid sequences of these antigen-presenting molecules may determine either protection from or susceptibility to IDDM. Recent studies indicate that several other genetic loci on different chromosomes show evidence of linkage to the disease.[21,22] This explains why IDDM tends to cluster in families but simple single-gene Mendelian inheritance is not observed. It is possible that in a genetically susceptible individual, exposure to an undefined environmental trigger (i.e., virus, food antigen) may then initiate the autoimmune process. As a result, there is gradual beta cell loss occurring over a period of years. Insulin release, which is normal early in this process, declines until finally hyperglycemia is present.

In the setting of pregnancy, if insulin is insufficiently available, it is impossible to properly balance the concepts of accelerated starvation and facilitated anabolism, which normally occur during pregnancy. This means that the heightened oscillations of glucose and other substrates that normally occur during a pregnancy cannot be properly regulated, because under normal pregnant conditions extra insulin is available to promote facilitated anabolism and to keep the phenomenon of accelerated starvation from being too severe.

Not only are special hormonal mechanisms necessary for the proper growth and development of the fetus, but undue damage to the mother is difficult to prevent because all of Cahill's rules are violated. Pregnancy does not allow glucose to be maintained within quite such narrow limits as in the nonpregnant state, but the absence of insulin in IDDM precludes glucose being maintained at anywhere near the appropriate levels. Because of the insulin lack, the optimal amount of glycogen will no longer be available as an emergency fuel, since the mother's glucose will be continually drained by the fetus. She also will be unable to maintain an optimal protein supply and to properly conserve it without the effect of insulin helping to offset the effect of hPL. Particular attention to the replacement regimen of insulin therapy is needed to mimic normal physiology as closely as possible.

LABOR

There is one late event in pregnancy that is also worthy of mention. This event is labor and it is of interest what happens to insulin requirements during that time. It has been emphasized that throughout pregnancy the insulin needs of the mother are increased. There is extra endogenous insulin available in normal pregnancies, as well as an extra exogenous requirement for insulin-dependent women. However, it has been shown that the maternal insulin requirement during labor dramatically diminishes.[23,24] Women in labor who are known to require insulin have been studied while on a continuously monitored system with an algorithm for infusing glucose and insulin as needed. Some of these patients have required no insulin for hours during labor, despite their clearly documented clinical state of insulin deficiency (IDDM). Part of this lack of insulin need has been ascribed to the increased consumption of glucose by both uterine and skeletal muscle. Nonetheless, it seems surprising that the insulin requirement would actually disappear, since this is not the usual state during nonpregnant exercise.

POSTPARTUM

It has long been known that within the first day of delivery, women with IDDM have a marked sensitivity to exogenous insulin. This change is particularly dramatic because their insulin requirements have gradually increased during their pregnancy and may be twice as great as in their prepregnant requirement. On the day of delivery, their insulin requirement is typically less than half of their prepregnant requirement, and thus an even smaller fraction of their insulin requirement from their last pregnant day. The reason for this sudden marked sensitivity to insulin is not clear.

It is obvious that at the time of delivery not only the fetus is expelled, but so is the placenta and, therefore, this source of hormonal production is lost. As stated earlier, both placental steroid and peptide hormones have contrainsulin properties. It is also known that human placental lactogen, estrogen, and progesterone rapidly clear the circulation after delivery and have greatly diminished concentrations or are even undetectable within hours.[25]

It has been suggested that women in the postpartum period are relatively hypopituitary. In fact, there are data showing that women in the immediate puerperium have blunted gonadotropin and growth hormone secretory responses when stimulation is attempted.[26] One possible explanation for this is the observation that growth hormone, placental lactogen, and prolactin have some similarity to one another and share structural and physiologic characteristics. It has been suggested that maternal growth hormone secretory capability is blunted because of the high levels of hPL and hPRL in the circulation. After delivery, the abrupt disappearance of hPL from the maternal circulation leaves the mother without its contrainsulin effect and in a relatively growth hormone deficient state not unlike hypopituitarism.

Also unclear and even less well studied is what may or may not happen to insulin expression at the cellular level. Studies of insulin receptor population and binding[27] have been done during pregnancy but the results of different investigators have been at variance with one another. Moreover, different tissues have been used to study this phenomenon. Not only are the conclusions about insulin receptor or postreceptor action during pregnancy inconsistent, but there are no studies of the immediate postpartum period in which the clinical phenomenon of marked insulin sensitivity is so obvious.

It seems fair to assume that the blunted maternal growth hormone response observed in response to a variety of stimuli, including hypoglycemia, both in diabetic and nondiabetic women, is the best explanation.

REFERENCES

1. Cahill GF. Physiology of insulin in man. Diabetes 20:785–799, 1971.
2. Freinkel N. Of pregnancy and progeny. Diabetes 29:1023–1035, 1980.
3. Bewley TA, Dixon JS, Li CH. Sequence comparison of human pituitary growth hormone, human chorionic somatomammotropin, and ovine pituitary growth and lactogenic hormones. Int J Peptide Protein Res 4:281–287, 1972.
4. Shome B, Parlow AF. Human pituitary prolactin (hPRL): The entire linear amino acid sequence. J Clin Endocrinol Metab 45:1112–1115, 1977.
5. Walker WH, Fitzpatrick SL, Barrera-Saldana HA, Reséndez-Pérez D, Saunders GF. The human placental lactogen genes: Structure, function, evolution, and transcriptional regulation. Endocrin Rev 12:316–328, 1991.
6. Handwerger S. Clinical counterpoint: The physiology of placental lactogen in human pregnancy. Endocrin Rev 12:329–336, 1991.
7. Samaan N, Yen SCC, Gonzalez D, Pearson OH. Metabolic effects of placental lactogen (hPL) in man. J Clin Endocrinol Metab 28:485–491, 1968.
8. Kalkhoff RK, Richardson BL, Beck P. Relative effects of pregnancy, human placental lactogen and prednisolone on carbohydrate intolerance in normal and subclinical diabetic subjects. Diabetes 18:153–163, 1969.
9. Williams C, Coltart TM. Adipose tissue metabolism in pregnancy: The lipolytic effect of human placental lactogen. Br J Obstet Gynaecol 85:43–46, 1978.
10. Freinkel N. Effects of the conceptus on maternal metabolism in pregnancy. In Leibel BS, Wrenshall GA (Eds): "On the Nature and Treatment of Diabetes." Amsterdam: Excerpta Medica Foundation, pp 679–691, 1965.
11. Felig P, Lynch V. Starvation in human pregnancy: Hypoglycemia, hypoinsulinemia, and hyperketonemia. Science 170:990–992, 1970.
12. Freinkel N, Metzger BE, Nitzan M, Daniel R, Surmaczynska BZ, Nagel TC. Facilitated anabolism in late pregnancy: Some novel maternal compensations for accelerated starvation. In Malaise WJ, Pirart J (eds): "Proceedings of the VIIIth Congress of the International Diabetes Federation." International Congress Series No. 312. Amsterdam: Excerpta Medica, pp 474–488, 1974.
13. Freinkel N, Metzger BE. Pregnancy as a tissue culture experience: The critical implications of maternal metabolism for fetal development. In: "Pregnancy Metabolism, Diabetes and the Fetus." Ciba Foundation Symposium No. 63. Amsterdam: Excerpta Medica, pp 3–23, 1979.
14. Gepts W, LeCompte PM. The pancreatic islets in diabetes. Am J Med 70:105–115, 1981.

15. Gepts W. Pathologic anatomy of the pancreas in juvenile diabetes mellitus. Diabetes 14:619–633, 1965.
16. Foulis AK, Liddle CN, Farquharson MA, Richmond JA, Weir RS. The histopathology of the pancreas in Type I (insulin-dependent) diabetes mellitus: A 25-year review of deaths in patients under 20 years of age in the United Kingdom. Diabetologia 29:267–274, 1986.
17. Palmer JP, Asplin CM, Clemons P, Lyen K, Tapati O, Raghu PK, Paquette TL. Insulin antibodies in insulin-dependent diabetics before insulin treatment. Science 222:1337–1339, 1983.
18. Baekkeskov S, Aanstoot H-J, Christgaus S, Reetz A, Solimena M, Cascalho M, Folli F, Richter-Olesen H, DeCamilli P. Identification of the 64k autoantigen in insulin dependent diabetes as the GABA-synthesizing enzyme glutamic acid decarboxylase. Nature 347:151–156, 1990.
19. Gianani R, Pugliese A, Bonner-Weir S, Shiffrin AJ, Soeldner JS, Erlich H, Awdeh Z, Alper CA, Jackson RA, Eisenbarth GS. Prognostically significant heterogeneity of cytoplasmic islet cell antibodies in relatives of patients with Type I diabetes. Diabetes 41:347–353, 1992.
20. Todd JA, Bell JI, McDevitt HO. A molecular basis for genetic susceptibility to insulin-dependent diabetes mellitus. Trends Genet 4:129–134, 1988.
21. Davies JL, Kawaguchi Y, Bennett ST, Copeman JB, Cordell HJ, Pritchard LE, Reed PW, Gough SCL, Jenkins SC, Palmer SM, Balfour KM, Rowe BR, Farrall M, Barnett AH, Bain SC, Todd JA. A genome-wide search for human type I diabetes susceptibility genes. Nature 371:130–135, 1994.
22. Hashimoto L, Habita C, Beressi JP, Delepine M, Besse C, Cambon-Thomsen A, Deschamps I, Rotter JI, Djoulah S, James MR, Froguel P, Weissenbach J, Lathrop GM, Julier C. Genetic mapping of a susceptibility locus for insulin-dependent diabetes mellitus on chromosome 11q. Nature 371:161–164, 1994.
23. Jovanovic L, Peterson CM. Insulin and glucose requirements during the first stage of labor in insulin-dependent diabetic women. Am J Med 75:607–612, 1983.
24. Golde SH, Good-Anderson B, Montoro M, Artal R. Insulin requirements during labor: A reappraisal. Am J Obstet Gynecol 144:556–559, 1982.
25. Falcone T, Little AB. Placental polypeptide hormones. In Tulchinsky D, Little AB (eds): "Maternal–Fetal Endocrinology." Philadelphia: W.B. Saunders, 1994, pp 16–32.
26. Tulchinsky D. The postpartum period. In Tulchinsky D, Little AB (eds): "Maternal–Fetal Endocrinology." Philadelphia: W.B. Saunders, 1994, pp 172–191.
27. Gratacos JA, Neufeld N, Kumar D, Artal R, Paul RH, Mestman J. Monocyte insulin binding studies in normal and diabetic pregnancies. Am J Obstet Gynecol 141:611–616, 1981.

CHAPTER 2

Gestational Diabetes

Aviva Lee-Parritz, MD and Linda J. Heffner, MD, PhD

INTRODUCTION

Gestational diabetes mellitus (GDM) is defined as carbohydrate intolerance of variable severity with onset or first recognition during pregnancy.[1] This diagnosis may include a small group of women with preexisting or incipient diabetes that is only discovered during laboratory examinations that are part of routine prenatal care.[2] Unlike overt diabetes, in which aggressive treatment during pregnancy has been shown to benefit mother and fetus, this form of carbohydrate intolerance seen in 3–5% of pregnancies demonstrates a far less clear benefit to treatment in the index pregnancy. Because the major immediate risk of GDM appears to be overgrowth of the fetus (macrosomia) and the control of fetal growth is complex and multifactorial, the exact relationship between glycemic control and fetal size is unclear. Fetal macrosomia can occur independently of maternal glycemic control. No absolute cutoff is apparent that defines a disease based on precise neonatal outcome variables. While there do appear to be long-term health implications for the woman who develops glucose intolerance during pregnancy and long-term effects may persist in her macrosomic offspring, the exact relationship of treatment during pregnancy to long-term outcome is unknown. This lack of a well-defined outcome variable has led to a lack of consensus within both the obstetric and diabetes communities on multiple aspects of screening for, diagnosis, and treatment of GDM.

PATHOPHYSIOLOGY

Early pregnancy is characterized by enhanced insulin sensitivity. Catalano and coworkers[3] studied insulin response longitudinally in normal

Diabetes Complicating Pregnancy: The Joslin Clinic Method, Edited by Florence M. Brown, MD and John W. Hare, MD.
ISBN 0-471-11031-0 © 1995 John Wiley & Sons, Inc.

pregnant women and found a 60% decrease in insulin sensitivity by 36 weeks gestation. Insulin release to a glucose load is increased up to 2.5 times over that in nonpregnant women.[4]

Steroid and peptide hormones appear to play important roles in the insulin resistance of normal pregnancy. Progesterone can directly affect glucose metabolism.[5] Kalkoff and coworkers[6] increased basal and stimulated levels of insulin by infusing progesterone into nonpregnant women. Estrogen has weak antiinsulin properties but stimulates production of cortisol-binding globulin, which increases maternal production of cortisol. Human chorionic somatomammotropin (HCS) (also known as human placental lactogen) stimulates insulin release and inhibits peripheral glucose uptake.[7] These hormones rise with growth of the conceptus and work in concert to ensure a steady flow of nutrients to the developing fetus.

The specific mechanisms by which exaggerated glucose intolerance develops in pregnancy remain to be defined. Conflicting reports of altered insulin-binding affinity in adipocytes and skeletal muscle exist;[8] however, most authors do not feel there is enough evidence to consider this an important factor. Most do propose a postinsulin receptor defect, which needs to be further elucidated. Insulin degradation has not been shown to be altered in GDM.

There is good evidence to support theories of disordered insulin secretion as a primary defect in GDM. Fasting plasma-insulin levels are much higher in pregnancy, both in normal women and women with GDM; however, they are higher still in obese women with GDM.[9] In response to a glucose load, there is a temporal delay in the peak plasma-insulin concentration in women with GDM compared to normal pregnant women, as well as a decreased insulin response per unit glycemia.[10]

Several studies have implicated lowered beta cell sensitivity in the pathogenesis of gestational diabetes. Altered first-phase insulin release, which is the release of stored preformed insulin from beta cell stores, is one of the first abnormalities seen in the development of Type II diabetes and may also be seen in GDM. Ryan et al[11] performed hyperinsulinemic–euglycemic clamp studies on nonpregnant women, normal pregnant women, and women diagnosed with GDM. A stepwise decrement in insulin sensitivity was found among the three groups, respectively. Failure to control the study for varying maternal weights and gestational age weakens the conclusions.

Buchanan et al[12] examined insulin sensitivity and beta cell responsiveness in nonpregnant women, normal pregnant women and women with GDM using the minimal-model technique. This technique utilizes frequent blood sampling of glucose and insulin concentrations during an intravenous glucose-tolerance test coupled with a computer-generated model to quantitate insulin sensitivity. Insulin sensitivity was reduced by 70% in normal pregnant women and women with GDM compared to nonpregnant controls. Normal pregnant women were able to compensate for reduced insulin sensitivity with a three-fold increase in first-phase beta cell responsiveness. Women with GDM were different, and demonstrated a 75% decrease in first-phase beta cell responsiveness compared to normal pregnant women. Maternal body habitus did not significantly alter the abnormal beta cell responsiveness of GDM. Second-phase beta cell response, which represents ongoing insulin synthesis and release, was normal in women with GDM. The loss of compensation for altered insulin sensitivity may contribute to the pathogenesis of glucose intolerance in women diagnosed with GDM.

Catalano and coworkers[13] longitudinally studied women with normal carbohydrate tolerance and women at high risk for developing GDM. The testing was performed prior to conception, in early pregnancy, and in late pregnancy, using an oral glucose tolerance test (OGTT), intravenous glucose tolerance test (IVGTT), and a hyperinsulinemic–euglycemic clamp technique. Their findings confirmed that pregnant women with GDM exhibit a significant decrease in first-phase insulin release and that there does not appear to be a notable increase in insulin resistance above that of normal pregnancy. In addition, women with GDM demonstrated impaired suppression of hepatic glucose production compared to those with normal carbohydrate tolerance.

In summary, the normal insulin resistance of pregnancy coupled with altered first-phase insulin response may be responsible for postprandial hyperglycemia. Impaired suppression of hepatic glucose production is responsible for fasting hyperglycemia when present. Much work remains to be done to understand the altered physiology of glucose metabolism in normal pregnancy, as well as the pathophysiology of GDM. Because insulin resistance increases normally with gestational age, the diagnosis is made more easily in late gestation; however, subtle disorders of insulin secretion and action may be present earlier in gestation. A better understanding of the pathophysiology of GDM may lead to more timely and appropriate therapeutic approaches.

MATERNAL OUTCOME

Gestational diabetes poses little or no direct risk to the mother during pregnancy. A modest overall health risk is present because of the higher cesarean section rate occurring in GDM as a result of fetal macrosomia.

Cesarean deliveries are associated with both increased maternal morbidity and mortality. The association between pregestational diabetes and hypertension, both chronic and preeclampsia, is well documented. The association between pregnancy-induced hypertension and gestational diabetes has been less clearly demonstrable. Suhonen and Teramo[14] prospectively followed 81 women with gestational diabetes and 327 healthy women as controls, as well a group of 203 women labeled "borderline," with only one abnormal value on the OGTT. There were no differences in parity between the groups; however, the women in the GDM and borderline groups tended to be older and heavier than those in the control group. Women with GDM had significantly more chronic hypertension (2.5% versus 0.3%) and pregnancy-induced hypertension/preeclampsia (19.8% versus 6.1 %) than did the control women. Gestational age at delivery was slightly lower in the GDM group; however, there was no difference in birth weight among the groups.

RECURRENCE RISK

Philipson and Super[15] followed 36 women with a pregnancy complicated by GDM who were tested in the same institution in a subsequent pregnancy. Twenty of the 36 patients had abnormal glucose tolerance in the subsequent pregnancy. When the maternal characteristics of the women diagnosed with GDM in the subsequent pregnancy were examined, significantly increased body mass index was found compared to those with subsequent normal glucose testing. Gaudier et al[16] studied 90 women with GDM and found that 52% had recurrence in the following pregnancy. They found that those women with recurrence were more likely to require insulin and have a large-for-gestational-age baby during the index pregnancy and to have greater body mass index. Neither of these studies reported interval glucose testing; therefore, the influence of underlying diabetes cannot be determined.

POSTPARTUM GLUCOSE TOLERANCE

The disordered glucose intolerance of gestational diabetes is reversible in most but not all patients. Clearly, patients with previously unrecognized Type I or Type II diabetes will have persistent glucose intolerance. For the more common patient with true pregnancy-induced glucose intolerance, the time frame for restoration of normal glucose tolerance is unclear. Initially, normal glucose tolerance was thought to return within 24 hours of delivery. Oats and Beischer[17] performed a 2 hour (75 g) OGTT on 270 women diagnosed with GDM and 100 normal women within seven days postpartum. Among the women with GDM, more of the women who were delivered by cesarean section displayed abnormal glucose testing immediately postpartum than those who delivered vaginally. Breastfeeding did not alter the rate of abnormal puerperal glucose testing in this study. The authors suggest that there may be some utility in performing glucose testing in the immediate postpartum period in women with an adverse neonatal outcome who did not undergo prenatal screening.

Kjos and coworkers[18] also examined postpartum resolution of GDM. Two-hour glucose tolerance tests were performed 5–8 weeks postpartum in 246 women. Seventy-four percent of the women tested were obese. Overall, 81% of the women had normal glucose testing postpartum, 10% had impaired glucose testing, and 9% had overt diabetes. Fasting hyperglycemia during pregnancy glucose testing and early diagnosis of GDM were risk factors for abnormal glucose testing postpartum. Fasting hyperglycemia during pregnancy was a very high risk characteristic; 44% of the women with a fasting blood glucose of greater than 140 mg/dl were diagnosed with overt diabetes at the postpartum examination.

In O'Sullivan and Mahan's original work,[19] 37% of their patients in the level II test group developed diabetes within 8 years. Many studies subsequently have been performed to address the risk of overt diabetes mellitus after GDM. Unfortunately, very few studies use the same diagnostic criteria or equivalent time spans for follow-up, resulting in a wide reported range of risk (6–62%)[20] for developing diabetes after GDM. Two studies that included women who met the World Health Organization (WHO) definition of diabetes and a control population[21,22] revealed a diabetes rate between 18–36% in women with GDM compared with a rate between 0–5% in women without GDM. Clearly, some patients diagnosed with GDM have overt diabetes, thus prompting a need for immediate postpartum glucose testing to identify such individuals.

Damm et al[23] followed 241 women diagnosed with diet-controlled GDM and 57 control women for up to 11 years, in order to identify predictive factors for developing diabetes mellitus. They found fasting hyperglycemia, preterm delivery, and abnormal glucose testing two months postpartum were predictors for developing overt diabetes over the study interval. In addition, a low insulin response during the OGTT during pregnancy was an independent risk factor for developing diabetes mellitus. In contrast to previous studies, maternal body habitus was not an independent risk factor.

In summary, GDM is clearly a marker for future risk of carbohydrate intolerance. The magnitude of GDM as a single risk factor alone remains unclear. Studies are currently underway to examine the role of early intervention to prevent complications of diabetes in this identified high-risk population.

PERINATAL OUTCOME

Although early studies suggested that perinatal mortality was higher in women with GDM, more recent work has failed to show an association between reversible glucose intolerance in pregnancy and increased perinatal mortality. O'Sullivan and coworkers[24] compared perinatal mortality rates between 187 women with gestational diabetes and 259 controls with a normal 3-hour OGTT. The perinatal mortality rate was significantly higher in the group diagnosed with gestational diabetes than for controls (6.4% versus 1.5%). In this study 66% of the patients were over the age of 25 years, and the perinatal mortality was exclusively in this group. Maternal obesity also increased the risk of perinatal death among the GDM group. Pettitt and coworkers[25] found an increased perinatal mortality rate among Pima Indians with an abnormal 75 g 2-hour OGTT, and the rate positively correlated with an elevated glucose concentration at the 2-hour time point.

Infants born to women with GDM share some of the perinatal complications, such as macrosomia and related birth trauma, attributed to diabetes antedating pregnancy. Whether they share any of the other morbidity seen with preexisting diabetes (increased intrapartum hypoxia, respiratory distress syndrome, neonatal hypoglycemia, hypocalcemia, polycythemia, and hyperbilirubinemia) has not been clearly shown. Hod et al[26] assessed neonatal morbidity in a retrospective study of 878 women diagnosed with gestational diabetes compared to 380 control pregnancies. Despite tight metabolic control, the incidence of neonatal morbidity was increased in the group with GDM, independent of diet or insulin therapy. Other studies have shown that women with gestational diabetes that is well controlled, either by diet or insulin therapy, have the same risk of neonatal complications as the general population.[27]

Increased risk of respiratory distress syndrome (RDS) in infants of women with pregestational diabetes is well described and thought to be the result of fetal hyperinsulinemia suppressing surfactant production.[28] The prevalence of this complication in pregnancies complicated by gestational diabetes is less clear. In a study by Kjos and coworkers,[29] three different tests for fetal lung maturity were applied to 584 women with diabetes, 90% of whom were diagnosed with gestational diabetes. Five hundred and twenty six women were delivered within 5 days of the amniocentesis. There were 18 cases of RDS, only five of which could be attributed to surfactant deficiency and all of the cases occurred in gestations of less than 34 weeks. The remaining cases were attributed to transient tachypnea of the newborn, hypertrophic cardiomyopathy, pneumonia, and meconium aspiration.

Neonatal Morbidity Other Than Macrosomia

The mechanisms of neonatal morbidity remain to be elucidated. Although hyperglycemia plays an important role, alterations of other metabolic fuels need to be considered. Salvesen and coworkers[30] examined fetal metabolic characteristics by cordocentesis prior to delivery at term in women with pregestational and gestational diabetes. Findings included a significantly lower venous pH and increased PCO_2, lactate, erythropoietin, hemoglobin concentration, and erythroblast count in fetuses of women with diabetes compared to gestational-age norms. Fetal blood PO_2 was similar. The erythropoietin levels did not correlate with measurements of long-term glucose control in the mother; however, there was a correlation between maternal glucose concentration and fetal glucose, pH, and lactate measurements. The authors postulate that maternal hyperglycemia causes fetal hyperglycemia and fetal hyperinsulinemia leading to increased metabolism and relative tissue hypoxia. Thus, fetal blood pH may be a marker for short-term maternal hyperglycemia.

MACROSOMIA

Macrosomia is the main adverse neonatal outcome attributed to gestational diabetes. Whereas the perinatal mortality rate in GDM has been significantly reduced, there has been little change in the macrosomia rate over the last two decades. Langer et al[31] studied the recorded birth weight in 75,363 consecutive deliveries and found that birth weights greater than 4000 g occurred in 26% of pregnancies complicated by diabetes versus 8% of women without diabetes. In spite of the higher risk of a macrosomic fetus in GDM, recognized glucose intolerance accounts for only 15% of macrosomic infants.

Macrosomia describes a large baby but poorly defines a neonatal outcome. It is difficult to compare many studies addressing this issue because some use a relative definition of birth weight greater than the 90th percentile for gestational age, others use an absolute birth weight greater than or equal to 4000 g, and still others use a 4500 g limit. Some use either criterion. Percentile rank takes gestational age into account, whereas a static limit of 4000 g does not.

The impact of macrosomia on perinatal outcome is largely through birth injury. Two studies[32,33] have shown a two-fold increase in mortality rate in neonates with birth weights greater than 4500 grams. The mechanism of birth trauma in macrosomia is largely related to the dreaded obstetric complication known as shoulder dystocia. Shoulder dystocia occurs when, following the delivery of the fetal head, the anterior fetal shoulder does not deliver with gentle traction due to impaction behind the pubic symphysis. Complications include asphyxia, brachial plexus injury, as well as perinatal death. Brachial plexus injury is thought to be the result of lateral traction on the fetal head and can result in permanent neuromuscular disability.

Substantive data indicate that the combination of maternal diabetes and a large infant predisposes to shoulder dystocia. Acker and coworkers[34] retrospectively examined this relationship and demonstrated that women with diabetes were five times more likely to experience a shoulder dystocia than women without diabetes. Of the nondiabetic women who delivered vaginally, those with neonates weighing 4000–4499 g and 4500+ g experienced shoulder dystocia rates of 10.0% and 22.6% respectively. Those women with diabetes undergoing vaginal delivery were shown to have a shoulder dystocia rate of 23.1% if the birth weight was 4000–4499 g and 50% if the birth weight was greater than 4500 g.

The increased risk of birth injury in the macrosomic infant appears not to be just a matter of birth weight alone, but also related to the body habitus of the fetus. Modanlou et al[35] studied the anthropometric characteristic among macrosomic infants (>4000 g) of women with and without diabetes. Infants of nondiabetic women who experienced shoulder dystocias had significantly greater shoulder-to-head circumference ratios than those without dystocia. Infants of diabetic mothers not only weighed more despite a lower mean gestational age at delivery but, more importantly, demonstrated increased shoulder-to-head circumference ratios than their nondiabetic weight-matched counterparts. It may be these anthropometric differences that put infants of women with diabetes at an increased risk of shoulder dystocia for their weight.

The pathophysiology of fetal macrosomia is complex. Several factors have been implicated in fetal macrosomia, including gender, maternal parity, race, prepregnancy weight and weight gain during pregnancy. The factors most consistently predictive of fetal weight are maternal weight followed by maternal weight gain.[36] However, as maternal obesity increases, particularly greater than 135% ideal body weight (IBW), the influence of maternal weight gain decreases. Women with gestational diabetes tend to be older, shorter and heavier than women with normal carbohydrate tolerance. Insulin is the key fetal growth-promoting hormone during intrauterine development. Animal studies have demonstrated insulin binding as early as the blastocyst stage.[37] in 1954, Pederson[38] postulated that maternal hyperglycemia leads to fetal hyperglycemia, which causes fetal hyperinsulinemia and subsequent fetal overgrowth. Freinkel[39] modified this hypothesis to include abnormal fetal metabolism of other metabolic fuels including proteins and lipids. Animal models confirm the critical role of insulin in fetal growth. In a Rhesus monkey model using streptozotocin-induced pancreatic ablation, offspring were macrosomic.[40] Susa and coworkers[41] implanted osmotically driven mini-pumps to deliver insulin in fetal Rhesus monkeys during the last third of gestation. Hyperinsulinemia was comparable to that of fetuses of diabetic mothers. Although glucose concentration was not controlled, the offspring were euglycemic at birth. The offspring were macrosomic and exhibited organomegaly in the pattern typical of the human infant of a diabetic mother.

The degree to which the level of maternal glycemic control contributes to macrosomia has been the subject of much debate. Several studies have found a positive correlation between macrosomia and glucose control.[42–44] Langer and Mazze[45] prospectively followed 246 women with GDM, and stratified them into three groups by mean plasma glucose to determine the influence of glycemic control on birth weight. He found a positive correlation between glycemic control and birth weight. Other studies have disputed this.[46,47] Jacobson and Cousins's[48] population-based study of perinatal outcome in women with GDM concluded that plasma glucose levels were not predictive of birth weight. Treatment with either diet or diet plus insulin did not normalize birth weight. The only significant predictor of birth weigh was maternal weight at the time of delivery. The birth trauma rate was not higher in the women with GDM in this study.

The argument relating macrosomia to glycemic control ignores the contribution of abnormal levels of other metabolic fuels that stimulate fetal insulin secretion. In addition to elevated serum glucose concentration, GDM is also characterized by elevated serum free fatty acids[49,50] and amino acids.[51,52] Milner et al[53] demonstrated that human fetal islet cells secrete insulin considerably earlier to an amino-acid than to a glucose stimulus. This finding suggests that increased levels of amino acids in diabetic pregnancies may prime the fetal islet cells to produce an exaggerated response to later glucose stimulation, of even a modest degree.

LONG-TERM IMPLICATIONS

In addition to neonatal complications, there are good epidemiologic and animal data to suggest long-term physiologic alterations due to exposure to the diabetic state in utero. Freinkel[39] formulated a hypothesis of "fuel-mediated teratogenesis" to describe the long-term impact of fetal hyperglycemia–hyperinsulinemia on the fetal pancreatic beta cell.

Studies of nondiabetic rats, in which a hyperglycemic intrauterine environment was created either by glucose infusion during the last week of pregnancy[54] or streptozotocin-induced diabetes[55] demonstrated altered glucose homeostasis and insulin secretion in the subsequent generation. In the work of Gaugier et al,[54] progressive glucose intolerance and altered insulin secretion were exhibited with increasing age as compared to control animals. In addition, when pancreatic function was assessed in an in vitro model of isolated pancreas perfusion, glucose regulation was not significantly altered, suggesting defective neuroregulation of insulin secretion.

Related studies performed in a Rhesus monkey model[39] involved in utero placement of a minipump into fetal monkeys creating a chronic exogenous hyperinsulinemic–euglycemic intrauterine environment. Offspring were found to be macrosomic and displayed altered insulin secretion to glucose and glucagon challenges at least through one year of age.[56]

Epidemiologic evidence of the long-term health effects of exposure to hyperinsulinemia in utero includes several studies of the Pima Indians, who have a high prevalence of underlying Type II diabetes. A significant increase in childhood obesity[57] and risk of developing Type II diabetes was present in the offspring of women diagnosed with diabetes during pregnancy compared to offspring born of women who developed diabetes after pregnancy or who did not develop diabetes at all.[58]

DIAGNOSIS OF GDM

Current diagnostic practices are based on work done by O'Sullivan and Mahan in the early 1960s.[19] An OGTT was performed on an unselected population of women attending a prenatal clinic. Whole blood glucose concentrations exhibited a Gaussian distribution at each time point. Test levels I, II, and III were defined as exceeding the mean by 1, 2, or 3 standard deviations at each time point of the test. Classification in each test level required two or more values at or above the threshold to minimize the influence of laboratory error. Follow-up for eight years demonstrated a correlation between severity of classification and subsequent development of overt diabetes. The authors proposed a conservative threshold, choosing test level II (two standard deviations above the mean) to define the abnormal state because it best approximated the prevalence of diabetes in the community at the time.

Some authors have criticized the OGTT as a diagnostic test for GDM because the original definition of abnormal was not based on perinatal outcome. Perinatal mortality was not described in the original work. However, later work by O'Sullivan[22] indicated an increased perinatal mortality rate among women with a positive OGTT. Proponents of the OGTT definition of disease point to studies that show improved perinatal outcome with intervention.[59] However, improved perinatal outcome over the years since O'Sullivan's original work may reflect advances in obstetric care. Today, the perinatal mortality rate is sufficiently low, so that to redefine an abnormal test in terms of perinatal mortality would require an inordinately large number of subjects. New studies must focus on long-term pediatric morbidity, which is subtle and more difficult to measure.

The National Diabetes Data Group (NDDG) threshold for diagnosing diabetes mellitus in adults is fasting hyperglycemia greater than 140 mg/dl. This is a reproducible test that is specific but not very sensitive. The glucose tolerance test is more sensitive, but in the nonpregnant population has been shown to lack reproducibility.[60] Harlass et al[61] investigated the reproducibility of the OGTT during pregnancy. Sixty-four patients with a 50-g glucose screen greater than 135 mg/dl underwent two 100-g OGTTs one to two weeks apart. Using the NDDG criteria to diagnose GDM (see below) the reproducibility was 78%. Catalano and coworkers[62] also evaluated the reproducibility over one week of the 100-g OGTT in 38 women with a 50-g glucose screen greater than 135 mg/dl and obtained similar results. The intraassay coefficient of variation of the glucose measurements was less than 2%, between the two tests one week apart, and reproducibility of the test was 76%. The authors postulated that maternal stress may have been responsible in a significant number of women who exhibited abnormal testing followed by normal testing.

DIAGNOSTIC CRITERIA FOR GDM

NDDG criteria[63] were formulated by extrapolating from O'Sullivan and Mahan's original data, with a correction for a change from whole blood to plasma glucose measurements. The NDDG criteria are currently recommended by both the American College of Obstetricians and Gynecologists and the American Diabetes Association.

Recommendations regarding administration of the 100-g oral glucose tolerance test are as follows:

1. The test should be performed in the morning.
2. The patient should be instructed to consume an unrestricted diet including at least 150 g of carbohydrates per day for the three days preceding the test.
3. Patients should fast overnight for 8–12 hours before the test.

4. Patients should refrain from smoking prior to the test.
5. The test should be performed with the patient seated.
6. Two or more values above the NDDG threshold criteria constitute a positive test.

Carpenter and Coustan[64] derived a set of diagnostic criteria by taking the O'Sullivan and Mahan criteria and subtracting 5 mg/dl, to account for the difference between the Symogi-Nelson and glucose oxidase methods of glucose measurement in the same medium. Table I compares the various sets of diagnostic criteria for the 3-hour OGTT.

The World Health Organization and many countries in Europe use a 75-g glucose challenge test. There are clinical situations in which a patient may be unable to tolerate an oral glucose tolerance test. An intravenous glucose tolerance test (IVGTT), which tests the glucose disappearance rate as a measure of glucose intolerance, may be an alternative. As with the original criteria suggested by O'Sullivan, none of these tests have been correlated with perinatal outcome.

SCREENING FOR GDM

The 50-g oral glucose load test was proposed as a screening test for GDM by O'Sullivan and coworkers in 1973.[65] Utilizing a whole-blood threshold value of 130 mg/dl (plasma value of 140 mg/dl), the authors found a sensitivity of 79% and a specificity of 87% in predicting a subsequent abnormal OGTT. The threshold value necessitating further testing with the formal 3-hour oral glucose tolerance test has been debated in the literature. Some have advocated lowering the threshold[61] to increase the sensitivity. Espinosa et al[66] examined the reproducibility of the 50-g glucose screen by performing the test on two consecutive days, with four

TABLE I.

	O'Sullivan[19] Criteria (whole blood)	Carpenter and Coustan[64] Criteria (plasma)	NDDG[63] Criteria (plasma)
Fasting	90 mg/dl	95 mg/dl	105 mg/dl
1 hour	165 mg/dl	180 mg/dl	190 mg/dl
2 hour	145 mg/dl	155 mg/dl	165 mg/dl
3 hour	125 mg/dl	140 mg/dl	145 mg/dl

permutations of the fed and fasted states: fast–fast, fed–fed, fast–fed, and fed–fast. In all groups except the fed–fed state, there was a significant difference between the two serum glucose measurements, and the glucose measurement on day one was consistently higher than on day two.

Some authors have suggested the use of a mixed-nutrient meal as a screening test. Coustan and coworkers[67] examined women with known GDM and women with normal carbohydrate tolerance and found reduced specificity with little gain in sensitivity compared to the 50-g glucose load. Cheney et al[68] also studied a mixed-meal challenge in both lean and obese women with GDM compared to controls. They concluded that there was a heterogeneous response in the peak and timing of insulin response that correlated with maternal body habitus, with obese women as a group exhibiting hyperinsulinemia and lean women displaying relative insulin deficiency.

The Second International Workshop Conference on Gestational Diabetes Mellitus in 1985 recommended universal screening of pregnant women because several studies demonstrated that screening of women using risk factors alone missed approximately 50% of those with abnormal glucose testing. The American College of Obstetrics and Gynecology recommends glucose screening for women under 30 years of age with risk factors and all women over 30 years of age.

There is some disagreement on timing of the glucose screen in pregnancy, with most advocating screening between 24–28 weeks. Super and coworkers[69] showed, in a small series of patients, that two-thirds of 15 patients that developed GDM could be identified earlier than 20 weeks gestation. Berkowitz et al[70] screened 2776 women at their first prenatal visit, 354 of whom were diagnosed with gestational diabetes using the Carpenter and Coustan criteria. Twenty-nine percent of these women had an abnormal test prior to 24 weeks. Patients diagnosed with GDM early in pregnancy were more likely to have one of the traditional risk factors, notably increased maternal age and obesity.

MANAGEMENT

The goal for treatment of any type of diabetes in pregnancy traditionally has been to achieve euglycemia. The levels of hyperglycemia in GDM above which perinatal morbidity and mortality increases are not known. Normal mean maternal fasting plasma glucose is lower than in the non-pregnant state at 68 ± 1.5 mg/dl, and postprandial levels do not exceed 120–130 mg/dl.[71] The American College of Obstetricians and Gynecologists and the American Diabetes Association have recommended that the therapeutic goals for glycemic control are fasting plasma glucose below 105 mg/dl and 2-hour postprandial plasma glucose of less than 120 mg/dl. However, most studies show that glycemic control alone cannot predict fetal outcome,[43] and the role of other stimulants of fetal insulin production, such as amino acids, may need to be considered. The role of other metabolic fuels in stimulating fetal insulin release is currently under investigation; however, their measurement is not useful in clinical management at this time.

DIET

Dietary modification is the cornerstone of all diabetes management. It involves caloric restriction as well as caloric redistribution to foods that may decrease extremes in glycemic excursions by improving target-organ insulin sensitivity. Since 60–80% of women diagnosed with gestational diabetes are obese, they suffer from both the insulin resistance of obesity and the disordered insulin action of GDM. Studies in normal women and nonpregnant patients with Type II diabetes have documented enhanced insulin sensitivity with as little as two weeks of dietary modification.

Most authors recommend a diet of 30–36 kcal/kg for lean or normal weight GDM patients, and 24 kcal/kg for obese patients. (see Chapter 5) The diet should be 40–50% carbohydrates, 20–25% protein, and 20–30% fats. Concentrated sugars should be avoided. High-fiber foods are encouraged because delayed gastrointestinal absorption helps reduce glycemic excursions. The length of trial of dietary management is dictated by the clinical situation and includes attention to both the degree of hyperglycemia and the gestational age of the fetus. For example, a patient with marked hyperglycemia, (> 200 mg/dl) is unlikely to respond to dietary modification, and would benefit from an expedient move to insulin therapy. A patient close to term may benefit from delivery of the fetus rather than institution of short-term insulin therapy.

Glucose monitoring should include daily fasting and 2-hour postprandial measurements. The widespread availability and reliability of portable reflectance meters makes them ideal for home blood-glucose monitoring. Measurement of a fasting and 2-hour postprandial glucose in a reference laboratory once a week should corroborate the patient's determinations. Continuation of frequent daily home blood-glucose measurements, once a patient has been shown to be adequately controlled on a diet, is controversial, as there are no data on the efficacy of multiple daily glucose measurements on pregnancy outcome in GDM. Clinical circumstances should determine its appropriateness. For patients with only minimal disturbances in their OGTT, coupled with an excellent and consistent response to diet modification, measurement of a weekly fasting and two-hour postprandial blood sugar in the office should suffice. Glycosylated hemoglobin concentrations, which are indispensable in the management of pregestational diabetes, have not exhibited enough sensitivity to be clinically useful.[72]

In the past, patients have been discouraged from weight reduction during pregnancy due to potential adverse fetal effects of maternal ketonemia. This fear was based on rodent studies that showed ketosis to be teratogenic. There are little human data to support this concern. The few studies that suggested impaired intellectual development of offspring in the setting of ketosis[73,74] have had confounding variables. Rizzo and coworkers[75] found an inverse correlation between third trimester β-hydroxybutyrate levels and performance on a standardized test of intellectual growth. However, the Dutch Famine study failed to find differences in intellectual performance among recruits born during the famine compared to those not exposed to famine conditions. Buchanan[76] measured glucose, insulin, free fatty acids, and 3-hydroxybutyrate in obese women with and without GDM after a 12-hour and an 18-hour fast. Although glucose concentration fell more quickly in women with GDM, there was no difference in levels of 3-hydroxybutyrate between the two groups. The authors concluded that obese women with GDM are not more prone to ketosis after a fast. Knopp et al[77] randomized obese women diagnosed with GDM to hypocaloric diets (50% or 33% calorie restriction) or insulin management, and examined their effect on maternal metabolic status. Both dietary programs improved glycemic status 10–20%, and reduced levels of triglycerides. There was a 50% increase in ketonuria in the 50% calorie restricted group, but no significant increase in the 33% restricted group. The insulin treated group demonstrated little improvement in glycemic control, but also had little ketonuria. Fetal effects of these treatments were not measured. Dornhurst et al[78] compared a group of women with GDM who were calorie restricted at 1200–1800 kcal to two control groups: women with a normal glucose screen and those with an abnormal glucose screen but normal OGTT. The calorie-restricted women with GDM had the same rate of macrosomia (>4000 g) as the glucose screen negative group and less than the screen positive control group. No babies born to the calorie-restricted women weighed less than the 10th percentile.

INSULIN

Current management of gestational diabetes dictates that after dietary modification, if the fasting glucose exceeds 105 mg/dl or 2-hour postprandial values are greater than 120 mg/dl, then insulin therapy should be instituted.

With the widespread availability of human recombinant insulin, there is no rationale for starting pregnant women on any other insulin. Dosing can be either calculated or empiric. The calculated dose of 0.7 U insulin/kg is based on the current pregnancy weight, and given as two-thirds of the total insulin dose in the morning (2:1 intermediate acting/regular) and one-third of the total dose in the evening (1:1 intermediate/regular). As with pregestational diabetes, occasionally a patient may require that the evening dose be split by taking the short-acting insulin at supper time and the intermediate-acting insulin at bedtime. In empiric insulin dosing, the patient is started on 20 U NPH/10 U regular insulin in the morning and 10 U NPH insulin at supper time. For the lean woman with GDM, careful titration of the insulin dose is indicated.

The rationale for tight glycemic control has been that it appears to reduce the risk of macrosomia. Interestingly, insulin therapy may exert an additive effect in this regard. O'Sullivan's group[79] demonstrated that women with GDM randomly assigned to 10 units of NPH insulin daily had a reduced rate of macrosomia compared to women treated with diet alone. Coustan and Lewis[80] randomized women with abnormal OGTTs but normal postprandial blood-glucose concentrations to treatment with either diet or diet plus prophylactic insulin. The macrosomia rate was reduced but the difference in mean birth weight among the two treatment groups did not meet statistical significance. In 1984 Coustan and Imrah[81] studied prophylactic insulin to determine its effect on fetal outcome. Women diagnosed by OGTT with GDM but normal blood glucose levels treated with prophylactic insulin and diet were compared to women treated with diet alone and women not receiving any treatment for their GDM. Women treated with insulin had a significantly reduced number of macrosomic infants (>4000 g) than the diet group or the untreated group: 7.0% versus 18.5% and 17.8%, respectively. There was also a reduction in operative delivery rates and birth trauma among the insulin treated group. However, because this was not a randomized or blinded study, other factors besides insulin therapy may have influenced outcome variables. Women who accepted prophylactic insulin may have represented a group of women more committed to dietary compliance. In addition, the insulin treated group had a significantly higher fasting plasma glucose concentration and degree of glucose test abnormality.

Roversi et al[82] treated 280 women with GDM with the maximal tolerated insulin dose but did not have a dietary management group for comparison. The macrosomia rate in the insulin treated GDM group (fasting blood glucose > 105 mg/dl) was close to that of the pregestational diabetic group (including those with a fasting blood glucose > 130 mg/dl, White classes B and C). Opperman and Camerini-Davalos[83] divided a group of 243 women with GDM on the basis of fasting hyperglycemia (> 95 mg/dl), then treated half of each group with diet or diet and insulin therapy. The macrosomia rate was more dependent on the presence of fasting hyperglycemia than on insulin therapy. Maternal obesity was the strongest predictor of neonatal macrosomia.

Persson's[84] Swedish group randomized 202 women with GDM to small doses of insulin and diet or diet alone and found no difference in the macrosomia rate between the two groups. Leiken et al[85] examined a group of 181 women diagnosed with GDM and 1850 women with normal glucose screens. Women with normal fasting plasma glucose levels were treated with diet alone, and those with fasting hyperglycemia were given insulin and diet therapy. Women with fasting euglycemia on diet therapy and lean women with fasting hyperglycemia treated with diet and insulin exhibited macrosomia rates comparable to control women. Obese women with fasting hyperglycemia did not have a significant reduction in the macrosomia rate with insulin therapy. Thompson and coworkers[86] randomized 108 women to diet or diet plus insulin therapy. Neonatal outcome variables were measured after removing those patients who either failed diet therapy and went onto insulin treatment, or were initially treated with insulin and required increased doses. Among those remaining patients with good glycemic control by either method, there were no cases of perinatal mortality or birth trauma. The birth weight and macrosomia rate were significantly reduced in the insulin treated group, but the operative delivery rate was the same. The authors demonstrated that insulin therapy was associated with a larger reduction in birth weight among the heavier women, postulating that this group may benefit the most from this therapy.

Several studies have shown that even mild levels of hyperglycemia may impact on fetal growth. Tallarigo et al[87] studied women with normal 3-hour OGTTs and divided them into three groups based on their glucose value at the 2-hour time point. The higher the glucose concentration at 2 hours, the higher the rate of macrosomia. Langer et al[88] found that women who had only one abnormal value on a 3-hour OGTT, which is considered a normal test by current standards, exhibited the same mean birth weight as control subjects but had an increased rate of macrosomia. Leikin et al[85] found that women with abnormal glucose screens had a higher rate of macrosomia compared to women with normal glucose screens.

Some authors have questioned whether extreme glycemic control can be deleterious to the fetus. Langer and coworkers[89] found that when the mean blood-glucose concentration is greater than 87 mg/dl, 10% of the fetuses were small for gestational age (SGA). When the mean glucose concentration was below this level, the SGA rate was 23%.

EXERCISE

There is increasing evidence that exercise and physical training are beneficial in Type II diabetes, presumably due to the increased sensitivity to insulin (see Chapter 6). Both fasting and postprandial glucose concentrations can be lowered[90,91] and the effect can last up to a week following a full training session. The application of exercise to the management of gestational diabetes has been hampered by the lack of consensus regarding the impact of exercise in pregnancy. Although no study has demonstrated fetal loss, alterations in fetal heart rate, risk of uterine contractility leading to premature labor, and possible decreased birth weight have been inconsistently found among studies. The American College of Obstetricians and Gynecologists supports exercise for women who exercised prior to conception, but not for those who were not previously exercising.

Jovanovic-Peterson et al[92] studied the effect of exercise in the setting of GDM. Twenty women were randomized to diet alone or diet therapy plus an exercise protocol for 6 weeks. The exercise protocol consisted of arm ergonometry for 20 minutes three times per week. Arm ergonometry was chosen because it is not associated with uterine contractions or fetal bradycardia. The exercise group exhibited decreased fasting plasma glucose by 4 weeks, and a significant decrease in 1-hour glucose response to a 50-g challenge after 6 weeks. Glycosylated hemoglobin levels fell in both groups during the duration of the study, and the decrease was significantly greater in the exercise group at 6 weeks. Neonatal outcomes were not evaluated. Bung and coworkers[93] randomized 41 women who failed dietary modification to insulin therapy or an exercise program of 45 minutes on a recumbent bicycle three times per week. The two treatment groups did not differ in glycemic control, birth weight, macrosomia rate, or operative delivery rates. The authors suggest that an exercise program under supervision can be an adjunct or even option to insulin therapy.

OBSTETRIC MANAGEMENT

Fetal Surveillance

There are no studies examining the benefit of antepartum fetal surveillance in gestational diabetes. Neonatal complications in diet-controlled women without other medical or fetal complications are comparable to the general population. Patients with other complications, such as chronic hypertension, should be monitored appropriately. Coustan[94] advocates fetal testing with weekly nonstress tests (NST) starting at 40 weeks. Although not studied in a randomized manner, most experts agree that women who require insulin, or have poor glycemic control, should be managed similarly to women with pregestational diabetes, with weekly fetal testing starting no later than 32 weeks. Methods of fetal testing (nonstress test, biophysical profile, or contraction stress test) are based on the resources of the institution.

Timing of Delivery

The low perinatal mortality rate associated with diet-controlled gestational diabetes allows these women to be managed as normal patients, including postdates testing when appropriate. For GDM requiring insulin therapy to maintain euglycemia, most practitioners follow similar guidelines as for women with pregestational diabetes, which is to deliver the fetus at 38–40 weeks gestation following documentation of fetal lung maturity.

Gestational diabetes is associated with fetal macrosomia. The combination of macrosomia (birth weight >4000 g) and diabetes predicted 73% of women with shoulder dystocia according to Acker's data.[34] This finding raises the question of early delivery for women with diabetes in order to reduce the risk of macrosomia and birth injury. Recently, Kjos et al[95] addressed the question of timing of delivery in a randomized trial of active induction of labor at 38 weeks versus expectant management in 200 women with insulin requiring GDM and class B pregestational diabetes with an estimated fetal weight less than 3800 grams. There was no difference in cesarean section rate between the two groups in spite of a higher birth weight and macrosomia rate (>90th percentile) in the expectantly managed group. There were three shoulder dystocias, none of which led to a permanent birth injury, in the expectant management group and none in the induction group. There was no other significant perinatal morbidity in either group.

Most studies of macrosomia and birth injury are based on birth weight, but obstetrical decisions must be made without knowledge of the exact birth weight. Most decisions are made based on an ultrasound estimate of fetal weight, which has 10–15% error. Some investigators have tried to define predictors of macrosomia other than estimated weight. The biparietal diameter has not been a good predictor, because there does not appear to be an increase in this measurement among infants of diabetic mothers. Abdominal circumference may be a better predictor, because subcutaneous fat and hepatic glycogen deposition are under the influence of insulin, and can enlarge the fetal liver.[96] Landon and coworkers[97] demonstrated that ultrasound measurement of growth of the abdominal circumference (AC) was accelerated after 32 weeks gestation in diabetic women delivering a large-for-gestational-age (LGA) infant. An increase in AC of more than 1.2 cm/week detected a LGA infant with 84% sensitivity and 85% specificity. Bochner et al[98] also examined the AC as a predictor of macrosomia-related complications and found that fetuses with an AC >90th percentile at 30–33 weeks gestation had an increased rate of shoulder dystocia at term versus those with an AC < 90th percentile.

Mode of Delivery

The major risk of GDM is fetal macrosomia and consequent birth injury, and prediction of those infants at greatest risk and delivery by cesarean section is a desirable goal. It is, however, very difficult to achieve for several reasons, which include the inaccuracy of ultrasound estimates of fetal weight, the continuum of risk for shoulder dystocia, which shows no specific fetal weight below which the risk approaches zero, and the influence of other factors such as maternal parity and pelvimetry. For these reasons, institutions and individuals vary appreciably in their approach to the upper limits of estimated fetal weight for which a trial of labor is offered. Currently, an estimated fetal weight of 4000 g or more in a woman known to have GDM is a threshold at which many practitioners offer a cesarean delivery without a trial of labor. However, this is not a universal standard and clinical judgment is necessary in managing the labor and delivery of all infants of mothers with glucose intolerance during pregnancy.

SUMMARY

GDM is currently treated with the goal of improved perinatal outcome, especially avoidance of birth injuries, while screening and diagnostic criteria were developed with the goal of identifying the long-term maternal risk of developing carbohydrate intolerance. Treatment targets glycemic control, while other abnormalities of fuel metabolism may be operative in fetal overgrowth. Conflicting information is available on the impact of treatment during pregnancy and on the long-term risk of developing overt diabetes. The development of diagnostic criteria that use both maternal and fetal outcome variables to redefine the disease and treatment plans that address both maternal and fetal risks will do much to clarify this interesting, but very confusing pregnancy disorder.

REFERENCES

1. Freinkel, N, Gabbe SG, Hadden R, et al: Summary and Recommendations of the Second International Workshop-Conference on Gestational Diabetes Mellitus. Diabetes 34 (Suppl):123–126, 1985.
2. Hare JW: Diabetes and pregnancy. In Kahn CR and Weir G (eds): "Joslin's Diabetes Mellitus." 13th ed. Philadelphia: Lea and Febiger, 1994, pp 889–899.
3. Catalano PM, Tyzbir ED, Roman NM, Amini SB, Sims EA: Longitudinal changes in insulin release and insulin resistance in nonobese pregnant women. Am J Obstet Gynecol 165:1667–1672, 1991.
4. Spellacy WN, Goetz FC: Plasma insulin in normal late pregnancy. N Eng J Med 268:988–991, 1963.
5. Hiriis-Nielsen J, Nielsen V, Molsted-Pedersen L, et al: Effects of pregnancy hormones on pancreatic islets in organ culture. Acta Endocrinol 111:336–341, 1986.
6. Kalkoff RK, Jacobson M, Lemper D: Progesterone, pregnancy and the augmented plasma insulin response. J Clin Endocrinol Metab 31:24–28,1970.
7. Gaspard VJ, Sandront HM, Luyckx AS, et al: The control of human placental lactogen (HPL) secretion and its interrelation with glucose and lipid metabolism in late pregnancy. In Camerini-Davalos RH, Coles HS (eds): "Early Diabetes in Early Life." New York: Academic Press, 1975, pp 273–278.
8. Damm P, Handberg A, Kuhl C, Beck-Nielsen H, Molsted-Pedersen L: Insulin receptor binding and tyrosine kinase activity in skeletal muscle from normal pregnant women and women with gestational diabetes. Obstet Gynecol 82:251–259, 1993.
9. Hornnes PJ, Kuhl C, Lauritsen KB: Gastrointestinal insulinotropic hormones in normal and gestational-diabetic pregnancy: Response to oral glucose. Diabetes 30:504–509, 1981.
10. Kuhl C, Holst JJ: Plasma glucagon and insulin: Glucagon and the insulin : glucagon ratio in gestational diabetes. Diabetes 25:16–23, 1976.
11. Ryan EA, O'Sullivan MJ, Skyler JS: Insulin action during pregnancy: Studies with the euglycemic clamp technique. Diabetes 34:380–389, 1985.
12. Buchanan TA, Metzger BE, Freinkel N, Bergman RN: Insulin sensitivity and B-cell responsiveness to glucose during late pregnancy in lean and moderately obese women with normal glucose tolerance or mild gestational diabetes. Am J Obstet Gynecol 162:1008–1014, 1990.
13. Catalano PM, Tyzbir ED, Wolfe RR, Calles J, Roman NM, Amini SB, Sims EAH: Carbohydrate metabolism during pregnancy in control subjects and women with gestational diabetes. Am J Physiol 264:E60–E67, 1993.
14. Suhonen L, Teramo K: Hypertension and pre-eclampsia in women with gestational glucose intolerance. Acta Obstet Gynecol Scand 72:269–272, 1993.
15. Philipson EH, Super DM: Gestational diabetes mellitus: Does it recur in subsequent pregnancy? Am J Obstet Gynecol 160:1324–1331, 1989.
16. Gaudier FL, Hauth JC, Poist M, deLacee C, Cliver SP: Recurrence of gestational diabetes mellitus. Obstet Gynecol 80:755–758, 1992.
17. Oats JN, Beischer NA: The persistence of abnormal glucose testing after delivery. Obstet Gynecol 75:397–401, 1990.

18. Kjos SL, Buchanan TA, Greenspoon JS, Montoro M, Bernstein GS, Mestman JH: Gestational diabetes mellitus. The prevalence of glucose intolerance and diabetes mellitus in the first two months postpartum. Am J Obstet Gynecol 163:93–98, 1990.
19. O'Sullivan JB, Mahan CM: Criteria for the oral glucose tolerance test in pregnancy. Diabetes 13:278–285, 1964.
20. O'Sullivan, JB: Diabetes mellitus after GDM. Diabetes 40 (Suppl 2):131–135, 1991.
21. Damm PD, Molsted-Pedersen, LMP, Kuhl CK: High incidence of diabetes mellitus and impaired glucose tolerance in women with previous gestational diabetes mellitus. (Abstract) Diabetologia 32:479A, 1989.
22. O'Sullivan, JB: The Boston Gestational Diabetes Studies: Review and perspectives. In Sutherland HW, Stowers JM, Pearson DWM, (eds): "Carbohydrate Metabolism in Pregnancy and the Newborn." Vol. 4. London: Springer-Verlag, 1989, pp 287–294.
23. Damm P, Kuhl CK, Bertelsen A, Molsted-Pedersen L: Predictive factors for the development of diabetes in women with previous gestational diabetes mellitus. Am J Obstet Gynecol 167:607–616, 1992.
24. O'Sullivan JB, Charles D, Mahan CM, Dandrow RV: Gestational diabetes and perinatal mortality rate. Am J Obstet Gynecol 116:901–904, 1972.
25. Pettitt DJ, Knowler WC, Baird HR, Bennett PH: Gestational diabetes: Infant and maternal complications of pregnancy in relation to third trimester glucose tolerance in Pima Indians. Diabetes Care 3:458–464, 1980.
26. Hod M, Merlob P, Friedman S, Schoenfeld A, Ovadia J: Gestational diabetes mellitus: A survey of perinatal complications in the 1980's. Diabetes 40 (Suppl 2):74–78, 1991.
27. Maresh M, Beard RW, Bray CS, Elkeles RS, Wadsworth JW: Factors predisposing to and outcome of gestational diabetes. Obstet Gynecol 74:342–346, 1989.
28. Stubbs WA, Stubbs SM: Hyperinsulinism, diabetes mellitus and respiratory distress of the newborn: A common link? Lancet 1(8059):308–309, 1978.
29. Kjos SL, Walther FJ, Montoro M, Paul RH, Diaz F, Stabler M: Prevalence and etiology of respiratory distress in infants of diabetic mothers: Predictive value of fetal lung maturation tests. Am J Obstet Gynecol 163:898–903, 1990.
30. Salvesen DR, Brudenell M, Proudler AJ, Crook D, Nicolaides KH: Fetal pancreatic B-cell function in pregnancies complicated by maternal diabetes mellitus: Relationship to fetal acidemia and macrosomia. Am J Obstet Gynecol 168:1363–1369, 1993.
31. Langer O, Berkus M, Huff R: Should the fetus with an estimated weight >4000 g be delivered by Cesarean section? Presented at the 11th Annual meeting of the Society of Perinatal Obstetricians, San Francisco, California, 1991.
32. Modanlou HD, Dorchester WL, Thorosian A, Freeman RK: Macrosomia: Maternal, fetal and neonatal implications. Obstet Gynecol 55:420–424, 1980.
33. Spellacy WN, Miller S, Winegar A, Peterson PQ: Macrosomia–maternal characteristics and infant complications. Obstet Gynecol 66:158–161,1985.
34. Acker DB, Sachs BP, Friedman EA: Risk factors for shoulder dystocia. Obstet Gynecol 66:762–768, 1985.
35. Modanlou HD, Komatsu G, Dorchester W, Freeman RK: Large-for-gestational-age neonates: Anthropometric reasons for shoulder dystocia. Obstet Gynecol 60:417–423, 1982.
36. Eastman NJ, Jackson E: Weight relationships in pregnancy. I. The bearing of maternal weight gain and pre-pregnancy weight on birth weight in full term pregnancies. Obstet Gynecol Surv 23:1003–1025, 1968.
37. Rosenblum IY, Mattson BA, Heyner S: Stage-specific insulin binding in mouse preimplantation embryos. Devel Biol 116:761–763, 1986.

38. Pedersen J: Weight and length at birth of infants of diabetic mothers. Acta Endocrinol 16:330–342, 1954.
39. Freinkel N. Banting Lecture: Of pregnancy and progeny. Diabetes 29:1023–1035, 1980.
40. Cheek DB, Hill DE: Changes in somatic growth after ablation of maternal or fetal pancreatic beta cells. In Cheek DB (ed): "Fetal and Postnatal Cellular Growth." New York: Wiley, 1975, p 311.
41. Susa JB, Neave C, Segal P, Singer DB, Zeller WP, Schwartz R: Chronic hyperinsulinemia in the fetal rhesus monkey: Effects of physiologic hyperinsulinemia on fetal growth and composition. Diabetes 33:656–660, 1984.
42. Forsbach G, Contreras-Soto JJ, Fong G, Flores G, Moreno O: Prevalence of gestational diabetes and macrosomic newborns in a Mexican population. Diabetes Care 11:235–238, 1988.
43. Madsen H, Ditzel J: The influence of maternal weight, smoking, vascular complications and glucose regulation on the birth weight of infants of type I diabetic women. Eur J Obstet Gynecol Reprod Biol 39:175–179, 1991.
44. Jovanovic-Peterson L, Peterson CM, Reed GF, Metzger BE, Mills JL, Knopp RH, Aarons JH: Maternal postprandial glucose levels and infant birth weight: The Diabetes in Early Pregnancy Study. The National Institute of Health and Human Development. Am J Obstet Gynecol 164:103–111, 1991.
45. Langer O, Mazze R: The relationship between large-for-gestational-age infants and glycemic control in women with gestational diabetes. Am J Obstet Gynecol 159:1478–1483, 1988.
46. Goldman M, Kitzmiller JL, Abrams B, Cowan RM, Laros RK: Obstetric complications with GDM. Effects of maternal weight. Diabetes 40:79–82, 1991.
47. Leiper JM, Small M, Talwar D, Robb D, Lunan CB, MacCuish AC: Fetal glycemic control and neonatal complications in diabetic pregnancy. Diabetes Res 8:143–146, 1988.
48. Jacobson JD, Cousins L: A population based study of maternal and perinatal outcome in patients with gestational diabetes. Am J Obstet Gynecol 161: 981–986, 1989.
49. Gillmer MD, Beard RW, Oakley NW, Brooke FM, Elphick MC, Hull D: Diurnal plasma free fatty acid profiles in normal and diabetic pregnancies. Br Med J 2:670–673, 1977.
50. Persson B, Lunell NO: Metabolic control in diabetic pregnancy. Variations in plasma concentration of glucose, free fatty acids, glycerol, ketone bodies, insulin and human chorionic somatomammotropin during the last trimester. Am J Obstet Gynecol 122:737–745, 1975.
51. Metzger BE, Phelps RL, Freinkel N, Navickas IA: Effects of gestational diabetes on diurnal profiles of plasma glucose, lipids and individual amino acids. Diabetes Care 3:402–409, 1980.
52. Kalkoff RK, Kandaraki E, Mitchell T, Kasdorf G, Borkowf HI: Maternal plasma fuel disturbances in mild non-obese and obese gestational diabetes mellitus. In Proc lnt Workshop-Conf Gestational Diabetes, 3rd, Chicago IL, 9 November 1990.
53. Milner RDG, Ashworth MA, Barson AJ: Insulin release from human fetal pancreas in response to glucose, leucine and arginine. J Endocrinol 52:497–505, 1972.
54. Gaugier D, Bihoreau MT, Picon L, Ktorza A: Insulin secretion in adult rats after intrauterine exposure to mild hyperglycemia during late gestation. Diabetes 40 (Suppl 2):106–108, 1991.
55. Van Assche FA, Aerts L, Holemans K: Metabolic alterations in adulthood after intrauterine development in mothers with mild diabetes. Diabetes 40 (Suppl 2):106–108, 1991.
56. Susa JB, Boylan JM, Sehgal P, Schwartz R: Persistence of impaired insulin secretion in

infant rhesus monkeys that had been hyperinsulinemic in utero. J Clin Endocrinol Metab 75:265–269, 1992.
57. Pettitt DJ, Baird HR, Alice K, Bennett PH, Knowler WC: Excessive obesity in offspring of Pima Indian women with diabetes during pregnancy. N Engl J Med 308: 242–245, 1983.
58. Pettitt DJ, Nelson RG, Saad MF, Bennett PH, Knowler WC: Diabetes and obesity in the offspring of Pima Indian women with diabetes during pregnancy. Diabetes Care 16:310–314, 1993.
59. Gyves MT, Rodman HM, Little AB, Faranoff AA, Merkatz IR: A modern approach of management of pregnant diabetics: A two year analysis of perinatal outcomes. Am J Obstet Gynecol 128:606–616, 1977.
60. Rushforth NB, Bennett PH, Steinberg AG, Miller M: Comparison of the value of the two- and one-hour glucose levels of the oral GTT in the diagnosis of diabetes in Pima Indians. Diabetes 24:538–546, 1975.
61. Harlass FE, Brady K, Read JA: Reproducibility of the oral glucose tolerance test in pregnancy. Am J Obstet Gynecol 164:564–568, 1991.
62. Catalano PM, Avallone DA, Drago NM, Amini SB: Reproducibility of the oral glucose tolerance test in pregnant women. Am J Obstet Gynecol 169:874–881, 1993.
63. National Diabetes Data Group: Classification and diagnosis of diabetes mellitus and other categories of glucose intolerance. Diabetes 18:1039–1057, 1979.
64. Carpenter MW, Coustan DR: Criteria for screening tests for gestational diabetes. Am J Obstet Gynecol 144:768–773, 1982.
65. O'Sullivan JB, Mahan CM, Charles D, Dandrow RV: Screening criteria for high risk gestational diabetic patients. Am J Obstet Gynecol 116:895–900, 1973.
66. Espinosa de los Montero A, Parra A, Carino N, Ramirez A: The reproducibility of the 50-g, 1-hour glucose screen for diabetes in pregnancy. Obstet Gynecol 82:515–518, 1993.
67. Coustan DR, Widness JA, Carpenter MW, Rotondo L, Pratt C: The "breakfast tolerance test": Screening for gestational diabetes with a standardized mixed nutrient meal. Am J Obstet Gynecol 157:1113–1117, 1987.
68. Cheney C, Shragg P, Hollingsworth D: Demonstration of heterogeneity in gestational diabetes by a 400-kcal breakfast meal tolerance test. Obstet Gynecol 65:17–23, 1985.
69. Super DM, Edelberg SC, Philipson EH, Hertz RH, Kalhan SC: Diagnosis of gestational diabetes early in pregnancy. Diabetes Care 14:288–294, 1991.
70. Berkowitz GS, Roman SH, Lapinski RH, Alvarez M: Maternal characteristics, neonatal outcome and the time of diagnosis of gestational diabetes. Am J Obstet Gynecol 167:976–982, 1992.
71. Phelps RL, Metzger BE, Freinkel N. Carbohydrate metabolism in pregnancy. XVII. Diurnal profiles of plasma glucose, insulin, free fatty acids, triglycerides, cholesterol and individual amino acids in late normal pregnancy. Am J Obstet Gynecol 140:730–736, 1981.
72. Grandis AS, Morris MA, Litton JC: Gestational diabetes: Maternal response to diet and insulin therapy as reflected by glycosylated hemoglobin concentration. Am J Obstet Gynecol 157:1118–1121, 1987.
73. Churchill JA, Berendes HW, Nemore J: Neuropsychological deficits in children of diabetic mothers. A report from the Collaborative Study of Cerebral Palsy. Am J Obstet Gynecol 105:257–268, 1969.
74. Stehbens JA, Baker G, Kitchell M: Outcome at age 1, 3 and 5 years of children born to diabetic women. Am J Obstet Gynecol 127:408–413, 1977.
75. Rizzo T, Metzger BE, Burns WJ, Burns K: Correlations between antepartum maternal metabolism and intelligence of offspring. N Engl J Med 325:911–916, 1991.
76. Buchanan TA, Metzger BE, Freinkel N: Accelerated starvation in late pregnancy: A

comparison between obese women with and without gestational diabetes mellitus. Am J Obstet Gynecol 162:1015–1020, 1990.

77. Knopp RH, Magee MS, Raisys V, Benedetti T: Metabolic effects of hypocaloric diets in management of gestational diabetes. Diabetes 40 (Suppl 2):165–171, 1991.
78. Dornhurst A, Nicholls JSD, Probst F, Paterson CM, Hollier KL, Elkeles RS, Beard RW: Calorie restriction for treatment of gestational diabetes. Diabetes 40 (Suppl 2):161–164, 1991.
79. O'Sullivan JB, Mahan CM, Dandrow RV: Medical treatment of the gestational diabetic. Obstet Gynecol 44:817–821, 1974.
80. Coustan DR, Lewis SB: Insulin therapy for gestational diabetes. Obstet Gynecol 51: 306–310, 1978.
81. Coustan DR, Imrah J: Prophylactic insulin treatment of gestational diabetes reduces the incidence of macrosomia, operative delivery and birth trauma. Am J Obstet Gynecol 150:836–842, 1984.
82. Roversi GD, Gargiulo M , Nocolini U, Ferrazzi E, Pedretti E, Gruft L, Tronconi G: Maximal tolerated insulin therapy in gestational diabetes. Diabetes Care 3:489–494, 1980.
83. Opperman W, Camerini-Davalos RA: Early diabetes during pregnancy. Diabetes Care 3:465–467, 1980.
84. Persson B, Stangenberg M, Hansson U, Nordlander E: Gestational diabetes mellitus (GDM). Comparative evaluation of two treatment regimens, diet versus insulin and diet. Diabetes 34 (Suppl 2):101–105, 1985.
85. Leiken E, Jenkins JH, Graves WL: Prophylactic insulin in gestational diabetes. Obstet Gynecol 70:587–592, 1987.
86. Thompson DJ, Portter KB, Gunnells DJ, Wagner PC, Spinnato JA: Prophylactic insulin in the management of gestational diabetes. Obstet Gynecol 75:960–964, 1990.
87. Tallarigo L, Giampietro O, Penno G, Miccoli R, Gregori G, Navalesi R: Relationship of glucose tolerance to complications of pregnancy in non-diabetic women. N Engl J Med 315:989–992, 1986.
88. Langer O, Brustman L, Anyaegbunam A, Mazze R: The significance of one abnormal glucose tolerance test value on adverse outcome in pregnancy. Am J Obstet Gynecol 157:758–763, 1987.
89. Langer O, Levy J, Brustman L, Anyaegbunam A, Merkatz R, Divon M: Glycemic control in gestational diabetes mellitus—how tight is tight enough: Small for gestational age versus large for gestational age? Am J Obstet Gynecol 161:646–653, 1989.
90. Bjorntorp P, De Jounge K, Sjostrom L, Sullivan L: The effects of physical training on insulin production in obesity. Metabolism 19:631–638, 1970.
91. Bjorntorp P, Fahlen M, Grimby G, Gustafson A, Holm J, Renstrom P, Schersten T: Carbohydrate and lipid metabolism in middle aged physically well trained men. Metabolism 21:1037–1042, 1972.
92. Jovanovic-Peterson L, Durak EP, Peterson C: Randomized trial of diet versus diet plus cardiovascular conditioning on glucose levels in gestational diabetes. Am J Obstet Gynecol 161:415–419, 1989.
93. Bung P, Artal R, Khodiguian N, Kjos S. Exercise in gestational diabetes. An optional therapeutic approach. Diabetes 40 (Suppl 2):182–185, 1991.
94. Coustan DR: Management of gestational diabetes. Clin Obstet Gynecol 34:558–564, 1991.
95. Kjos SL, Henry OA, Montoro M, Buchanan TA, Mestman JH: Insulin-requiring diabetes in pregnancy: A randomized trial of active induction of labor and expectant management. Am J Obstet Gynecol 169:611–615, 1993.
96. Brans YW, Shannon DL, Hunter MA: Maternal diabetes and neonatal macrosomia. II. Neonatal and anthropometric measurements. Early Human Dev 8:297–305, 1983.

97. Landon MB, Mintz M, Gabbe SG: Sonographic evaluation of fetal abdominal growth: Predictor of large-for-gestational-age infant in pregnancies complicated by gestational diabetes mellitus. Am J Obstet Gynecol 160:115–121, 1989.
98. Bochner CJ, Medearis AL, Williams J, Castro L, Hobel CJ, Wade ME: Early third-trimester ultrasound screening in gestational diabetes to determine the risk of macrosomia and labor dystocia at term. Am J Obstet Gynecol 157:703–708, 1987.

SECTION II

MEDICAL CONSIDERATIONS

CHAPTER 3

Medical Management

Florence M. Brown, MD and John W. Hare, MD

INTRODUCTION

Long before the results of the Diabetes Control and Complications Trial demonstrated that excellent diabetes control significantly reduces the incidence of long-term diabetic complications,[1] it was known that the outcome of the diabetic pregnancy was highly dependent on the level of blood-sugar control. Karlson and Kjellmer showed that mothers with average third trimester blood sugars of 100 or less had lower perinatal mortality rates than women whose blood sugars were more than 150 mg/dl—3.8% versus 24%, respectively.[2] Other studies have revealed that excellent control of diabetes in the second and third trimesters of pregnancy reduces infant morbidities such as respiratory distress syndrome, hypoglycemia, and macrosomia.[3–5] In addition, numerous studies have demonstrated that congenital abnormalities and spontaneous abortions are more common in women who have poor control of diabetes during the 1st trimester[6,7,8,9,10] (see Chapter 12).

Since most congenital abnormalities related to diabetes occur before the seventh week postconception,[11] it is imperative that blood sugars are controlled during this critical time. The Diabetes in Early Pregnancy Trial (DIEP) revealed that women with insulin-dependent diabetes mellitus (IDDM) who were enrolled for intensification of insulin therapy early in pregnancy had fewer congenital malformations than did women who were enrolled later in pregnancy.[12] Nevertheless, the congenital malformation rate among the early enrollees was 5%,[12] which is more than double the 2% rate seen in a nondiabetic control population. Many centers, including our own, report rates of major congenital malformations of 5–10%. In order to reduce these rates further, efforts must be aimed at obtaining optimal glycemic control prior to pregnancy. Preconception counseling

Diabetes Complicating Pregnancy: The Joslin Clinic Method, Edited by Florence M. Brown, MD and John W. Hare, MD.
ISBN 0-471-11031-0 © 1995 John Wiley & Sons, Inc.

and establishment of excellent diabetes control prior to pregnancy reduce the risk of spontaneous abortion and major congenital abnormalities to the level close to what is seen in the general nondiabetic population.[13–15] Women in preconception counseling groups have lower glycohemoglobin levels at their first prenatal visits than do women who do not receive preconception counseling. More importantly, excellent diabetes control is established prior to organogenesis, a time when many women are not yet aware that they are pregnant. It must be pointed out that, for ethical reasons, randomization was not performed in any of the above studies, so that women who entered these studies before pregnancy were likely to be a self-selected, highly motivated, well-informed group compared to the women who entered the studies postconception.

Efforts should be made to inform all women of childbearing age of the importance of prepregnancy blood-sugar control. It has been our policy to discuss this issue with every potentially fertile woman, at the time of her first general medical office visit and yearly thereafter, even if she is not anticipating pregnancy in the near future. However, this policy still does not address the need to inform the many women who do not receive their diabetes care at specialized institutions. It has been proposed that a warning label stating that "poor control of diabetes may cause birth defects" be included with insulin, syringes, glucose test strips, and meters.[16] This would indeed inform many women.

Inherently unstable diabetes and lack of maternal motivation to control blood sugars are the ultimate nemeses of our goal to reduce congenital abnormalities, spontaneous abortions, and poor perinatal outcome. Many women find it difficult to comply with the demands of testing and adjusting insulin until pregnancy is a reality. A few women continue to neglect their diabetes during their pregnancies because they really don't believe that there will be an adverse outcome. Rarely, some have knowingly-falsified the results of their blood-sugar testing (see Chapter 13).

For women who have uncomplicated IDDM, the risks of pregnancy to the mother are few. Perhaps the greatest risk to these women is severe hypoglycemia. While animal studies have demonstrated teratogenicity following severe prolonged hypoglycemia,[17] human studies do not confirm this finding.[13] Therefore, ideal blood-sugar control during pregnancy is a fine line separating hypoglycemia, with excessive risk to the mother, from hyperglycemia, with excessive risk to the fetus. For women with "brittle" diabetes, swings in blood sugars may occur even when activity, diet, and insulin administration are highly regimented. The American Diabetes Association (ADA) has proposed goals for glycemic control during pregnancy. Goals from the Joslin Diabetes Center (JDC) are provided for comparison. These goals need not be followed absolutely, particularly if the mother has hypoglycemic unawareness (see Table I).

In practice, we educate women and their partners that the risk of hypoglycemia during pregnancy is great. All women and partners, if present, are taught how to administer glucagon. Women are encouraged to teach other family members or supportive friends and colleagues how to inject glucagon if they become unconscious or refuse to take anything by mouth. Play-acting a severe hypoglycemic reaction and allowing the partner to give a practice injection will improve the likelihood that glucagon will be administered if it becomes necessary. Finally, hypoglycemia becomes life-threatening if it occurs when the woman is operating a motor vehicle. Women should be advised to check their blood sugars immediately before they plan to drive and a snack should be readily available inside the car at all times.

CLASSIFICATION OF DIABETES IN PREGNANCY

A half century ago, Priscilla White of the Joslin Clinic proposed a classification for diabetes that bears her name and has achieved worldwide acceptance. She used a series of letters to separate the classes. The underlying rationale for her classification was that longer-term diabetes, or diabetes complicated by vascular disease, has increasingly adverse effects on maternal and fetal outcome, particularly the latter. The majority of the pregnant patients seen at the Joslin Clinic are women with IDDM and this has been the case for many years. Thus, except for Class A, which includes women with diet-controlled noninsulin-dependent diabetes mellitus (NIDDM), the White classification is particularly slanted toward women with IDDM. Placement of a woman into a class depends upon her age at the time of onset of diabetes and/or the duration of her diabetes. More-

TABLE I. Goals for Glycemic Control during Pregnancy

	ADA Goals (IDDM)	JDC Goals (IDDM)
Fasting	60–90 mg/dl	60–100
Premeal	60–105 mg/dl	—
1 hr postprandial	110–130 mg/dl	—
2 hr postprandial	90–120 mg/dl	80–120
2–6 am	60–120 mg/dl	—
Nocturnal	—	80–100

over, the emergence of a microvascular or macrovascular (coronary artery disease) complication places her in another class. The most recent revision of this classification was in 1980 (Table II).[18] At that time, gestational diabetes was given a separate category (see Chapter 2). Classes B, C, and D are generally assigned depending upon the woman's age of onset of diabetes and/or the duration. Whenever a criterion appears that places a women in the next lower class, it is the one that applies. For example, a woman whose diabetes began when she was 18 years of age and is now 22 would be considered Class C because her onset was under age 20, and not Class B because her duration was less than 10 years. It should also be pointed out that Class D includes not only women with an onset of diabetes under age 10 or duration of 20 years or more, but also women with background retinopathy or with hypertension (not pregnancy-induced). Class R diabetes is designated for women with proliferative retinopathy or vitreous hemorrhage. This category is also sometimes difficult to assign because of the increasing tendency to treat preproliferative or early pro-

TABLE II. White Classification (Revised)*

Gestational diabetes	Abnormal GTT[†], but euglycemia maintained by diet alone
	Diet alone insufficient, insulin required
Class A	Diet alone, any duration or onset age
Class B	Onset age 20 yr or older and duration less than 10 yr
Class C	Onset age 10–19 yr or duration 10–19 yr
Class D	Onset age under 10 yr, duration over 20 yr, background retinopathy, or hypertension (not preeclampsia)
Class R	Proliferative retinopathy or vitreous hemorrhage
Class F	Nephropathy with over 500 mg/day proteinuria
Class RF	Criteria for both Classes R and F coexist
Class H	Arteriosclerotic heart disease clinically evident
Class T	Prior renal transplantation

*All classes below A require insulin therapy. Class R, F, RF, H, and T have no onset/duration criteria but usually occur in long-term diabetes.The development of a complication moves the patient to the lower class.
[†]GTT = oral glucose tolerance test.
Reproduced from Hare JW, White P: Gestational diabetes and the White classification. Diabetes Care 3:394, 1980, with permission from the American Diabetes Association, Inc.

liferative retinopathy with laser photocoagulation. If one uses the need for laser therapy as a criterion for inclusion in Class R, a larger number of women will now fall into this category. Women with previously successfully treated or spontaneously remitted proliferative retinopathy are also included in Class R. The presence of significant proteinuria of over 500 mg/day or albuminuria of over 300 mg/day places women in Class F. The category FR is used for women who have both proliferative retinopathy and significant proteinuria due to their diabetes. Since retinopathy commonly clinically precedes nephropathy, a great many women with renal disease will fall into this category. If their retinopathy is only background, they are still considered Class F. If they have or have had proliferative retinopathy, they are considered Class FR. Women who have progressed to renal failure and have had a kidney transplant are considered to be Class T. The presence of coronary artery disease places the woman in Class H. (For a more complete discussion of maternal complications of diabetes and Classes F, T, and H or R, see Chapters 7 and 8.)

Consideration has been given to changing the White classification. Reasons for modifying it include the fact that Class A is an almost nonexistent category. The metabolic stresses of pregnancy lead to the need for exogenous insulin in almost all women with diet-controlled NIDDM, thus moving these women into at least Class B status. Furthermore, the distinction between normotensive Class B and Class C diabetes is negligible due to universal good maternal and fetal outcomes in both of these categories. The utility of the White classification is apparent with Classes D, R, and F patients. Each of these confers increased risk to the fetus, as a result of overt microvascular disease. In addition, Class H diabetes is associated with maternal mortality. In order for a new classification to improve upon the White classification, there must be better prediction of both fetal and maternal morbidity and mortality. Since complications of diabetes are important determinants of outcome independent of diabetes control, a newer classification has been suggested. No letters or numbers have been assigned in order to avoid confusion with the White classification or Types (I and II) of diabetes. Instead the use of DM (uncomplicated) or DM + complications has been used[19] (Table III). In one study, early pregnancy urinary protein excretion of 190–499 mg/24 hours was shown to be associated with a greater risk of preeclampsia.[20] This level of proteinuria represents incipient nephropathy, which has been shown to predict progression to overt diabetic nephropathy in nonpregnant patients with IDDM. However, in another study, first-trimester urinary albumin excretion of 40–250 μg/mg creatinine was not associated with increased risk of preeclampsia but did predict small-for-gestational-age infants.[21] Further stud-

TABLE III. Classification of Diabetes Mellitus and Pregnancy

Category	Abbreviation
Uncomplicated	DM
Complicated	DM+
Microvascular disease	
Retinopathy	
Background	BDR
Proliferative	PDR
Nephropathy	
Overt, macroalbuminuria	K-W
Microalbuminuria	MA
Hypertension	
Preexisting	HTN
Pregnancy-induced	PIH
Preeclampsia/toxemia	PET
Macrovascular disease	
Coronary artery disease	CAD
Autonomic neuropathy	AN
Discovered during gestation	GDM

Reprinted with permission from Hare JW: Diabetes and pregnancy. In Kahn CR, Weir G (eds): "Joslin's Diabetes Mellitus." Philadelphia: Lea and Febiger, 1994.

ies should be performed to determine whether or not urinary albumin excretion rates better stratify risk than the present White classification.

Management of Diabetes in Pregnancy

The management of diabetes in pregnancy ideally starts prior to conception (see Chapter 4). Prepregnancy counseling stresses the importance of good diabetes control and the use of folic acid beginning prior to pregnancy. Maternal and fetal risks are also discussed with the patient in advance of pregnancy. Notably, women with renal disease have a higher incidence of preeclampsia, premature delivery, and increased perinatal mortality rate (see Chapter 10). Moreover, women with proteinuria, particularly those aged 35 and older, may also have a greater incidence of coronary artery disease (see Chapter 8).

Once pregnancy is established, a team approach becomes the cornerstone of management and requires the cooperation of a variety of disciplines that include not only diabetologists but perinatologists, nurse educators, nutritionists, and social workers. Moreover, all of these people are conveniently present in one place and at one time weekly, when the patients are seen. As the pregnancy progresses, if medical, obstetrical, nutritional, or psychological issues are noted that require attention, they can be promptly addressed. At the time of the first visit in the pregnancy clinic, all of these professionals see the patient. A medical and obstetrical history is obtained and the patient is examined. For those women with hypertension, antihypertensive therapy that is safe for use in pregnancy is substituted (see Chapter 8). If the patient has a history of thyroid disease or if a goiter is noted on physical exam, thyroid function tests are ordered. The nursing assessment is made and teaching instituted in the management of diabetes. A dietary history is taken and a meal plan prepared. A psychosocial assessment is also performed. At the second visit, laboratory data obtained at the first visit are reviewed. This includes a glycohemoglobin level to retrospectively assess the degree of control in the early weeks of pregnancy and the risk of malformation. Other routine tests include a complete blood count (CBC), a urine culture to detect asymptomatic bacteriuria, a serology for syphilis, a Papanicolaou smear, a culture for gonorrhea, and a determination of blood type, as well as a screen for minor antibodies not in the ABO/Rh system. A 24-hour urine for protein, creatinine, and creatinine clearance is collected on women who have detectable proteinuria (i.e., 30 mg/dl or greater) on dipstick. A morning urine microalbumin is performed on women whose urine is dipstick negative. If significant proteinuria is detected, this is followed up with repeat monthly determinations. Initial historical and laboratory information is recorded on a flow sheet (Fig. 1). Data from subsequent weekly visits are also recorded. Routine dilated ophthalmologic evaluations are planned for each trimester of pregnancy or more frequently if significant diabetic retinopathy is present. If none is detected in the first trimester in a woman with short-term diabetes, further evaluation is not needed. Hospitalization is recommended for those women with poorly controlled diabetes for whom expeditious outpatient control of blood sugars may be difficult.

After the patient is informed of her risk of having an infant with a congenital anomaly (see Chapter 12), it is her choice whether or not to continue her pregnancy. It is pointed out that subsequent ultrasonography at 18 weeks is helpful at identifying neural tube defects as well as major cardiac and renal abnormalities. However, mild or progressive cardiac, pulmonary, renal, and limb abnormalities may not be noted as readily.

onset: | age at onset: 28
DOB: 12-4-58 | pres. age: 34 | dur:
COMA/DKA:
severe hypoglycemia:
? convulsions:
eyes:
ALLERGIES: BEE STINGS
problems:
height: 64½" | Soc. Serv consult:

FOB bld type:
HBS Ac NEGATIVE 5-28-94
RPRCT NON-REACTIVE 2-16-94
PAP SM
GC cult
Uricult
Feto Prot
Rubella
TSH
T4
T3RU
TT3

24 URINES

dates:
tot vol
creat cl
ur creat
tot prot
ur gluc

phone #
work #
OB MD:

PAST PREGNANCIES

date	outcome	wt	type del.
4-14-92	♀	9 lb 2 oz	VAG.
5-27-93	MISC.		

INFANT

del. dt: | wt: | sex:
name:

Dates			11/9	11/16	11/23	11/30	12/7	12/14	12/21	12/28	1/4	1/11	1/18	1/25	2/1	2/8	2/15	2/22
Gest wk	5	6	7	8	9	10	11	12	13	14	15	16	17	18	19	20	21	22
B P			115/60			100/60	90/65	98/50	96/48			117/66	92/60	108/58		80/40	90/48	
Sono																		
Weight			124¼	125½	125¼	125¾	128	126¾	127				130½	134		136½	138½	138
Edema																		
Insulin			22.5	36		48	42	42	28	[illegible]		49						47
Bun/Creat																		
Bld Gluc			234	236	106	128	261	178	201			71	226	193	41	80	179	193
Ur Prot			30	0	0	0	0	0	0			0	0	0	0	0	TR	TR
Ac/DAc			0	0	0	0	0	0	0			0	0	0	0	0	0	0
Glyco AI			7.6				7.1					7.4				7.0		
Hct			36.7				35.2					36.4				36.5		

Dates	3/1	3/8	3/15	3/22	3/29	4/5	4/12	4/19	4/26	5/3	5/10	5/17	5/24	5/31	6/7	6/14	6/21	6/28
Gest wk	23	24	25	26	27	28	29	30	31	32	33	34	35	36	37	38	39	40
B P	102/58	98/60	98/54	108/58		94/54	100/60	100/80	110/70	106/68	108/66	108/64	110/70	[illegible]/68	[illegible]/70			
Sono																		
Weight	141½	141½	142½	145¼	146	147½	147½	150	151	153	155	156½	157½	159¼	161¾			
Edema																		
Insulin		55		68.5	70	72		88.5	60.5		99	116.5	106	117				
Bun/Creat																		
Bld Gluc		180	116	169	125	75	132	127	143	186	149	158	184	181	123			
Ur Prot	30	0	TR	0	0	30	TR	TR	TR	30	0	TR	0	30	30			
Ac/DAc	0	0	0	0	0	0	0	0	0	0	0	0	0	0	0			
Glyco AI		6.9				7.4				7.9				8.1				
Hct		34.9				33.1				32.8				33.5				

Fig. 1. The Joslin Pregnancy Clinic record sheet.

Current studies are investigating the use of transvaginal ultrasound in identifying these lesions earlier in gestation (L. Hornberger, personal communication).

Most women are seen weekly for the duration of their pregnancy. Some highly motivated and reliable women with stable Class B or C diabetes are seen biweekly, if all is going well. At each visit, a brief history is taken, as well as a brief review of systems. The blood pressure is taken and the retinal fundi are examined. Any previous historical physical findings of note are rechecked.

Attention is then focused on the blood-sugar values collected over the previous week. As noted in Chapter 4, our patients are asked to do four fingerstick glucoses a day: before breakfast and two hours after each meal. At the time of each week's visit, they are given a flow sheet that has a space for recording the glucose value, the time the meal was eaten, the time the glucose was measured and another column for indicating reactions. They are also asked to check for ketonuria in the morning, in order to ensure that nutrition is adequate. It should be pointed out that it is not uncommon for a normal pregnant woman to have some ketonuria after an overnight fast because of the phenomenon of accelerated starvation. It typically disappears as alimentation occurs. Testing for ketones later in the day, if the sugar is high (i.e., mid-200 range), is to prevent ketosis resulting from uncontrolled diabetes and to eliminate the development of ketoacidosis, which may lead to a poor fetal outcome. As a result of intensive home management, ketoacidosis has become quite rare in our population. The last time a fetal death occurred because of maternal ketoacidosis was 15 years ago.

Insulin Use

Since most patients in our pregnancy clinic have IDDM, they usually require three or four injections of insulin per day in order to achieve adequate glycemic control. Women with insulin-requiring gestational diabetes or NIDDM may be controlled with one or two injections per day. Women with IDDM, who present to the pregnancy clinic and are on a prebreakfast and presupper regimen of mixed short-acting and intermediate-acting insulins, are changed to a three-injection regimen: short-acting and intermediate-acting insulin before breakfast, short-acting insulin before supper, and intermediate-acting insulin at bedtime. This regimen decreases the risk of nocturnal hypoglycemia, since the intermediate-acting insulin will be peaking closer to morning rather than in the middle of the night. Some women may also require regular insulin before lunch, because insufficient action is obtained from their morning intermediate insulin by early afternoon but more than enough action is apparent by later afternoon or early evening.

Other regimens include the use of three injections of premeal regular and a fourth of intermediate-acting insulin at bedtime. In addition, ultralente, when used in equal, divided doses prebreakfast and presupper, provides fairly stable basal insulin levels. Premeal short-acting insulin eliminates postmeal excursions in blood sugars in these patients. The insulin pump, while not used very frequently in our pregnancy clinic, has its place in the management of patients with erratic schedules (i.e., shift workers) and in patients who have a prominent "dawn phenomenon." The dawn phenomenon refers to hyperglycemia occurring in the early morning hours (i.e., 4–8 a.m.), a result of the diurnal secretion of growth hormone and cortisol. These patients are predisposed to nocturnal hypoglycemia, prior to 4 a.m., and fasting hyperglycemia, when treated with intermittent injections. The advantage of an insulin pump is that it continuously delivers insulin subcutaneously and may be programmed for more than one basal insulin rate. A second-higher basal insulin rate (alternate basal) may, therefore, be used during the early morning hours to control hyperglycemia caused by relative insulin resistance. Premeal boluses of regular insulin are also delivered via the pump in order to prevent postprandial hyperglycemia. If a pump is to be initiated, the woman's total daily subcutaneous dose of insulin is summed. Roughly half of this is given as continuous basal insulin and half is given in divided doses premeals and presnacks. It is not uncommon for the prebreakfast bolus to be the largest one. This applies not only to the patients treated with pumps but also to those treated with premeal regular programs.

Whatever the method of insulin administration, patients are encouraged to make their own insulin adjustments if blood-sugar values rise prior to their next weekly visit. Algorithms for adjusting the insulin dose upward, in the case of hyperglycemia, and downward, in the case of hypoglycemia, are provided (see Chapter 4). The striking benefits derived from this autonomy are observed in the late second and early third trimesters of pregnancy, when the secretion of human placental lactogen by a growing placenta results in insulin resistance, fasting and postprandial hyperglycemia, and greater insulin needs before the next clinic visit. Women who are uncomfortable with insulin adjustments are encouraged to call our clinic as frequently during the week as necessary, in order to maintain good control of blood sugars during this period.

Adjustment of insulin doses is best done when one looks for the pattern of the patient's blood-sugar values. Because IDDM has an inherent instability, it is not wise to make an insulin adjustment after only one or two days' blood sugars have been reviewed. The exception to this would be the occurrence of a reaction with no explanation, such as a missed meal or increased exercise. At that point, the offending insulin should be immediately reduced. The essential principal for success with any insulin program is prospective use. Once a glucose pattern is established, the insulin dose is tailored to anticipate the next glucose level and not to react to a change in glucose. It is a rare patient whose diabetes requires a retrospective sliding scale as a mode of management. It should also be emphasized that elimination of hypoglycemia should occur before trying to correct any periods of hyperglycemia during the day. Hyperglycemia may be a direct result of the hypoglycemic event, either from overtreating an insulin reaction with sugar by mouth or because the counterregulatory hormones glucagon and epinephrine result in glycogenolysis and gluconeogenesis.[22,23] Too often, patients focus their concern on the secondary hyperglycemia rather than on the precipitating hypoglycemia, increasing their insulin dose instead of decreasing it, and thus potentiating the risk for more profound hypoglycemia.

There are typical changes in insulin requirements throughout pregnancy. During the first trimester, it is not uncommon for the insulin requirement to decrease by about 10% or so. A larger decrease suggests that the patient's diabetes was not optimally controlled before pregnancy, either because of poor diet or overinsulinization. Those who require increases in insulin doses probably had inadequate control of diabetes prior to pregnancy due to inadequate insulin administration. Diabetes tends to be more unstable than usual in the first trimester. This may lead to more difficulty with insulin reactions and more difficulty in achieving good control. Glucagon may be needed to treat severe hypoglycemic reactions during this time. On the other hand, some women who have stable diabetes may have no significant problems with insulin reactions.

Whatever a particular patient's inherent degree of instability is, after the first trimester has passed, it will improve and once delivered, she will revert to her prepregnancy status. There is a gradual increase in the insulin requirement during the middle trimester. This may not be readily apparent from week to week, but when one reviews the insulin requirements from the third to sixth or seventh month of pregnancy it is occasionally seen that it has doubled. The insulin requirements may rise more abruptly early in the third trimester. Interestingly, the degree of instability decreases. This phenomenon protects the patient from hypoglycemic reactions and subsequent rebound hyperglycemia, enabling the woman to achieve the best control of diabetes that she ever will. She rides the sea of diabetes like an ocean liner in the third trimester, as contrasted to a rowboat in the first. In the last month or so of pregnancy, there may be a decrease in the insulin requirement, particularly at night. This is because fetal siphonage of maternal glucose and amino acids continues at an ever increasing rate as fetal growth progresses. However, placental growth and, hence, the levels of its contrainsulin hormones level at about the 36th week, causing a decrease in maternal glucose, particularly at night when the fetus is continuously feeding and the mother is not. In some patients, this decrease may be dramatic and result in as much as a 20% or 30% diminution in insulin requirements. This is worth noting because, in the days before the availability of fetal monitoring, a falling insulin requirement of 50% was taken as an indication of a failing fetoplacental unit and necessitated emergency delivery. It is hard to know, in retrospect, how many of deliveries of healthy fetuses were precipitated by normal physiology rather than placental pathology.

Our general aim is to avoid hospitalization until delivery is imminent. Women with uncomplicated pregnancies and well-controlled blood sugars may remain at home until the day of their induction or planned C-section. The timing of delivery is individualized (see Chapter 9).

The management of diabetes during labor and delivery or caesarian section is discussed in Chapter 9. In brief, insulin requirements are minimal during this period and there is a marked sensitivity to insulin. In fact, insulin requirements decrease to zero during active stage 1 labor.[24] This insulin sensitivity may continue for up to 5 to 7 days postpartum. The physiology of this phenomenon is unknown. In preparation for delivery, the patient is asked to take nothing by mouth after midnight. For those patients who take intermediate-acting insulin, a small dose (one-third of their original prepregnancy dose) may be given. For patients who are using ultralente preparations, insulin may be held on the day of induction, due to the longer half-life of ultralente. Patients who take premeal regular and intermediate-acting insulin at bedtime may take a small dose of intermediate-acting insulin the morning of induction while holding their usual regular insulin. This provides minimal basal insulin requirements. Alternatively, subcutaneous insulin may be held and an intravenous insulin infusion may be started when the blood glucoses rise above 120 mg/dl. Dextrose (5%) and 0.5 Normal saline are administered at a continuous rate of 125 ml per hour or higher if hypoglycemia develops. Boluses of dextrose are not given.

Postpartum, insulin should be given in small doses, while titrating the blood glucose levels to between 200–300 mg/dl. This level of glycemic control is often difficult for patients to accept, since they are used to much more "tightly" controlled blood sugars. However, the risk of hypoglycemia is great if more aggressive treatment is given. Furthermore, there is no significant short-term risk to the mother of maintaining blood sugars in this range. As food intake increases postpartum and insulin sensitivity decreases, insulin requirements approach prepregnancy levels. Unfortunately, most women are discharged from the hospital before blood sugars have stabilized. We review parameters for increasing insulin doses at home and encourage patients to phone the on-call diabetologist for advice. After nine months of reviewing and adjusting insulin doses, many women are comfortable with this task. Patients may also be warned that the degree of stability of diabetes that they became accustomed to during the later part of their pregnancy will revert to the relative instability that they had prior to their pregnancy.

Breast feeding is encouraged for infants of women with IDDM, as it is for all infants in general. Whether to breast feed or bottle feed is a mother's personal decision. It is unclear whether exposure to cow's milk based formulas in genetically susceptible infants increases the risk of IDDM. This is reviewed in depth in reference 25. A prospective trial comparing breast feeding with cow's milk formula feeding in infants of diabetic mothers would help to clarify this issue. For women who choose to breast feed, a mechanical breast pump is used to provide the nipple stimulation necessary to induce lactation during the period of separation of infant and mother, while the infant is in the neonatal intensive care unit. Increased caloric requirements in women who breast feed are incorporated into the revised meal plan prior to hospital discharge (see Chapter 5).

Our patients are routinely seen six weeks postpartum for an obstetrical examination. They are also seen by the diabetologist who reviews their blood sugars and adjusts their insulin dosages. If they had hypertension due to preeclampsia during pregnancy, it should have resolved by this time. Since preeclampsia sometimes induces long-standing hypertension, the presence of an elevated blood pressure, at this postpartum visit, suggests that it is established hypertension and requires treatment. The patient, at this point, may resume her usual schedule of outpatient visits with her internist. If there were no complications of delivery, she needs no further visits with the obstetrician.

REFERENCES

1. The DCCT Research Group. The effect of intensive treatment of diabetes on the development and progression of long-term complications in insulin-dependent diabetes mellitus. N Engl J Med 329:977–986, 1993.

2. Karlsson K, Kjellmer J. The outcome of diabetic pregnancies in relation to the mother's blood sugar level. Am J Obstet Gynecol 112:213–220, 1972.
3. Jovanovic L, Druzin M, Peterson CM. Effect of euglycemia on the outcome of pregnancy in insulin-dependent diabetic women as compared with normal control subjects. Am J Med 71:921–927, 1981.
4. Coustan DR, Berkowitz RL, Hobbins JC. Tight metabolic control of overt diabetes in pregnancy. Am J Med 68:845–852, 1980.
5. Landon MB, Gabbe SG, Piana R, Mennuti MT, Main EK. Neonatal morbidity in pregnancy complicated by diabetes mellitus: Predictive value of maternal glycemic profiles. Am J Obstet Gynecol 156:1089–1095, 1987.
6. Leslie RDG, Pyke DA, John PN, White JM. Haemoglobin A1 in diabetic pregnancy. Lancet 2:958–959, 1978.
7. Miller E, Hare JW, Cloherty JP, Dunn PJ, Gleason RE, Soeldner JS, Kitzmiller JL. Elevated maternal hemoglobin A1c in early pregnancy and major congenital anomalies in infants of diabetic mothers. N Engl J Med 304:1331–1334, 1981.
8. Ylinen K, Alva P, Stenman U-H, Kesäniemi-Kuokkanen T, Teramo K. Risk of minor and major fetal malformations in diabetics with high haemoglobin A1c values in early pregnancy. Br Med J 289:345–346, 1984.
9. Führmann K, Reiner H, Semmler K, Fischer F, Fischer M, Glockner E. Prevention of congenital malformations in infants of insulin-dependent diabetic mothers. Diabetes Care 6:219–223, 1983.
10. Greene MF. Prevention and diagnosis of congenital abnormalities in diabetic pregnancies. Clinics in Perinatology 20:533–547, 1993.
11. Mills JL, Baker L, Goldman AS. Malformations in infants of diabetic mothers occur before the seventh gestational weeks. Diabetes 28:292–293, 1979.
12. Mills JL, Knopp RH, Simpson JL, Jovanovic-Peterson L, Metzger BE, Holmes LB, Aarons JH, Brown Z, Reed GF, Bieber FR, Van Allen M, Holzman I, Ober C, Peterson CM, Withiam MJ, Duckles A, Mueller-Heubach E, Polk BF, and the National Institute of Child Health and Human Development in Early Pregnancy Study. Lack of relation of increased malformation rate in infants of diabetic mothers to glycemic control during organogenesis. N Engl J Med 318:671–676, 1988.
13. Steel JM, Johnstone FD, Hepburn DA, Smith AF. Can prepregnancy care of diabetic women reduce the risk of abnormal babies? Br Med J 301:1070–1074, 1990.
14. Kitzmiller JL, Gavin LA, Gin GD, Jovanovic-Peterson L, Main EK, Zigrang WD. Preconception care of diabetes. Glycemic control prevents congenital abnormalities. JAMA 265:731–736, 1991.
15. Rosenn B, Miodovnik M, Combs CA, Khoury J, Siddiqi TA. Pre-conception management of insulin-dependent diabetes: Improvement of pregnancy outcome. Obstet Gynecol 77:846–849, 1991.
16. Greenspoon JS, Morgan BR. A product warning label to encourage prepregnancy control of diabetes. JAMA 266:2225, 1991.
17. Sadler TW, Hunter ES III. Hypoglycemia: How little is too much for the embryo? Am J Obstet Gynecol 157:190–193, 1987.
18. Hare JW, White P. Gestational diabetes and the White classification. Diabetes Care 3:394, 1980.
19. Hare JW. Diabetes and Pregnancy. In Kahn CR, Weir GC (eds): "Joslin's Diabetes Mellitus." Philadelphia: Lea and Febiger, 1994, pp 889–899.
20. Combs CA, Rosenn B, Kitzmiller J, Khoury J, Wheeler BC, Miodovnik M. Early-pregnancy proteinuria in diabetes related to preeclampsia. Obstet Gynecol 82:802–807, 1993.

21. Laffel LMB, Greene MF, Wilkins-Haug L. First trimester urinary albumin excretion predicts birth weight in diabetic pregnancies. Diabetes 41 (Suppl 1):133A, 1992.
22. Clutter WE, Rizza RA, Gerich JW, Cryer PE. Regulation of glucose metabolism by sympathochromaffin catecholamines. Diabetes Metab Rev 4:1–15, 1988.
23. Frizzell RT, Campbell PJ, Cherrington AD. Gluconeogenesis and hypoglycemia. Diabetes Metab Rev 4:51–70, 1988.
24. Jovanovic L, Peterson CM. Insulin and glucose requirements during the first stage of labor in insulin-dependent pregnant diabetic women. Am J Med 75:607–612, 1983.
25. Gerstein HC. Cow's milk exposure and type I diabetes mellitus. Diabetes Care 17:13–19, 1994.

CHAPTER 4

Home Management

Suzanne Z. Ghiloni, BSN, CDE

INTRODUCTION

Most women take a healthy pregnancy for granted. The wonder of natural body changes, the laughable food cravings, the "glow" this state induces, all serve to make pregnancy a wonderful and exciting time. But consider the woman who cannot take for granted what most women do—one who is considered at high risk. This is the woman whose pregnancy is complicated by diabetes. For her to achieve a healthy outcome, she must commit to a considerable investment of time and effort. "Controlled diabetes is essential to fetal welfare," Dr. Priscilla White, a pioneer in the field of diabetes and pregnancy, said in 1928. It is as pertinent now as it was then, but, fortunately, with medical advances, it is much easier.

The importance of patient education with a chronic disease such as diabetes cannot be overestimated. Achieving optimal control of diabetes requires balancing the meal plan, diabetes medication, and activity level. Education should aim to improve the patient's knowledge of diabetes and the skills for its management. Probably nowhere will the effects of education be so tangible as in the delivery of a healthy baby. The satisfaction of being involved in this wonderful endeavor is immense. An important outgrowth of the pregnancy experience is the opportunity for these women to see how well-controlled their diabetes can be. Many leave determined to keep their diabetes managed as never before. Working with the pregnant population is a rewarding experience. The motivation and willingness of these women are an inspiration to those who work with them.

A basic understanding of the relationship between good control of diabetes and a healthy baby should be reinforced in all women of childbearing age, long before they are considering pregnancy. Patients should be reminded periodically that the best chance for success comes with a

Diabetes Complicating Pregnancy: The Joslin Clinic Method, Edited by Florence M. Brown, MD and John W. Hare, MD.
ISBN 0-471-11031-0 © 1995 John Wiley & Sons, Inc.

planned pregnancy. The woman with diabetes should receive additional in-depth prepregnancy counseling when she has made the decision to become pregnant. Husbands and partners are strongly encouraged to participate in the planning, as it is important for them to be involved and aware of the seriousness of the endeavor. Prepregnancy counseling can be accomplished in a classroom setting or in an individual session with a diabetes educator specializing in pregnancy. While making those involved aware of the many facets of a diabetic pregnancy, this can be a wonderful means of establishing a relationship with the patient before meeting in the Pregnancy Clinic.

First and foremost, the woman must understand the rationale for this carefully planned pregnancy. Knowing why she must accomplish specific goals will be helpful in inducing compliance. A prepregnancy session with the diabetes educator is ideal and should include the following topics:

1. Rationale for tight control during pregnancy
2. Information about necessary management skills
3. Assessment of need for nutrition education
4. Maternal risks of diabetic pregnancy
5. Expense
6. Prenatal care

RATIONALE FOR TIGHT CONTROL DURING PREGNANCY

Infants of pregestational diabetic mothers are at higher risk for congenital anomalies. These anomalies are related to hyperglycemia, although the exact metabolic cause is not known. Since most defects occur within eight weeks after conception, early diabetes control is imperative. Poor control also carries with it a higher rate of spontaneous abortion. The threat of anomaly and miscarriage should not be presented in an overly alarming manner but the seriousness of the risk should be stressed. What should be emphasized are the statistics that demonstrate that when diabetes is well controlled, the risk for an anomaly approaches that of the general population.

Ideally, pregnancy planning for the diabetic woman begins six months before attempting to conceive. This can be considered "preventive medicine." Good metabolic control is desired before conception. Most authorities recognize the use of the glycosylated hemoglobin, or hemoglobin $A_1(A_1)$, as a satisfactory means of assessing control. This is a laboratory blood test that represents an average of blood-sugar control for the previous six to eight weeks. The values may vary among different laboratories; those at the Joslin Diabetes Center are as indicated in Table I.

TABLE I. Glycosylated Hemoglobin Values at the Joslin Diabetes Center Laboratory

A_1 values	Percentage	Approximate mean glucose level (mg/dl)
Normal	5.4–7.4%	90–120
Excellent	7.5–9%	120–160
Good	9–10%	160–180
Fair	10–11.5%	180–210
Poor control	Over 11.5%	>210

The woman planning a pregnancy is encouraged to aim for an A_1 in the "good" range, below 10%. This will place her at low risk for having an infant with an anomaly or a spontaneous abortion (see Chapter 12). Obviously it would be ideal to pursue an A_1 in the "normal" or "excellent" range; however, for many women with unstable insulin-dependent diabetes mellitus (IDDM), this would be very difficult to achieve. It is most important that each woman's goals be individualized and that they be safe and realistic. At the Joslin Diabetes Center, women are requested to contact the prepregnancy clinic six months before they plan to become pregnant. Follow-up contact (via visit or telephone) is maintained on a monthly basis. The educator can prompt contact by communicating A_1 results to the patient after each monthly lab visit and using this value to assist her with her management plan.

Once a woman has attained an A_1 in the desired range and finger-stick blood sugars are well controlled, she is given the green light to attempt conception.

Insulin Management

A crucial aspect of the management plan is the insulin regimen. A majority of the clinic patients are successful with a conventional split-mix regimen (fast-acting insulin and intermediate-acting insulin before breakfast and before supper), or a variation with the evening shot divided into presupper fast-acting insulin and bedtime intermediate insulin. The latter pattern benefits patients with nocturnal hypoglycemia.

Another option is a more intensive program such as twice daily long-acting insulin (ultralente) with premeal boluses of fast-acting (regular) insulin. This tends to work well for those patients who are more sophisticated and motivated but who have not done well with the traditional split-mix regimen. Ultralente is given twice daily in equally divided doses, before breakfast and before supper. Since ultralente has a broader peak than intermediate insulins, it provides good coverage for basal insulin requirements. Regular insulin is given one-half hour before meals, in order to prevent the glucose excursion following the ingestion of food. One concern, however, is that the full effect of an insulin adjustment on blood sugar is delayed due to ultralente's long half-life. Another intensive program, consisting of three injections of fast-acting (regular) insulin before meals and a bedtime injection of intermediate-acting (NPH or lente) insulin, works well for motivated patients who are willing to take four injections daily. Regardless of the insulin regimen used, all preparations with regular insulin must be taken at least 30 minutes before the appropriate meal. Failure to do so will lead to delayed absorption of insulin, high two-hour postprandial blood sugars, and hypoglycemia by three to four hours.

INFORMATION ABOUT NECESSARY MANAGEMENT SKILLS

Women should be prepared for the skills they will be expected to utilize in the future. These include home blood-glucose monitoring, urine ketone testing, glucagon administration, an understanding of the glycosylated hemoglobin, familiarity with guidelines for insulin adjustment and sick-day management, and exercise/activity recommendations. There is also a need to be able to recognize and treat acute complications such as hypoglycemia and hyperglycemia.

ASSESSMENT OF NEED FOR NUTRITION EDUCATION

A basic assessment of the patient's nutrition knowledge should be performed by asking several simple questions. How long has it been since she has been seen by a dietician? (It is recommended by the American Diabetes Association and other diabetes specialty groups that adults with diabetes consult with a dietician every 6–12 months.) Does she have an individualized meal plan? Is she following it? Is a weight problem apparent? Certainly, these are areas where referral to the specialist, a registered dietician, is most appropriate. Current recommendations also specify the inclusion of adequate folic acid intake prior to and early in pregnancy. This should be addressed in a prepregnancy session.

MATERNAL RISKS OF DIABETIC PREGNANCY

During pregnancy there is the potential for the exacerbation of preexisting complications, i.e., retinopathy, nephropathy, and neuropathy. Every patient should be made aware of these risks, for only then can an informed decision be made with respect to getting pregnant. To some women, the fear of worsening complications can be a great deterrent to pregnancy (see Chapters 7 and 8). However, on the positive side, it has also been found that, in general, complications revert to their prepregnancy status once the pregnancy has ended. Again, this is an area in which the specialist should be involved, and patients should be referred to the appropriate physician (ophthalmologist, diabetologist) before pregnancy for advice based on their individual situation. Since most women with 10 to 15 years of diabetes have at least the beginnings of chronic complications, there will be many who will face these maternal risks.

EXPENSE

While it is impossible to set a fixed price for a high-risk pregnancy, general agreement sets the cost at several thousand dollars, perhaps much more if there are complications that require lengthy hospitalization. The cost is typically covered by insurance to some degree, but since this does represent a financial investment, it would be unwise to neglect this area of concern. As financial considerations can add to the existing stress of a diabetic pregnancy, a recommendation should be made to (1) investigate present insurance coverage *before* pregnancy and (2) plan ahead for out-of-pocket expenses such as blood monitoring equipment and ketone testing strips.

PRENATAL CARE

Careful management is the key to a healthy pregnancy and outcome. Since it has been shown that skilled specialty centers specializing in high-risk pregnancies report the highest success rates, it stands to reason that the choice of a care giver is quite important. Most high-risk clinics have a team of professionals that include an obstetrician, endocrinologist, neonatologist, nurse educator, dietician, and social worker. This type of clinic also promotes a supportive atmosphere among the women who meet there each week. For those not fortunate enough to have access to this type of facility, this poses a problem. It is advisable, therefore, for the woman to consider ahead of time who will manage her care. Some places to turn to for a referral might be (1) a diabetologist or obstetrician, (2) the local chapter of the American Diabetes Association, or (3) a nearby teaching (university-affiliated) hospital.

During the session with the nurse educator, it is beneficial to allow women, their partners, and other interested family members to ask questions and voice concerns. In many cases, it allows for the separation of fact from fallacy, as there is an overabundance of misinformation connected to diabetic pregnancies. Some common myths are: inability of diabetic women to have children, extensive hospitalization during pregnancy, congenital diabetes, and proscription of vaginal delivery.

A frequent question of many potential parents is "Will my child develop diabetes?" While this is a possibility, it must be put into perspective. Heredity does play a role in determining who will be affected by this disease. In the general population, a person has a less than 1% chance of developing Type I diabetes. The offspring of a mother with Type I diabetes has less than a 5% lifetime risk of developing diabetes. If the father is affected the risk is less than 10%.[1] If both parents have Type I diabetes, the risk is elevated to about 30%.[2] The risk, in any case, is very low in infancy and early childhood. The genetic risks are much higher in Type II diabetes. The chances of someone in the general population developing Type II diabetes are 10%. If one parent has this type, the risk to the offspring is 30%. If both parents are afflicted, the risk increases to 50% or more.[3]

Since anxiety about the health of the baby is common, it is helpful for women to know that there are special diagnostic tests that are done to assess the status of the fetus (see Chapters 9 and 10). Information about the meaning and timing of these tests is beneficial.

It is not unusual for women who are not yet pregnant to voice apprehensions regarding labor, delivery, and the postpartum course. Discussing generalized information about these can provide a realistic view and perhaps reduce needless anxieties. In this area, the diabetes educator can be an excellent resource and referral guide to the woman and her partner.

Patients should be advised to be alert for signs of pregnancy, as early as possible. An appointment with the physician or clinic should be scheduled promptly after pregnancy is suspected. Unfortunately, some women do not plan well enough to have an ideal, unhurried, prepregnancy educational opportunity. Thus, all of the above information must be added to the management issues described in the next section.

THE INITIAL VISIT

The first visit to the Pregnancy Clinic is scheduled as soon as possible. Most women arrive at the Pregnancy Clinic excited, yet anxious. The pregnant woman may be seeing several practitioners of different disciplines in the space of a few hours. The diabetes educator should allow the patient time for verbalizing feelings at the first visit. By helping to allay fears and concerns, one can set a clearer path to learning.

There are many management issues to cover and the woman should be informed that she is not expected to retain everything that is taught the first day. A very useful resource is *A Guide for Women with Diabetes Who Are Pregnant . . . Or Plan to Be*,[4] a 165-page reference that contains a wealth of pertinent information for the diabetic woman. This is available to each new patient at her first visit. It is also helpful to assure the patient at the initial visit, that she is welcome to call the staff with any questions. The Clinic provides 24-hour telephone coverage to all its patients.

Individual assessment should be the first step. Some preliminary questions to consider in assessing a patient (time constraints may make an in-depth assessment difficult) are as follows: Has the patient had access to education previously? How long ago? Is she consistent about being seen at regular intervals by her physician? Do previous lab values indicate that diabetes has been well-managed? If the patient appears to be lacking in basic diabetes knowledge, she should be referred for further education.

HOME MONITORING

During pregnancy, it is necessary to assess the impact of the treatment program on a frequent basis. Patients do this by testing blood sugars at home. Home blood-glucose monitoring is one of the most important new developments in the management of all types of diabetes. Introduced in the late 1970s, most diabetes health experts have concluded that home blood-glucose monitoring is essential for, among others, pregnant women with diabetes. This procedure has been responsible for the patients' and doctors' ability to monitor the course of diabetes much more closely.

Because there is no doubt that glycemic levels during pregnancy affect perinatal outcome, it is best to be as well-informed as possible about blood-sugar levels at various times of day. Home blood-glucose monitoring has become, therefore, a standard and routine part of the pregnancy regimen, as it aids in daily management decisions and helps in the recognition of emergency situations. If monitoring is not being done already, it should be taught at the initial visit to the Pregnancy Clinic. Recommendations are that monitoring be done at least four times per day: fasting and two hours postprandially. A blood-glucose meter is utilized for monitoring in order to provide accurate glucose results. It is a portable, pocket-sized device that uses electronic capability to measure the blood sugar more accurately than the human eye. It requires a finger puncture and manual placement of blood on the test strip; however, the meter reads the strip and eliminates the guesswork. Most current meters have memory capacity. There are many meters competing in the market, such as One Touch II®, Accu-Chek Easy®, Companion 2®, and Glucometer Elite®. Each meter functions in a similar manner but there are variable features among them. An educator can assist the patient in choosing the one that best suits her needs. Meters, when used correctly, provide a reasonable range of accuracy. However, it cannot be overstated that proper training and consistent maintenance checks are of the utmost importance.

Most methods take one to two minutes for completion. Each method has steps specific to its use, but there are generalities that must be followed.

1. Follow manufacturer's directions exactly (i.e., if product calls for a wipe with a cotton ball, do not substitute any other item).
2. Wash hands thoroughly before puncture. Sugar from food or other sources may alter the reading.
3. Touch blood droplet, not finger, to test pad; especially, do not smear blood, as this may alter chemical composition of the separate pads.

Suggestions for Ease of Use

1. Wash hands with warm soapy water (blood is more difficult to obtain from cold hands).
2. Hang arm by side for 30 seconds to increase blood flow to fingertips.
3. Use side of fingertip for puncture, as there are less nerve endings there and, therefore, less discomfort.
4. Read product label for storage conditions and expiration date.
5. Investigate the various spring-loaded devices available that make puncturing easier. Many have two different end caps—one for shallow punctures and one for deep punctures.
6. Avoid reuse of lancets, as dull needles are more painful.
7. Rotate puncture sites to avoid repeated skin trauma and callus formation.

Tips for Meter Use

1. Blood droplets should cover the test pad, as the sensor may read uncovered portions as low.
2. The meter should be calibrated as often as the manufacturer recommends, using a checkstrip device and/or glucose control solution.
3. Meter accuracy can be gauged by checking a blood sugar simultaneously with a venous lab specimen. Meter result should be within 10–15% of the lab value.

Occasionally, for financial reasons, women will need to use a visual method of home blood-glucose monitoring. Chemstrip bG® are the strips of choice. Home blood-glucose monitoring for most people is easy to learn, but it should be emphasized that individual instruction by a trained professional is the preferred method of teaching. It is worthwhile to evaluate a patient's skill periodically, since accurate results are dependent on the user's skill. For women who are new to this technique, the educator should request that they save several of their used strips to be brought in the following week. The diabetes educator can then assess the patient's skill at reading the strip. Most strips are stable for up to seven days after use, if stored according to the manufacturer's directions.

All data should be carefully recorded. The Joslin Pregnancy Clinic uses a specially adapted record sheet (Fig. 1), which includes date, time meal ended, time of blood test result, insulin dose, fasting urine ketone result, and a remarks column to accommodate information such as reactions, unusual activity patterns, alterations in meal plans, etc. Since the treatment plan relies heavily on the patient's weekly monitoring record, keeping accurate data is essential. Patients should understand how their home blood-glucose monitoring results will be incorporated into their treatment plan so that they will bring records to each visit without fail.

Women are encouraged to maintain blood sugars as close to normal as possible during pregnancy. Goals for blood sugar at this time are: fasting, 60–100 mg/dl; two hours postprandial (after each meal), 80–120 mg/dl.[5] While euglycemia is strongly desired and to be worked towards, women with insulin-dependent diabetes will often have blood-sugar results outside the normal range. It can be very beneficial for the woman's stress and frustration level to be aware of this.

Some women express concern about the possibility of infection or decreased sensitivity of the fingertips with frequent testing. To prevent the occurrence of infection (the risk is low), thorough handwashing is stressed. Sensory decrease has not been found to be a side effect of multiple punctures, but thickened skin has been noted by many.

Another type of testing that women are taught to perform is for urine ketones (acetone). The ketone level is checked every morning with the first voided urine. Since there is an increased tendency toward ketosis during pregnancy, starvation or fasting will accelerate fat breakdown. After fasting all night, the possibility of ketonuria is increased. Since there may be a negative effect on the offspring's intelligence levels with consistently elevated ketone levels during pregnancy, this is considered a necessary part of the daily monitoring regimen.[6,7] Ketones in the morning urine, despite good blood-sugar control, indicate the need for a review of the meal plan to consider raising the calorie allotment at bedtime or

NAME: ______________________ DATE: ______________ TO: ______________________

DAY	FASTING		AFTER BREAKFAST		AFTER LUNCH		AFTER SUPPER		BEDTIME	INSULIN					REMARKS
OF WEEK	BLOOD SUGAR	URINE ACETONE (KETONES) TIME TAKEN	BLOOD SUGAR 2 HRS LATER	TIME MEAL ENDED TIME TAKEN	BLOOD SUGAR 2 HRS LATER	TIME MEAL ENDED TIME TAKEN	BLOOD SUGAR 2 HRS LATER	TIME MEAL ENDED TIME TAKEN	OR NIGHT BLOOD SUGAR TIME TAKEN	PRE-BREAK-FAST	PRE-LUNCH	PRE-SUPPER	BED-TIME	TOTAL 24 hr. Insulin Dose	
TUES															
WED															
THURS															
FRI															
SAT															
SUN															
MON															
TUES															

1. Test for urine acetone (ketones) before breakfast each morning.
2. Test for acetone anytime blood sugar is over 240 mg/dl, and record the level.
3. Do blood sugars fasting and 2 hours after meals daily. Blood sugar tests at additional times may be helpful.
4. Record time meal ends and time of blood test.
5. Record time of insulin reaction in "remarks" column. (Be sure to write a.m. or p.m.)
6. Record insulin dose(s) in appropriate columns
   Fast Acting (R)
   Intermediate Acting (N or L)
   Long Acting (U)

BRING YOUR RECORD AT EACH VISIT

Joslin Diabetes Center   One Joslin Place   Boston, Massachusetts 02215

Fig. 1. Diabetes monitoring record, Joslin Clinic.

throughout the day. Contact with the dietician is recommended if a woman has ketones in her urine for two or more consecutive days. There are several over-the-counter methods for ketone testing. Most patients are interested in a product that is simple, quick and convenient. Ketostix (Ames)® and Chemstrip K (Bio-Dynamics)® are two frequently used brands that provide these features. Again, one-to-one teaching for appropriate use is best.

In the last ten years, there has been a marked increase in the number of women referred to specialists when they have been diagnosed with gestational diabetes. The goal of treatment is the same for women with IDDM and gestational diabetes–normal blood sugar levels. For most women, the diagnosis of diabetes during pregnancy is unexpected and unsettling (see Chapter 2). Education about diabetes, for the woman with gestational diabetes, should begin as soon as possible after diagnosis by glucose tolerance test. She is generally started on diet therapy alone and, therefore, will meet with the nutritionist for an individual session on meal planning. She is then referred to the nurse educator to learn home blood-glucose monitoring and ketone testing. The monitoring pattern for these women is the same as for a woman with IDDM—fasting and 2 hours after each meal. However, the blood-sugar goals are slightly different. Fasting levels should be less than 105 mg/dl; postprandial levels should be less than 120 mg/dl.[8] If the woman is not able to maintain these levels consistently with dietary treatment, insulin therapy is indicated and she is referred again to the nurse educator for instruction regarding insulin use. Daily morning ketone testing is also recommended.

There is general agreement that when a woman is diagnosed with gestational diabetes (GDM), she is at risk for the development of diabetes in the next 10–15 years (usually Type II).[9,10] With this positive history, she is encouraged to make lifestyle changes to reduce her risk of future diabetes. Therefore, education should be directed towards potential prevention measures (i.e., weight loss and regular exercise).[11] Other considerations are an elevated risk of GDM in future pregnancies and contraception alternatives.[12]

HYPOGLYCEMIA

The first trimester can be especially difficult for the pregnant diabetic woman. After having the importance of good control early in pregnancy instilled in her, it is unfortunate that this tends to be the most unstable period of the pregnancy. In this three month period, the insulin dose may remain the same as before pregnancy or perhaps decrease slightly. Hypoglycemia in the first three months may be attributed to morning sickness and/or the emphasis on stricter blood-sugar control. It can also occur for the more obvious reasons—omitting or delaying a meal or snack, increasing the activity level without adequate preparation, or injecting too much insulin. Clinical research has found no evidence of detrimental effects of low blood sugar on the human fetus. The chief concern about hypoglycemia is the potential for maternal neuroglycopenia.

Women should be encouraged to assist in the prevention of hypoglycemia by: (1) eating meals and snacks on time or by covering delays, (2) compensating for extra activity by increasing food intake beforehand, and (3) carefully measuring insulin doses to prevent errors. Pregnant women must be cautioned about the possibility of altered symptoms of hypoglycemia, which is much more likely in this population.[13] This could lead to a delay in treatment and a potential for unconscious hypoglycemia. Women should be taught to be attentive to any sensation that may indicate a low blood sugar. If possible, blood sugar should be measured immediately to assess if hypoglycemia is occurring. If blood sugar cannot be checked at this time, a prudent course of action is to assume a reaction is occurring and treat immediately.

Preferred treatment is the immediate use of a simple, fasting-acting carbohydrate that will raise the blood sugar quickly. A delay in treatment tends to make the reaction more difficult to remedy. Several recommended choices for treating an insulin reaction are any one of the following: 4 oz regular soda, 4 tsp sugar, 4 oz fruit juice, 10 oz skim milk, 3 glucose tablets, or 4 dextrose tablets. After treatment, symptoms generally abate within 10–15 minutes. If they do not, the treatment should be repeated. If it is nearly time for a meal or snack, eating immediately should be adequate. However, if food is not due for 30 minutes or more, the patient should be counseled to have a fast-acting carbohydrate plus another slower complex carbohydrate (i.e., starch/bread exchange), to provide coverage until the next meal. If the next meal or snack is not scheduled for an hour or more, a protein/meat should also be included.

Since it is possible for reactions to occur without warning or recognition, patients should be encouraged to wear identification bracelets, and to educate family and friends as to the appropriate treatment for hypoglycemia. For women who know that they experience unrecognized hypoglycemia, more frequent blood-glucose monitoring is a must. In the event of an unconscious insulin reaction, glucagon can be used to treat at home. Glucagon is a naturally occurring pancreatic hormone that causes a rise in blood sugar by stimulating glycogenolysis and gluconeogenesis. It is extracted from bovine pancreas and is stable in a desiccated form. The husband, partner, or other family member should be taught its use at the first visit. If they are not present, the patient can be taught the procedure and instructed to provide teaching to the appropriate person at home. The Glucagon Emergency Kit® contains a syringe prefilled with diluting solution and a vial containing glucagon crystals. It is available at pharmacies by prescription. It should be stored at room temperature with an awareness of the expiration date (generally 1-2 years). The person administering this needs only to (1) inject the solution into the vial, (2) roll it to mix, (3) withdraw the fluid into the syringe, and (4) inject the medication into the unconscious person in the same manner as insulin. Because glucagon may cause vomiting, the patient should be turned on her side to prevent aspiration. Glucagon will generally arouse the person within 5–20 minutes. Once awake, the diabetic will require fast-acting carbohydrate to prevent a second episode. Physicians should be notified of the occurrence of unconscious hypoglycemia. If the partner is unwilling or unable to administer a glucagon injection, instructions should be given to have the patient brought to the local emergency room for treatment.

When an insulin reaction occurs, it is important that the woman review the circumstances to determine the cause of the reaction. It is assumed that an unexplained insulin reaction is due to an excess amount of insulin. For these unexplained insulin reactions, guidelines for reduction of insulin dose are provided (Figs. 2 and 3).[14] Women who are on an insulin pump or an intensive insulin management program should have individually tailored instructions from their physician, but the basic outline for adjusting insulin with an intensive program is demonstrated in Fig. 4 and 5.

INSULIN ADJUSTMENTS

During the second and third trimesters there is a definite change in insulin requirements. Even when the treatment program is followed carefully, blood sugars above recommended levels may be experienced. It is helpful to let the women know that a rise in blood sugars, and therefore in their insulin dose (perhaps twice their prepregnancy dose), is expected secondary to the physiological effects of pregnancy on diabetes.

At this stage the placenta produces hormones (especially human placental lactogen) that are necessary for a healthy pregnancy but antagonistic to insulin, thereby rendering it less effective. Also, increased caloric requirements during the third trimester of pregnancy increase the need for insulin. At each weekly visit to the Pregnancy Clinic the diabetologist will assess the previous week's blood-sugar results and adjust the insulin dose accordingly. But, in many cases, the blood sugar will rise above the re-

Guidelines for reducing insulin—conventional regimen.

Insulin dosage	When reactions occur	Changes to make
Single morning dose of intermediate-acting (usually NPH or lente)	Any time of the day	Reduce dosage by 1–2 units the next morning
Mixed morning dose of short-acting (usually regular) and intermediate-acting (usually NPH or lente)	Before noon	Reduce dosage of short-acting by 1–2 units the next morning
	Afternoon or evening	Reduce dosage of intermediate-acting by 1–2 units the next morning
Mixed dose of short-acting (usually regular) and intermediate-acting (usually NPH or lente) in the morning and intermediate-acting (usually NPH or lente) at bedtime	Before noon	Reduce dosage of short-acting by 1–2 units the next morning
	Noon to bedtime	Reduce dosage of intermediate-acting by 1–2 units the next morning
	During the night	Reduce dosage of intermediate-acting by 1–2 units the next evening
Mixed dose of short-acting (usually regular) and intermediate-acting (usually NPH or lente) in the morning and again at dinnertime	Before noon	Reduce dosage of short-acting by 1–2 units the next morning
	Noon to supper	Reduce dosage of intermediate-acting by 1–2 units the next morning
	Supper to bedtime	Reduce dosage of short-acting by 1–2 units the next evening
	During the night	Reduce dosage of intermediate-acting by 1–2 units the next evening

Fig. 2. From Folkman J, Hollerorth HJ (eds): "A Guide for Women with Diabetes Who Are Pregnant . . . Or Plan to Be." Revised edition. Boston: Joslin Diabetes Center, 1986, p. 117. Adapted with permission from the Joslin Diabetes Center.

Guidelines for reducing insulin—intensive regimen A.

Insulin dosage	When reactions occur	Changes to make
Regular and intermediate insulin (NPH or lente) before breakfast, regular before supper, intermediate at bedtime	Fasting/during the night	Reduce bedtime intermediate insulin by 1–2 units
	Before noon	Reduce prebreakfast regular insulin by 1–2 units
	Afternoon	Reduce morning intermediate insulin by 1–2 units
	Evening	Reduce presupper regular insulin by 1–2 units

Fig. 3.

commended parameters before the next clinic appointment. Because of this, the woman is taught to make adjustments in the treatment program so that she will be able to act quickly to return blood-sugar levels within the recommended range (Figs. 6–9).[14] Those on insulin pump or intensive management may require individually tailored instructions from their physician.

Before increasing the dosage, the woman must be sure that she is (1)

Guidelines for reducing insulin—intensive regimen B.

Insulin dosage	When reactions occur	Changes to make
a.m. and p.m. ultralente Regular insulin prebreakfast, prelunch, predinner	Fasting/during the night	Reduce each ultralente dosage by 1–2 units
	Before noon	Reduce prebreakfast regular by 1–2 units
	Afternoon	Reduce prelunch regular by 1–2 units
	Evening	Reduce predinner regular by 1–2 units

Fig. 4.

Guidelines for reducing insulin—intensive regimen C.

Insulin dosage	When reactions occur	Changes to make
Premeal regular insulin Intermediate (NPH or lente) at bedtime	Fasting/during the night	Reduce bedtime intermediate by 1–2 units
	Before noon	Reduce prebreakfast regular by 1–2 units
	Afternoon	Reduce prelunch regular by 1–2 units
	Evening	Reduce predinner regular by 1–2 units

Fig. 5.

following the meal plan, (2) consistent with activity, (3) not ill, (4) not having hypoglycemic reactions and rebounds, and (5) using testing equipment properly. If none of the above appear to be causing the elevations, she must look to the following criteria: Is the blood sugar elevated for two consecutive days (thereby indicating a pattern)? Is the elevation occurring at the same time of day? If both answers are yes, she may proceed as shown in Figs. 6–9.[14] (It is recommended that patients doing self-adjustment change only one insulin at a time.)

In the last few years, and especially since the 1993 publication of the results of the ten-year Diabetes Control and Complications Trial (DCCT), there has been increasing interest in intensive insulin management programs. In Figs. 10 and 11 insulin adjustment guidelines for intensive therapy are shown.

The insulin pump is a device that gives a continuous subcutaneous infusion of insulin by providing a basal (ongoing) rate of insulin supplemented by boluses of insulin before each meal. Although it is chosen by a minority of our patients during their pregnancy, it has a useful place in the array of management choices, especially among those with a strong dawn phenomena.

SICK DAYS

The protocol for illness is discussed early in pregnancy. This is not because it is necessarily expected that women will be prone to illness

Single morning dose of intermediate-acting (usually NPH or lente).

1. If your tests before taking insulin or eating in the morning are high for 2 days in a row, notify your physician. This may indicate the need for an evening dose of intermediate-acting insulin.
2. If your tests 2 hours after breakfast are high for 2 days in a row, notify your physician. This may indicate the need for a morning dose of short-acting insulin.
3. If your tests 2 hours after lunch are high for 2 days in a row, increase the amount of intermediate-acting insulin by 1–2 units the next morning.
4. If your tests 2 hours after dinner are high for 2 days in a row, increase the amount of intermediate-acting insulin by 2 units the next morning.

*These guidelines are usually appropriate. If, however, your total insulin dose is very high or very low, you may be given a different schedule to follow.

Fig. 6. Joslin Clinic guidelines for the self-adjustment of insulin. From Folkman J, Hollerorth HJ (eds): "A Guide for Women with Diabetes Who are Pregnant . . . Or Plan to Be," revised edition. Boston: Joslin Diabetes Center, 1986, pp. 111–112. Adapted with permission from the Joslin Diabetes Center.

Mixed morning dose of short-acting (usually regular)
and intermediate-acting (usually NPH or lente).

1. If your tests before taking insulin or eating in the morning are high for 2 days in a row, notify your physician. This may indicate the need for an evening dose of intermediate-acting insulin.
2. If your tests 2 hours after breakfast are high for 2 days in a row, increase the amount of short-acting insulin by 1–2 units the next morning.
3. If your tests 2 hours after lunch are high for 2 days in a row, increase the amount of intermediate-acting insulin by 1–2 units the next morning.
4. If your tests 2 hours after dinner are high for 2 days in a row, increase the amount of intermediate-acting insulin by 1–2 units the next morning.

*These guidelines are usually appropriate. If, however, your total insulin dose is very high or very low, you may be given a different schedule to follow.

Fig. 7. Joslin Clinic guidelines for the self-adjustment of insulin. From Folkman J, Hollerorth HJ (eds): "A Guide for Women with Diabetes Who are Pregnant . . . Or Plan to Be," revised edition. Boston: Joslin Diabetes Center, 1986, pp. 111–112. Adapted with permission from the Joslin Diabetes Center.

Mixed dose of short-acting (usually regular) and intermediate-acting (usually NPH or lente) in the morning and intermediate-acting (usually NPH or lente) before dinner or bedtime.

1. If your tests before taking insulin or eating in the morning are high for 2 days in a row, increase the intermediate-acting insulin by 1–2 units the next evening.
2. If your tests 2 hours after breakfast are high for 2 days in a row, increase the amount of short-acting insulin by 1–2 units the next morning.
3. If your tests 2 hours after lunch are high for 2 days in a row, increase the amount of intermediate-acting insulin by 1–2 units the next morning.
4. If your tests 2 hours after dinner are high for 2 days in a row, notify your physician. This may indicate the need for an evening dose of short-acting insulin.

The fasting blood sugar should be stabilized first.

*These guidelines are usually appropriate. If, however, your total insulin dose is very high or very low, you may be given a different schedule to follow.

Fig. 8. Joslin Clinic guidelines for the self-adjustment of insulin. From Folkman J, Hollerorth HJ (eds): "A Guide for Women with Diabetes Who are Pregnant . . . Or Plan to Be," revised edition. Boston: Joslin Diabetes Center, 1986, pp. 111–112. Adapted with permission from the Joslin Diabetes Center.

Mixed dose of short-acting (usually regular) and intermediate-acting (usually NPH or lente) in the morning and again at dinnertime or short-acting (regular) before dinner and intermediate at bedtime.

1. If your tests before taking insulin or eating in the morning are high for 2 days in a row, increase the intermediate-acting insulin by 1–2 units the next evening.
2. If your tests 2 hours after breakfast are high for 2 days in a row, increase the amount of short-acting insulin by 1–2 units the next morning.
3. If your tests 2 hours after lunch are high for 2 days in a row, increase the amount of intermediate-acting insulin by 1–2 units the next morning.
4. If your tests 2 hours after dinner are high for 2 days in a row, increase the amount of short-acting insulin by 1–2 units the next evening.

The fasting blood sugar should be stabilized first.

*These guidelines are usually appropriate. If, however, your total insulin dose is very high or very low, you may be given a different schedule to follow.

Fig. 9. Joslin Clinic guidelines for the self-adjustment of insulin. From Folkman J, Hollerorth HJ (eds): "A Guide for Women with Diabetes Who are Pregnant . . . Or Plan to Be," revised edition. Boston: Joslin Diabetes Center, 1986, pp. 111–112. Adapted with permission from the Joslin Diabetes Center.

Pre-meal doses of short-acting (usually regular) and long-acting (ultralente) in the morning and before dinner.

1. If your tests before taking insulin or eating in the morning are high for 3 days in a row, increase the amount of each long-acting (ultralente) insulin dose by 1–2 units.*
2. If your tests 2 hours after breakfast are high for 2 days in a row, increase the amount of short-acting insulin by 1–2 units the next morning.
3. If your tests after lunch are high for 2 days in a row, increase the amount of short-acting insulin by 1–2 units the next day before lunch.
4. If your tests after dinner are high for 2 days in a row, increase the amount of short-acting insulin by 1–2 units the next evening before dinner.

The fasting blood sugar should be stabilized first.

*It is beneficial to check the 2 a.m. blood sugar when a high fasting level is noted. If the 2 a.m. result is *low,* the high fasting may be due to a rebound and therefore a *decrease* in Ultralente may be needed.

Fig. 10. Joslin Clinic guidelines for the self-adjustment of insulin.

Pre-meal doses of short-acting (usually regular) and intermediate (NPH or lente) at bedtime.

1. If your tests before taking insulin or eating in the morning are high for 2 days in a row, increase the amount of evening intermediate (NPH or lente) by 1–2 units.
2. If your tests 2 hours after breakfast are high for 2 days in a row, increase the amount of short-acting insulin by 1–2 units the next morning.
3. If your tests after lunch are high for 2 days in a row, increase the amount of short-acting insulin by 1–2 units the next day before lunch.
4. If your tests after dinner are high for 2 days in a row, increase the amount of short-acting insulin by 1–2 units the next evening before dinner.

The fasting blood sugar should be stabilized first.

Fig. 11. Joslin Clinic guidelines for the self-adjustment of insulin.

during pregnancy, but because ketoacidosis, a complication of diabetes often precipitated by illness, can be fatal to the fetus and, therefore, must be avoided. Situations that may require the use of this protocol are: bacterial or viral infection, physical or emotional trauma, and surgery. When the body is physically or mentally stressed, contrainsulin hormones are released. There are basic guidelines to be followed when illness occurs.

1. The usual dose of insulin should always be taken, never omitted, even if unable to eat. It is not food intake that will raise blood-sugar levels when ill, but rather the stress of illness.

2. Blood sugar should be monitored every three to four hours while awake, and at least once during the night. Elevations in blood sugar can occur quite rapidly during an illness; therefore, blood sugar should be checked frequently.

3. If blood-sugar results are high (180 mg/dl or more), ketone levels should be checked. If the ketone test is clearly positive, it indicates the need for more insulin. Short-acting insulin is always used for these supplemental doses because quick results are desired. The amount of extra insulin to be taken will be 10–20% of the individuals daily dosage (Table II).

4. Fluids should be ingested at a rate of approximately 8 oz per hour to prevent dehydration. The type of fluid depends on the patient's situation. For those able to maintain their usual meal plan, sugar-free beverages (water, broth, diet soda) are recommended. The inability to eat solids is an indication of the need for sugared beverages (regular soda, fruit juice) to provide some nutrition, and in concert with insulin, blunt starvation ketosis.

After two consecutive applications of the supplemental doses, the patient must contact the internist for further instructions.

If the blood sugar is elevated due to illness but ketones are not present,

TABLE II. Sick Day Management*

Time	Blood sugar/ketones (mg/dl)	Action
6:30 a.m.	150/trace	Usual a.m. dose (4 regular 14 NPH)
10:30 a.m.	210/moderate	10% supplemental dose (3 units regular)
2:30 p.m.	280/moderate	20% supplemental dose (6 units regular)
6:30 p.m.	350/large	Notify MD

*Insulin dose: a.m., 4 units regular and 14 units NPH; p.m., 2 units regular and 10 units NPH. Total daily dose = 30 units; 10% = 3 units; 20% = 6 units.

the patient is instructed to modify the guidelines and use only 5% and 10% supplemental doses.

EXERCISE

Increasing interest in physical fitness, coupled with a renewed emphasis on the role of exercise as a part of the three-pronged approach (medication, diet, and exercise) to diabetes control, has made exercise during pregnancy a subject of much interest and concern. There has been much professional consideration of exercise for its role in maintaining physical conditioning during pregnancy and its value in improving glycemic control (see Chapter 6). More and more in recent years, women are requesting advice about its risks and benefits during gestation. The safety of the mother and baby is the priority in any exercise program at this time. As a general rule, guidelines for exercise should be considered on an individual basis (especially in a high-risk pregnancy) and should be discussed with the health care team. Usually activity/exercise that was part of the regimen prior to pregnancy can be continued into and throughout the pregnancy. However, it may be necessary to modify or replace an activity to make it safer or less taxing. Particular attention should be paid to meals, snacks, insulin doses, and timing because of the risk of hypoglycemia.

There has also been growing interest regarding the efficacy of exercise and its application as a part of therapy in the treatment of gestational diabetes.[15] Presently, it is recommended with physician approval, as an adjunct to dietary treatment. Women with gestational diabetes are also advised about its benefits in preventing or delaying the potential onset of future diabetes.[11]

In any case, an individualized session with an exercise physiologist may prove beneficial for the woman who desires a more in-depth or specialized regimen during this time.

REFERENCES

1. Warram JH, Krolewski AS, Gottlieb MS, Kahn CR: Differences in risk of insulin-dependent diabetes in off-spring of diabetic mothers and diabetic fathers. N Engl J Med 311:149–152, 1984.
2. Eisenbarth GS, Ziegler AG, Colman PA: Pathogenesis of insulin-dependent (Type I) diabetes mellitus. In Kahn CR, Weir GC (eds): "Joslin's Diabetes Mellitus," 13th ed. Philadelphia: Lea & Febiger, 1994, pp 216–239.
3. Warram JH, Rich SS, Krolewski AS: Epidemiology of diabetes mellitus. In Kahn CR, Weir GC (eds): "Joslin's Diabetes Mellitus," 13th ed. Philadelphia: Lea & Febiger, 1994, pp 201–215.

4. Folkman J, Hollerorth HJ (eds): "A Guide for Women with Diabetes Who are Pregnant . . . Or Plan To Be," Revised edition. Boston: Joslin Diabetes Center, 1986.
5. Hare JW: Diabetes and pregnancy. In Kahn CR, Weir GC (eds): "Joslin's Diabetes Mellitus," 13th ed. Philadelphia: Lea & Febiger, 1994, pp 889–899.
6. Rizzo T, Metzger BE, Burns WJ, et al: Correlations between antepartum maternal metabolism and child intelligence. N Engl J Med 325(13):911–916, 1991.
7. Silverman BL, Rizzo T, Green OC, et al: Long-term prospective evaluation of offspring of diabetic mothers. Diabetes 40 (Suppl 2):121–125, 1991.
8. American Diabetes Association—Clinical Practice Recommendations. Diabetes Care 16 (Suppl 2):5–6, 1993.
9. O'Sullivan JB: Diabetes Mellitus after GDM. Diabetes 40 (Suppl 2):131–135, 1991.
10. Gandier FL, Hauth JC, Poist M, et al: Recurrence of gestational diabetes. Obstet Gynecol 80(5):755–758, 1992.
11. Horton ES: Exercise in the treatment of NIDDM. Applications for GDM? Diabetes 40 (Suppl 2):175–178, 1991.
12. Molsted-Pedersen L, Skouby SO, Damm P: Preconception counseling and contraception after gestational diabetes. Diabetes 40 (Suppl 2):147–150, 1991.
13. Diamond MP, Regee EA, Caprio S, Jones TW, et al: Impairment of counterregulatory hormone responses to hypoglycemia in pregnant women with IDDM. Am J Obstet Gynecol 166:70–77, 1992.
14. Hollerorth HJ (ed): "Diabetes Teaching Guide," Revised edition. Boston: Joslin Diabetes Center, 1986.
15. Bung P, Artal R, Khaliguian N, Kjos S: Exercise in gestational diabetes. An optional therapeutic approach? Diabetes 40 (Suppl 2):182–185, 1991.

CHAPTER 5

Nutritional Management

Anna Maria Bertorelli, MBA, RD

INTRODUCTION

Women usually become concerned about their diet and nutritional well-being upon learning that they are pregnant. It is well established that nutrition and diet play an integral role in fetal outcome for all women. For the woman with diabetes who becomes pregnant or the woman who develops diabetes during pregnancy, proper diet and nutrition add another dimension—that of optimizing diabetes control for the healthy outcome of the infant.

Proper nutritional management is crucial for all women with diabetes who become pregnant. Diet and meal planning must take into account the normal metabolic changes that occur during pregnancy and their effects on diabetes management. The woman's lifestyle and daily habits, financial resources, and education must be considered. Nutrition education must also be sensitive to psychosocial, cultural, and religious issues.

For nutritionists who counsel women with diabetes, there remain many unanswered questions and controversies relating to: optimal caloric requirements during pregnancy; the ideal percentage of dietary protein, carbohydrate, and fat; the distribution of nutrients; the caloric intake and weight gain for the obese individual; and the effects of nonnutritive sweeteners and caffeine on the fetus.

This chapter initially addresses recommendations for preconception counseling, alterations in fuel metabolism during pregnancy, and recommendations for the normal pregnancy, followed by nutritional recommendations for diabetes in pregnancy, with special considerations for insulin-dependent diabetes mellitus (IDDM), noninsulin-dependent diabetes mellitus (NIDDM), and gestational diabetes mellitus (GDM). Finally, postpartum concerns, including breastfeeding and lactation, are addressed.

Diabetes Complicating Pregnancy: The Joslin Clinic Method, Edited by Florence M. Brown, MD and John W. Hare, MD.
ISBN 0-471-11031-0 © 1995 John Wiley & Sons, Inc.

PRECONCEPTION COUNSELING

In order to prevent major congenital anomalies in infants of diabetic mothers, all pregnant women should establish optimal diabetes control prior to conception. This can be accomplished through early intervention, diabetes education, and management.[1] Women who do not have or are not following a meal plan are strongly advised to meet with a nutritionist specializing in diabetes management. Each woman should have a complete nutritional assessment. An individualized meal plan should be provided, the use of food lists or other instructional material reviewed and discussed, and goals for diabetes management shared and established. The diet should be designed to enable the woman to reach and maintain a desirable body weight, achieve optimal blood-glucose control, prevent ketonemia, and ensure adequate nutrition.[2]

In addition to using a meal plan, our clinic advises all women who are planning to become pregnant to consume a folic acid supplement of 400 μg per day, beginning at least one month prior to conception. This, along with a properly varied diet, may reduce the risk of neural tube defects.[3] Women must be advised to avoid alcoholic beverages. They should be instructed to record their blood-sugar levels on a regular basis and to make any necessary adjustment in their diet, activity, and/or insulin regimens.

If a woman becomes pregnant prior to obtaining preconception counseling, she should see a nutritionist at the time of her first prenatal visit. This usually occurs at 4–6 weeks gestation.

FUEL METABOLISM

Beginning early in the normal pregnancy, glucose reaches the fetus by facilitated diffusion; that is, glucose crosses the placenta at a rate faster than would be expected by passive transfer.[4,5] Amino acids are actively transported to the fetal circulation against a concentration gradient. Of note is the significant decrease in the maternal plasma concentration of the gluconeogenic amino acid alanine. Thus, the maternal loss of glucose and gluconeogenic substrate to the fetus occur concomitantly and conspire to cause maternal hypoglycemia, described by Freinkel as one aspect of the phenomena of "accelerated starvation."[4,5] These factors make meal planning a crucial part of early pregnancy.

Metabolic alterations become more evident during the second half of pregnancy. During mid-gestation, insulin requirements gradually increase.[4] The mother's main fuel source becomes lipids, derived from either circulating fats or stored adipose tissue. The conversion from a primarily glucose-based to a lipid-based fuel source allows glucose and protein to be spared for fetal growth. In late pregnancy, the basal insulin needs are higher than in the nongravid state, and eating produces a two-to-three-fold greater requirement for insulin.[4] For women with IDDM, this problem is further compounded by inadequacies in current insulin delivery systems. Subcutaneously administered short-acting insulin does not peak until two to four hours after injection. This delay must be compensated for with dietary modifications, usually the inclusion of snacks two to three hours after meals, in order to prevent profound hypoglycemia before the next meal. These issues are addressed later in this chapter under "Special Considerations: Insulin-Dependent Diabetes Mellitus."

CURRENT NUTRITIONAL RECOMMENDATIONS

Current nutritional recommendations for pregnant women with diabetes are based on acceptable guidelines for nutrition during normal pregnancy[6,7] and nutrition principles for the management of diabetes.[2] This section reviews current recommendations for weight gain, energy and protein needs during pregnancy, vitamin and mineral requirements and supplementation, and the use of caffeine, alcohol and nonnutritive sweeteners during pregnancy.

Weight Gain Recommendations

Weight gain during pregnancy reflects growth of both fetal and maternal tissues as outlined in Table I. Current recommendations for weight gain are based on a woman's prepregnancy height and weight status. The National Academy of Science (NAS) recommends using prepregnancy body mass index (BMI), since it is a better indicator of nutritional status than weight alone. The BMI can be calculated (Table II) or determined by the use of a chart (Table III).[6]

Weight gain in women giving birth to healthy infants is highly variable. It has been suggested that underweight women with prepregnant BMIs of <19.8 kg/m^2 (<90% ideal body weight [IBW]) achieve a gain of 28–40 pounds; women who begin pregnancy with a BMI of 19.8–26.0 kg/m^2 (IBW) achieve a gain of 25-35 pounds; overweight women with BMIs of 26.0–29.0 kg/m^2 (>120% IBW) gain 15–25 pounds; and obese women with BMIs >29.0 kg/m^2 (>135% IBW) gain at least 15 pounds by term.[6]

The recommended rate of weight gain for women who enter pregnancy at a normal prepregnancy weight is 2–5 pounds during the first trimester with a linear weight gain rate of approximately 1 pound per week thereafter.[6] If a woman is underweight, it is suggested that she gain slightly more than a pound (1.1 lb) per week, and if she is overweight, slightly less

TABLE I. Average Composition for Pregnancy Weight Gain[a]

Tissue	Weight (pounds)
Fetal	
Fetus	7.5
Placenta	1.0
Amniotic fluid	2.0
Uterus[b]	2.5
Total	13.0
Maternal	
Breast tissue[b]	3.0
Blood volume[c]	4.0 (1500 ml)
Maternal stores	4.0–8.0
Total	11–15
Total fetal plus maternal	24–28

[a]Adapted from: Maternal nutrition and the course of pregnancy. NAS, 1970, with permission.
[b]Weight increase.
[c]Increase in volume (ml).

TABLE II. Calculating Body Mass Index

$$\frac{\text{Body weight (kilograms)}}{\text{Height (meters)}^2} = \text{BMI}$$

Example: Your patient is 5′4″ (64 inches) and weight 130 lbs:

$$\frac{59.1}{(1.60\text{ m}) \times (1.60\text{ m})} = 23.1$$

To calculate a patient's BMI follow these steps:

1. Convert pounds to kilograms (kg) by dividing the pound figure by 2.2. — $130\text{ lb} \div 2.2 = 59.1\text{ kg}$
2. Convert inches to meters (m) by multiplying the inch figure by 0.025. — $64\text{ in.} \times 0.025 = 1.60\text{ m}$
3. Square the figure of the height in meters. — $1.60 \times 1.60 = 2.56$
4. Divide the weight in kilograms by the square of the height in meters. — $\frac{59.1}{2.56} = 23.1$

23.1 represents a BMI in the normal range and suggests an optimal total weight gain during pregnancy of 25–35 pounds.

TABLE III. Chart for Estimating Body Mass Index (BMI) Category and BMI*

Directions: To find BMI category (e.g., obese), find the point where the woman's height and weight intersect. To estimate BMI, read the bold number on the dashed line that is closest to this point.

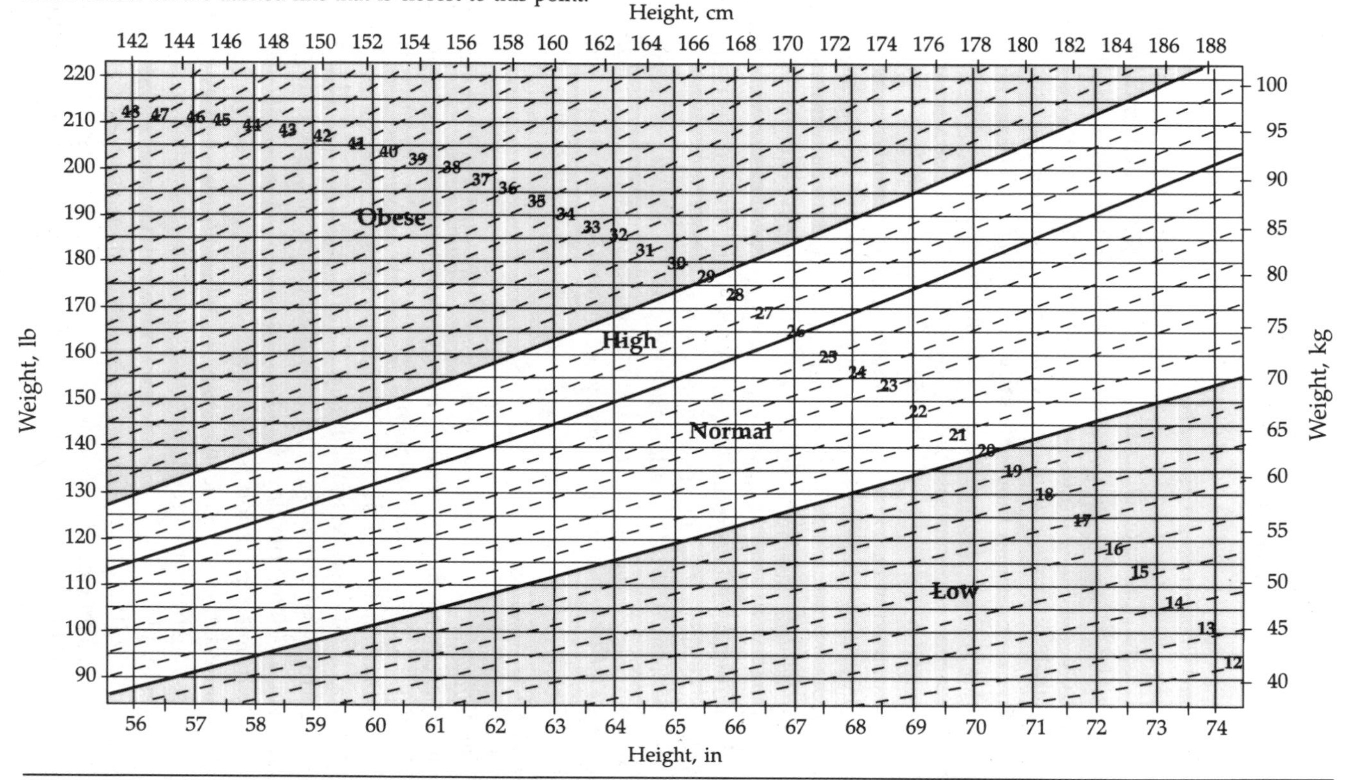

*Reprinted with permission from Nutrition During Pregnancy and Lactation: An Implementation Guide. Copyright 1992 by the National Academy of Sciences. Courtesy of the National Academy Press, Washington, D.C.

than a pound (0.7 lb) per week in the last two trimesters (Table IV). Additional research is necessary to determine appropriate weight gain patterns for obese women.[6]

Energy and Protein Requirements

Recently, the American Diabetes Association established recommended energy intake levels for the pregnant woman with diabetes.[8] Recommendations from various institutions throughout the country are generally around 30–38 kilocalories per kilogram of ideal prepregnancy weight daily.[4,9,10,11] The Joslin Clinic generally recommends 30 kilocalories per kilogram of ideal body weight in the first trimester, increasing to 36–38 kilocalories per kilogram of ideal body weight in the second and third trimesters (Table V).

Based on theoretical calculations, the National Research Council (NRC) recommends an additional intake of 300 kcal per day during the second and third trimesters.[7] This has been debated, with others estimating that the daily caloric increments should be only 150–200 kcal/day.[6] Since the precise increase in calories needed during pregnancy varies from individual to individual, it is emphasized that meal planning and the monitoring of calorie requirements be specific for each woman.

The recommended daily allowance for protein during pregnancy is an additional 10–14 g/day. Most American women routinely consume the allowance of 60 g of protein per day recommended during pregnancy.

Vitamins and Minerals

Supplementation—Calcium, Iron, and Folic Acid. All vitamins and minerals are needed in increased amounts during pregnancy, as indicated in Table VI. However, requirements for calcium, iron, and folic acid increase substantially and deserve special attention.

A report by the Centers for Disease Control supports that all women of child-bearing years take a folic acid supplement of 400 μg per day, though not to exceed 1.0 mg per day.[3] Folic acid is needed for DNA synthesis and cell growth and replication (see Chapter 12). During pregnancy, dietary requirements rise to meet the increased demands for the vitamin as a result of increased maternal erythropoiesis, uterine and mammary tissue growth, and placental and fetal growth. Greater urinary losses of the vitamin during pregnancy increase requirements further. Adequate folic acid for pregnancy can be obtained by regular consumption of fruits and vegetables in a well-selected diet. Since pregnant women in the United

TABLE IV. Prenatal Weight Gain Chart*

Prepregnancy BMI <19.8 (- - -); prepregnancy BMI 19.8–26.0 (Normal Body Weight) (– –); prepregnancy BMI >26.0 (—).

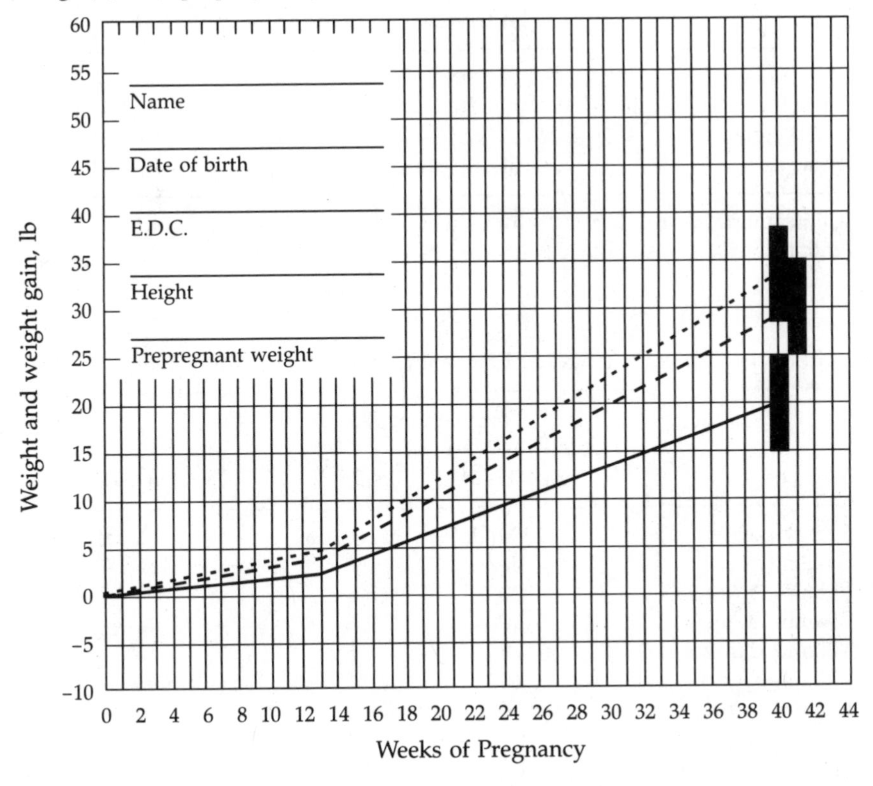

Date	Weeks of gestation	Weight	Notes

*Reprinted with permission from Nutrition During Pregnancy and Lactation: An Implementation Guide. Copyright 1992 by the National Academy of Sciences. Courtesy of the National Academy Press, Washington, D.C.

TABLE V. Caloric Requirements (cal/kg/DBW unless noted)*

	1st trimester	2nd trimester	3rd trimester
Underweight	30	36–40	36–40
Desirable body weight	30	36	36–38
Overweight	24 cal/kg/present	24	24
Obese	24 cal/kg/present	24	24

*Clinical judgment will be a factor as well in the calculation of calories.
From Joslin Diabetes Centers, Policy and Procedure Manual, 1994, with permission.

TABLE VI. Nutrient Changes of Pregnancy for An Adult Woman Age 19–50*

	Nonpregnant RDA		
Nutrient	Age 19–24	Age 25–50	Pregnant RDA
Energy (kcal)	2200/day	2200/day	+300 cal/day
Protein (g)	46	50	60
Vitamin A (μg RE)	800	800	800
Vitamin D (μg)	10	5	10
Vitamin E (mg TE)	8	8	10
Vitamin K (μg)	60	65	65
Vitamin C (mg)	60	60	70
Thiamin (mg)	1.1	1.1	1.5
Riboflavin (mg)	1.3	1.3	1.6
Niacin (mg NE)	15	15	17
Vitamin B-6 (mg)	1.6	1.6	2.2
Folate (μg)	180	180	400
Vitamin B-12 (μg)	2.0	2.0	2.2
Calcium (mg)	1200	800	1200
Phosphorus (mg)	1200	800	1200
Magnesium (mg)	280	280	320
Iron (mg)	15	15	30
Zinc (mg)	12	12	15
Iodine (μg)	150	150	175
Selenium (μg)	55	55	65

*Adapted with permission from: Food and Nutrition Board, National Research Council, National Academy of Sciences: "Recommended Dietary Allowances," 10th edition. Washington, DC: National Academy Press, 1989.

States tend to consume less than the current RDA of 400 μg per day, routine supplementation of at least 400 μg of folic acid is now being routinely prescribed.

The Subcommittee on Dietary Intake and Nutrient Supplements recommends the routine daily use of an iron supplement (ferrous iron, 30 mg) beginning at about 12 weeks gestation.[6] This amount of ferrous iron is provided by 150 mg of ferrous sulfate, 300 mg of ferrous gluconate, or 100 mg of ferrous fumarate. Iron is absorbed more completely from tablets when taken alone, rather than as part of a multivitamin/mineral supplement, and when taken between meals with liquids other than milk, tea, or coffee. Fewer gastrointestinal side effects occur when the iron supplement is taken at bedtime. Women who cannot tolerate an iron supplement should ensure an adequate intake of red meats, Vitamin C, and iron-fortified cereal products. Doses of ferrous iron above 30 mg may impair the absorption of zinc and should be reserved for the treatment of iron deficiency anemia. Anemia is defined as a hemoglobin concentration of less than 11 g/dl during the first or third trimesters or below 10.5 g/dl during the second trimester. Anemia accompanied by a serum ferritin concentration of <12 μg/dl can be presumed to be due to iron deficiency and requires treatment with ferrous iron, 60–120 mg.[6]

The Recommended Daily Allowance for calcium during pregnancy and lactation is 1,200 mg per day, irrespective of age.[7] It has been suggested that pregnant adolescents receive 1200–1500 mg per day to ensure adequate bone deposition.[6] Calcium is deposited in the fetus mainly in the last trimester, but the efficiency of maternal intestinal absorption is increased by at least the second trimester.[7] Women at risk for inadequate calcium intake are those under age 25, in whom some mineral is still being added to their own bones, and women with lactose intolerance. Ethnic groups in which calcium intake has been observed to be low include Blacks, Hispanics, and American Indians. For those with a low calcium intake (600 mg or less per day) calcium rich food, such as milk, yogurt and cheese, should be encouraged. Otherwise, addition of a supplement providing at least 600 mg per day is necessary.[7] Calcium carbonate tablets, such as Tums™, have the least amount of lead contamination of any calcium supplement, whereas bone meal has the most.[12]

Caffeine, Alcohol, and Nonnutritive Sweeteners

The use of caffeine-containing products remains controversial. In a recent study of 430 women, no evidence was shown that moderate amounts (<300 mg per day) of caffeine consumption increased the risk of spontaneous abortion, intrauterine growth retardation (IUGR), or microcephaly, after adjusting for other risk factors, particularly smoking and maternal age.[13] Studies have limitations due to the difficulty in determining the amount of caffeine in a foodstuff because of differences in preparation. Data evaluating pregnancy outcome with the use of very large doses are not available. Since data are limited and because caffeine crosses the placenta, it seems prudent to limit consumption to 300 mg per day or about two to three 5-ounce cups of regular coffee per day (Table VII).

The adverse effects of excessive alcohol consumption on fetal development have been clearly demonstrated.[14] The lower limit of safety for fetal exposure to alcohol has not been established. Therefore, total abstinence from alcohol is recommended during pregnancy. Women who are planning to become pregnant should also abstain from alcohol, since terato-

TABLE VII. Caffeine Content of Food and Beverages

	Milligrams of caffeine	
Item	Average	Range
Coffee (5-oz cup)		
Brewed, drip method	115	60–180
Brewed, percolator	80	40–170
Instant	65	30–120
Decaffeinated, brewed	3	2–5
Decaffeinated, instant	2	1–5
Tea (5-oz cup)		
Brewed, major U.S. brands	40	20–90
Brewed, imported brands	60	25–110
Instant	30	25–50
Iced (12-oz glass)	70	67–76
Some soft drinks (6 oz)	18	15–30
Cocoa beverage (5 oz)	4	2–20
Chocolate milk beverage (8 oz)	5	2–7
Milk chocolate (1 oz)	6	1–15
Dark chocolate, semisweet (1 oz)	20	5–35
Baker's chocolate (1 oz)	26	26
Chocolate-flavored syrup (1 oz)	4	4

Sources: U.S. Food and Drug Administration and National Soft Drink Association.

genesis begins before eight weeks gestation—a time when some women are not yet aware that they are pregnant.

Currently, there are three nonnutritive sweeteners (referred to as intensive, low-calorie, or alternative sweeteners) approved by the Food and Drug Administration (FDA) for use in the United States. They are: saccharin, aspartame, and acesulfame potassium (acesulfame-K). The FDA assigned an Acceptable Daily Intake (ADI) to aspartame and acesulfame-K. This is the amount of food additive that can be safely consumed on a daily basis over a person's lifetime without adverse effects. It includes a 100-fold safety factor.

Aspartame is the most popular artificial sweetener and it is approved for use in a wider variety of foods than saccharin or acesulfame-K. Aspartame is marketed under the brand name NutraSweet™ in food products or as Equal™ or Sweet Mate™ as a table-top sweetener. Aspartame is a methyl ester of aspartyl phenylalanine, which is metabolized in the small intestine into methanol and two amino acids, aspartic acid and phenylalanine. It is a nutritive sweetener, yet because it is 180–200 times sweeter than sucrose; only very small amounts are needed to achieve equivalent sweetness. Consequently, its caloric contribution to a food is insignificant. For persons with diabetes, the average aspartame consumption ranges from 2 to 4 mg/kg/day, well below its ADI of 50 mg/kg/day (Table VIII).[2,15] Recent reports of the American Diabetes Association and The American Dietetic Association imply that aspartame is safe for use during pregnancy, though there are no specific recommendations for intake levels.[2,15]

TABLE VIII. Content of Nonnutritive Sweeteners in Select Food Items

Aspartame (approximate)	
Diet soft drink, 12 oz	170 mg
Powdered drink, 8 oz	100 mg
Gelatin Dessert, 4 oz	80 mg
Aspartame-sweetened fruit yogurt, 8 oz	124 mg
Tabletop sweetener, 1 packet	35 mg
Acesulfame potassium	
Sweet One™, 1 packet	35 mg
Saccharin	
Sweet'n Low™, 1 packet	40 mg

Adapted from: Position of the American Dietetic Association: Use of nutritive and nonnutritive sweeteners. Journal of the American Dietetic Association 93:816–821, 1993.

Saccharin is 300–400 times as sweet as sucrose and has essentially no caloric value. Though saccharin can cross the placenta, there is no evidence of harm to the fetus from maternal saccharin ingestion.[2] In addition, current intake of saccharin is comparably lower than that of aspartame.

Acesulfame potassium, the most recently FDA-approved sweetener, is 200 times sweeter than sucrose. It is a derivative of acetoacetic acid that imparts a clean, sweet taste and is stable at high temperatures and can be used in cooking and baking. Its ADI is 15 mg/kg of body weight. It is marketed under the brand name Sunnette™ and as Sweet-One™ or Swiss Sweet™ tabletop sweeteners. Although acesulfame-K crosses the placenta, multigenerational reproduction studies in rats reported no adverse effect on fertility or their fetuses.[2] No specific recommendations on acesulfame-K use during pregnancy have been published (Table VIII).

SPECIAL CONSIDERATIONS

Insulin-Dependent Diabetes Mellitus

The nutritionist counseling the woman with IDDM should take into account various factors during her initial assessment. Did the woman plan this pregnancy and have nutrition counseling prior to conception? If not, when was the last time she saw a nutritionist? At some point in their diabetes history, most women will have seen a nutritionist. Therefore, it is important to assess her understanding of diabetic meal planning, especially as it pertains to pregnancy.

The nutrition assessment should also consider current food practices, cultural or religious impact on food choices, timing of meals and snacks, where meals are eaten, and the level of physical activity. The woman's diet should be assessed for protein, calories, vitamins and minerals, caffeine, alcohol, and nonnutritive sweeteners. Twenty-four hour recalls and food frequency cross-checks are utilized for assessment purposes, as is a history of nausea and vomiting, food aversion or intolerance (taste or smell), and change in bowel habits.

For the woman with IDDM who is pregnant, fluctuating blood sugars during the first trimester are not uncommon. The importance of eating regular, consistent meals should be stressed. Snacks, sometimes unnecessary prior to pregnancy, become crucial in preventing hypoglycemia during pregnancy. Nausea or vomiting may result in decreased food intake or absorption, further affecting blood-sugar control. During this time, regular sweetened beverages and foods such as sodas, gelatins, sherbets and popsicles may be used to replace the usual carbohydrates. Constipation, often associated with pregnancy, may require additional fluids and fruit as well as increased activity, all possibly affecting diabetes control. In addition, fatigue and frequent napping can lead to changes in activity, and meal, snack, and insulin-injection times. Ideally, these common occurrences are discussed with patients prior to conception, so that they can anticipate and plan for prevention and treatment of blood-sugar fluctuations. Adjustments in insulin dose will need to be made and the client should be advised to be in close contact with her physician and diabetes educator should problems or questions arise.

A meal plan consisting of three meals per day and three snacks per day is usually well tolerated. Our patients are advised to space meals four to five hours apart with snacks approximately two to three hours after meals. Generally, women can be expected to eat a meal or snack every two to three hours. The meal plan is individualized, with nutrient caloric distribution, on average, consisting of 45–55% carbohydrates, 25–35% fat, and the balance protein.

Women should be advised that the bedtime snack is extremely important. If starvation ketosis occurs, it will be during prolonged periods of fasting, i.e., when the woman is sleeping. Thus, it is recommended that at least 25 grams of carbohydrate be consumed with the bedtime snack.

Noninsulin-Dependent Diabetes Mellitus

Since most women who develop NIDDM are more than 40 years of age and are postmenopausal, they are less likely to become pregnant and, therefore, are seen less frequently at our institution. Some United States populations, such as Mexican Americans and Native American Indians, have a higher prevalence of Type II diabetes. Many of these women tend to be overweight or obese at conception and, therefore, weight control during pregnancy is often an issue. Weight gain guidelines should be provided to these patients and their weight gain monitored. Many of them do well with a 15–20 pound weight gain. Insulin is substituted for oral agents prior to conception in planned pregnancies, or as soon as pregnancy is determined in unplanned pregnancies. Once this occurs, their treatment is similar to women with IDDM. As in the case of IDDM women, in order to prevent hypoglycemia and glucose excursion, these women are scheduled three meals and three snacks per day. A review is made of carbohydrate-containing foods, portion size, lowfat meal plans, and behaviors that promote blood glucose and weight control. Moderate forms of exercise, such as walking, should be encouraged.

Women with IDDM and NIDDM need to meet with a dietitian prior to each trimester to review individual nutrition needs. A registered dietitian should be available to answer questions on a weekly basis.

Gestational Diabetes Mellitus

The role of diet and nutrition in the treatment of GDM is still under investigation. Controversies exist with respect to optimal daily caloric intake, ideal weight gain, and the use of hypocaloric diets in order to control blood sugar levels. The goal of optimum nutritional therapy is to provide adequate calories without hypoglycemia and ketonemia.

The diet for the woman with gestational diabetes needs to be highly individualized. It is the practice of some institutions to use three meals with only a bedtime snack, while others prefer to use more frequent, smaller meals with three snacks. In addition, some institutions believe it is important to restrict carbohydrates, especially at breakfast. At the Joslin Diabetes Center, the patient's meal plan is based on blood sugar and urine ketone results, weight gain during her pregnancy, activity level, and degree of motivation to make dietary changes. Generally, three meals with one to three snacks per day are provided. A bedtime snack is usually planned, with additional snacks based on patient preference and blood-glucose control. A maximum of 45 grams of carbohydrates is provided at breakfast with juices omitted. Carbohydrates and calories are distributed based on 2-hour blood-glucose results until desired levels are achieved. Insulin injection may need to be initiated, if blood-sugar goals cannot be achieved after a short trial with diet.

Recent research has suggested that for obese clients with diabetes, caloric restriction can be advised without adverse pregnancy outcomes.[16,17] It appears that the use of hypocaloric diets may improve diabetes control and reduce the baby's weight at birth, thus lessening the magnitude of macrosomia. However, the minimum caloric intake for obese pregnant women with gestational diabetes is controversial. Studies that used caloric restriction for the treatment of gestational diabetes included relatively small numbers of patients and should not be interpreted as the current standard of care. In one study by Knopp and associates at the University of Washington, effects of a 50% and 35% caloric restriction were investigated for use with obese women with GDM. Study participants were given equivalent 2400 calorie diets during the first week on the metabolic ward. Then, during subsequent weeks, subjects were given either a 1200 caloric or 1600–1800 calorie diet. Results of the study showed improved glycemic status by 10–20% in both groups, but there was a significant difference in ketone production between groups. Ketone production was increased twofold in the 50% calorie-restricted group, but showed no increase in the 35% calorie-restricted group. These researchers concluded that the 35% restriction (1600–1800 calories) is sufficient to normalize glycemia without apparent adverse metabolic effects.[16] Additional studies are warranted to evaluate the efficacy of this therapy and the safety of its outcomes.

In general, caloric restriction that results in weight loss or inadequate weight gain, and/or ketonuria is not recommended.[10,11,18] Instead, insulin therapy may need to be initiated to achieve normal blood-glucose levels.[10,11,18]

All of our pregnant patients with preexisting or gestational diabetes are instructed to test their urine for ketones each morning by using one of the popular dipstick methods. The presence of moderate to large ketone levels for two consecutive days with normal or low blood-glucose levels may reflect starvation ketosis and requires adjustment in dietary calories, possibly at bedtime or throughout the day.

Breastfeeding and Lactation

Breastfeeding is recommended for all infants, including children of women with diabetes.[8] Women with diabetes should be encouraged to breastfeed if they choose to. Mother–infant bonding may be enhanced and the metabolic control of diabetes is made easier.[19]

During lactation, a woman's calorie, fluid, protein, vitamin, and mineral requirements increase. For women who exclusively breastfeed, the energy demands of lactation exceed prepregnancy demands by approximately 640 kcal/day during the first 6 months postpartum.[7] An additional 500 calories per day is recommended while breastfeeding. The balance of the calories (100–150 calories) theoretically can come from maternal fat stores, allowing for a slow weight loss.[7] This is particularly important for the women who may have started pregnancy overweight. One study found that women need to consume at least 31 kilocalories per kilogram maternal body weight each day for successful lactation.[20] No clinical data are available regarding the distribution of calories on metabolic control during lactation.[19]

The breastfeeding mother should be encouraged to drink 2–3 liters (8–12 cups) of caffeine-free liquid per day to ensure adequate fluids. A good practice is for the woman to drink a beverage each time she nurses.

A woman's blood-glucose levels should be tested more frequently during lactation. Factors that can affect blood-glucose control include the amount of milk produced and the frequency at which the baby is consuming. Hypoglycemia is more likely to occur between meals or shortly after nursing. Therefore, it is important to include snacks before or during breastfeeding to prevent reactions. Women should be advised that their usual signs and symptoms of low blood sugar may be altered during lactation. Treatment for low blood sugar reactions (such as glucose tablets or Lifesavers) should be kept at hand so that nursing does not have to be interrupted.

Factors that can affect success include: feeding frequency, infant condition, gestational age, development of mastitis, metabolic control, and dietary intake.[20] Women with diabetes should be encouraged to nurse as soon as possible after delivery. An electric breast pump may simulate suckling while the baby is in the intensive care nursery. Mothers with preterm infants may need additional support and encouragement if latching onto the breast and proper suckling does not occur at first. A list of organizations that provide ongoing lactation support should be made available. The signs and symptoms of mastitis and its prevention and treatment should be reviewed. Women should be encouraged to call their physician or nurse clinician, especially if fever develops.

Low-income diabetic women should be referred to programs like "WIC" (Women, Infants and Children Supplemental Food), which provide basic nutrition education and supplemental food throughout the prenatal and lactation periods. Other resources for food include food stamps and local food pantries.

In summary, nutrition management of the diabetic pregnancy requires a motivated individual, a registered dietitian with expertise in diabetic pregnancies, and a supportive and involved health care team. This chapter reinforces the important role of nutritional management in pregnancy, especially the one complicated by preexisting or gestational diabetes. Diet remains a cornerstone for diabetes control and optimizes the chance for a healthy outcome for both the mother and the child.

REFERENCES

1. Kitzmiller JL, Gavin LA, Gin GD et al: Preconception care of diabetes: Glycemic control prevents congenital anomalies. JAMA 265(6):731–736, 1991.
2. Franz MJ, Horton ES, Bantle JP et al: Nutrition principles for the management of diabetes related complications. Diabetes Care 17:490–518, 1994.
3. Centers for Disease Control: Recommendations for the use of folic acid to reduce the number of cases of spina bifida and other neural tube defects. MMWR 41(RR-14):1–7, 1992.
4. Abrams RS: Prepregnancy counseling for women with diabetes. Practical Diabetology 7: 1–3, 1988.
5. Metzger BE, Freinkel N: Diabetes and pregnancy: Metabolic changes and management. Clinical Diabetes 8:1–10, 1990.
6. Committee on Nutritional Status During Pregnancy and Lactation, Food and Nutrition

Board, Institute of Medicine, National Academy of Sciences: Nutrition during Pregnancy. Washington, DC: National Academy Press, 1990.

7. National Academy of Sciences: Recommended Dietary Allowances, 10th edition. Subcommittee on the Tenth Edition of the RDAs, Food and Nutrition Board, Commission on Life Sciences, National Research Council. Washington, DC: National Academy Press, 1989.
8. Medical Management of Pregnancy Complicated by Diabetes. Alexandria, VA: American Diabetes Association, 1993.
9. Sweet Success: California Diabetes and Pregnancy Program, Guidelines for Care. State of California, Department of Health Services, Maternal and Child Health Branch, 1992.
10. Jovanovic-Peterson L, Peterson CM, Wilkins M: Management of the obese gestational diabetic pregnant woman. Diabetes Professional (Fall):6–13, 1990.
11. Hollander P: Gestational diabetes: The diabetes of pregnancy. Practical Diabetology 7:14–19, 1988.
12. Bourgoin BP, Evans DR, Cornett JR et al: Lead content in 70 brands of dietary calcium supplements. Am J Public Health 83:1155–1160, 1993.
13. Mills JL, Holmes LB, Aarons JH et al: Moderate caffeine use and the risk of spontaneous abortion and intrauterine growth retardation. JAMA 269:593–597, 1993.
14. Hanson JW, Streissguth AP, Smith DW. The effects of moderate alcohol consumption during pregnancy on fetal growth and morphogenesis. J Pediatrics 92:457, 1978.
15. Position of The American Dietetic Association: Use of nutritive and nonnutritive sweeteners. Journal of The American Dietetic Association 93:816–821, 1993.
16. Knopp RH, Magee MS, Raisys V et al: Metabolic effects of hypocaloric diets in management of gestational diabetes. Diabetes (Suppl 2):165–171, 1991.
17. Dornhorst A, Nicholls JDS, Probst F et al: Calorie restriction for treatment of gestational diabetes. Diabetes (Suppl 2):161–164, 1991.
18. Abrams RS, Coustan DR: Gestational diabetes update. Clinical Diabetes 8:1–30, 1990.
19. Ferris AM, Reece EA. Postpartum management and lactation. In: Reece EA, Coustan DR (eds): "Diabetes Mellitus in Pregnancy: Principles and Practice." New York: Churchill Livingstone, 1988, pp. 623–634.
20. Ferris AM, Jensen RG: Lactation outcome in insulin-dependent diabetic women. J Am Dietetic Assoc 88:317–322, 1988.

CHAPTER 6

Exercise

Catherine A. Mullooly, MS

INTRODUCTION

Exercise has not been a traditional recommendation for pregnant women with diabetes. The unknown effects on the developing fetus and the additional challenge of metabolic control prevented women from safely participating in exercise. History reveals a time when women needed to be hospitalized and confined to bedrest in order to increase the chances of a successful delivery. Without today's technology to monitor blood-sugar fluctuations and fetal growth and activity, the risks associated with exercise placed both the mother and fetus in jeopardy. Now, research is busy identifying a new role for exercise. There is evidence that exercise is a safe modality that can be included during most pregnancies. The most recent recommendations of the American Diabetes Association[1] and the American College of Obstetricians and Gynecologists (ACOG)[2] reflect this conclusion.

The changing role of women in society has required this scientific exploration into the effects of exercise on the outcome of pregnancy. Women are now employed in job classifications that range from sedentary to extremely physical. More women are also participating in exercise and sport for health, recreation, or competitive purposes. Whether they are deemed sedentary or active, when a woman becomes pregnant her ability to safely participate in exercise needs to be examined. It is imperative that a thorough medical assessment is performed to determine if any contraindications do exist for exercise before embarking on, or continuing in, a program.

Diabetes Complicating Pregnancy: The Joslin Clinic Method, Edited by Florence M. Brown, MD and John W. Hare, MD.
ISBN 0-471-11031-0 © 1995 John Wiley & Sons, Inc.

MEDICAL ASSESSMENT

There are very specific contraindications which would exclude any woman from exercising while she is pregnant. The ACOG[2] identifies pregnancy-induced hypertension, preterm rupture of membranes, a past or present history of preterm labor, incompetent cervix/cerlage, persistent second- or third-trimester bleeding and intrauterine growth retardation as conditions that would exclude a woman from initiating or continuing with an exercise program. Special consideration is also given to chronic hypertension, and active thyroid, cardiac, vascular, or pulmonary diseases when establishing whether or not exercise can be performed safely. Any potential risks must be identified from the onset. Additionally, women with preexisting diabetes may have hypoglycemia unawareness, neuropathy, nephropathy, retinopathy, or poor glycemic control. Women with gestational diabetes may encounter problems associated with obesity or a decreased level of fitness. Each woman will need to be instructed as to which types of exercise she should avoid, how to prevent hypoglycemia, and when to terminate an exercise session. By carefully modifying the program to meet each woman's needs, exercise can be approached in an effective and safe manner.

PHYSIOLOGICAL ADAPTATIONS TO PREGNANCY

Pregnancy results in many changes in the female body. Some are very obvious, while others are more complex to identify. Subtle physiological adaptations occur during the course of a pregnancy in the cardiovascular, pulmonary, thermoregulatory, metabolic, and biomechanical systems, as the maternal and fetal demands placed on the body are met. Inevitably, these changes also influence the ability to participate in exercise;[3] some changes may be beneficial while others may require certain modifications to be safe.

Cardiovascular

The cardiovascular system undergoes many changes during the course of a pregnancy. The resting heart rate dramatically increases, during the first four weeks of gestation, by seven beats per minute and will eventually reach a resting rate of 15 beats per minute higher than prepregnancy.[4] Increases in venous return and aortic capacity, coupled with a reduced peripheral vascular resistance, result in a larger stroke volume.[5,6] This combination of an increased resting heart rate and larger stroke volume is then responsible for the increased cardiac output that occurs during pregnancy.

Another maternal physiological change is a 40–60% increase in the blood volume.[6,7] While an increase in blood volume, combined with an increased cardiac output, has raised concerns of an associated increase in blood pressure, this has not been seen to occur.[8] Reduced peripheral vascular resistance helps to offset these hemodynamic influences and results in a blood pressure that remains the same, or is slightly decreased, during pregnancy.

During submaximal exercise, the heart rate response has been reported to be significantly higher compared to that of a nonpregnant woman.[9] It is unclear what occurs during higher-intensity workloads. While some studies report a decrease in the maximal heart rate response,[10,11] other studies have found no significant changes.[12,13]

Pulmonary

As the fetus develops and the uterus grows in size, the diaphragm is shifted by as much as 4 cm upward into the thoracic cage. In order to compensate for this reduced pulmonary space, the angle of the lungs within the thoracic cage increases by approximately 35°, and the circumference of the thoracic cage is increased by 5–7 cm.[14] These adaptations provide enough compensation with only a modest reduction in total lung capacity.

There are some measurable changes in resting lung volumes during pregnancy. Most notable is a progressive increase in the minute ventilation. By the end of term, it can reach volumes of up to 50% greater than before conception. This occurs with no change in the respiratory rate but is attributed exclusively to a larger tidal volume.[14]

The arterial pH during pregnancy is moderately elevated to levels of approximately 7.46, due to a decrease in the arterial P_{CO_2}. This mild respiratory alkalosis allows the maternal blood supply to promote CO_2 exchange across the placenta, thus preventing the accumulation of CO_2 in the fetal blood supply.[15]

There is contradictory evidence regarding V_{O_2max} during pregnancy. While the oxygen uptake (l/min) does increase during pregnancy, studies have not yet clarified its effect on aerobic work capacity. At present there are studies that have measured increases,[16] decreases,[11] and no significant changes[13] in V_{O_2max}. Determining the impact on aerobic work capacity has been complicated due to the changes that occur in weight, body composition, and heart rate during pregnancy.

Thermoregulatory

The first trimester of pregnancy places the developing fetus at risk for defects that can be linked to increases in the maternal core temperature. Animal studies reveal that increases exceeding 1.5 °C can cause the neuronal mitotic cell growth to be disrupted in the ependymal layer of the brain.[17] This may explain why maternal exposure to environmental factors (i.e., sauna, hot tub) during early pregnancy has resulted in an increased incidence of neural tube defects.[18]

Increases in the maternal core temperature occur when exercise is performed. It is not yet undertood what risk this side effect of exercise has on fetal development during the first trimester. It is hypothesized that thermoregulatory adaptations are enhanced with pregnancy. Rectal temperatures were found to decrease by 0.3 °C in the first 8 weeks of pregnancy, and continued to fall 0.1 °C each succeeding month in a population of fit women. Shunting of cooled blood from the periphery, a lowered sweat threshold, increased blood flow to the skin, and an increased minute ventilation may combine to dissipate the heat production of exercise and offset its influence on the maternal core temperature through exercise.[19]

Metabolic

Metabolic needs increase during pregnancy. The Recommended Dietary Allowance is based on the total increased energy requirements during this time of 80,000 kcal. Therefore, an additional 300 kcal per day is recommended during the second and third trimesters.[20] The metabolic pathway of providing fuel to meet the increased energy demands is also altered during pregnancy. A higher percentage of carbohydrate is utilized for energy production at both rest and during exercise.[21]

Biomechanical

The obvious influence on mechanical changes stems from the enlargement of the uterus and breasts. This change in weight distribution causes an upward and forward shift in the center of gravity. This results in a progressive form of lordosis which usually leads to lower back pain. As the pregnancy progresses, the increase in body mass affects the ability to maintain balance, makes many movements difficult to perform, and places a great deal of strain on the lower body with knee pain sometimes occurring.[22]

A less obvious mechanical change is due to increased levels of relaxin and progesterone. These hormones cause significant relaxation of the joints and ligaments, thus increasing the range of motion and flexibility. This can predispose the pregnant woman to ligament injuries and muscle trauma, if stretching movements are not modified.[23]

FETAL IMPLICATIONS

In all likelihood, maternal adaptations have evolved through time, in an effort to nurture growth and development of the fetus and to protect it from harm. Yet the potential for birth defects and spontaneous abortion is a real risk that still exists during the gestation period. Theoretically, maternal exercise could upset the delicate balance that influences growth and development and results in a higher rate of birth defects and spontaneous abortion.

There are four implications of maternal exercise that may increase risk. First, blood flow is redistributed during exercise. Studies have found that this redistribution may reduce the blood flow to the uterus and placenta. If periods of hypoxia occur to the fetus during frequent exercise sessions, neurological damage could result.[24] Second, increased maternal utlization of carbohydrates during exercise could reduce the availability of glucose to the fetus. This reduced fuel supply could lead to malnutrition, growth retardation, and reduced birth weight.[25] Next, the aforementioned thermoregulatory response to maternal exercise may increase the incidence of neural tube defects in the first trimester.[18] Finally, exercise could be responsible for the onset of premature contractions or preterm labor. Norepinephrine levels increase wlth exercise and can act as a stimulant for the uterus to begin contractions.[26]

BENEFITS

Exercise can help to prevent many problems that occur during pregnancy. It can help to control excessive weight gain, maintain aerobic and muscular fitness, alleviate back discomfort, improve posture, enhance self-image, reduce anxiety, and combat depression.

A limited number of studies in healthy, nondiabetic women have been performed to explore the specific differences between those who exercise and who do not during pregnancy. One such example is a study which investigated the risk of spontaneous abortion in pregnant women. A control group was compared to groups of exercising participants. The runners and aerobic dancers had 8% and 7%, respectively, fewer pregnancies terminated than the controls.[27] A review of current literature does not reveal any evidence that contraindicates exercise for healthy women.

Pregnancies complicated by diabetes have specific benefits associated with exercise. The nature of these benefits depends on whether the pregnancy is complicated by gestational or Type I diabetes, with the role of exercise approached very differently in each of the two cases.

Gestational Diabetes

One of the most impressive benefits of exercise is its potential role in maintaining euglycemia in women diagnosed with gestational diabetes. One clinical trial investigated the use of exercise as a method of overcoming peripheral insulin resistance. Nineteen women participated in the study. Nine followed a standard diet protocol. The remaining ten followed the same diet protocol plus exercise for 20 minutes three times each week. After six weeks the diet-only group had an average fasting blood sugar of 87.6 mg/dl and an average one-hour value of 187.5 mg/dl. The exercise group had fasting and one-hour values of 70.1 and 105.9 mg/dl, respectively.[28]

While this study identifies exercise as a possible alternative to insulin initiation, it may also have other important implications. Women diagnosed with gestational diabetes have a 50–60% chance that it will recur in future pregnancies.[29,30] Exercise has been proposed as one means of preventing the return of gestational diabetes in these predisposed women.[31] Furthermore, statistics indicate that 40–60% of these women will develop Type II diabetes within 15 years.[32] Research is now being initiated through the National Institutes of Health to study the role of exercise in preventing the eventual onset of diabetes in this high-risk population.

Type I

Women who intend to become pregnant may choose to utilize exercise to achieve improved glucose control prior to conception, preferably as early as possible. This will provide information in advance concerning the effect that exercise has on glucose levels. Although these responses may differ after gestation begins, these women will have the confidence and experience needed to make the necessary adjustments to prevent exercise-related hypoglycemia. If an exercise physiologist/CDE has been consulted, they will also have a diabetes professional who is familiar with their needs and can assist them in achieving their goals.

EXERCISE PRESCRIPTION

The physiological adaptations to pregnancy require that specific modifications be made to the exercise prescription. The cardiovascular, respiratory, thermoregulatory, metabolic and biomechanical changes must all be factored into the development of an exercise program that meets the needs of the pregnant woman. This requires advising her of the recommended guidelines regarding mode of exercise, frequency, duration, and intensity. Diabetes management skills must also be integrated into the exercise program. Learning to prevent hypoglycemia and coordinating the timing of exercise with insulin regimens must be determined before initiating an exercise program.

Mode

New exercise programs should not be started during the first trimester. By the second trimester, the threat of neural tube defects has passed, and thermoregulatory adaptations to pregnancy can safeguard the fetus during exercise.[17] Studies suggest that nonweight-bearing aerobic exercises (arm ergometer, swimming) are the preferred options. One study examined the effect of different types of exercise equipment on maternal blood pressure, fetal heart rate, and uterine contraction. The researchers concluded that upper-body exercise proved to have the least effect on these factors.[33] This, combined with the fact that nonweight-bearing activities can also be sustained throughout the duration of the pregnancy,[34] makes it the preferred option for exercise at present.

If the patient had been exercising prior to conception, she may already be performing weight-bearing activities (walking, tennis, running). As long as no contraindications exist, these aerobic programs may be continued. However, many women experience a significant decline in exercise performance, and only half are able to continue their weight-bearing exercise program through the third trimester.[35] Biomechanical influences also need to be taken into consideration after 20 weeks. At this point low-impact forms of weight-bearing exercise make better options than higher-impact activities.

Frequency and Duration

Guidelines for the frequency and duration of exercise should meet those requirements established to develop and maintain fitness.[36] At least three aerobic exercise sessions a week should be performed for a minimum of 20 minutes. Each exercise session is to be preceded with an adequate warm-up period of 5–10 minutes. This is necessary to reduce the increased risk of injury that exists with pregnancy-induced joint laxity. A 5–10 minute cool-down period should follow each session.

Intensity

Since both the resting and maximal maternal heart rates change with pregnancy, attempting to use exercise heart rate ranges may not be feasible. It may be better to use alternative methods of monitoring exercise intensity. A rating of perceived exertion (RPE) is a subjective quantifier of exercise intensity. Patients should be instructed to maintain a rating of 13–14 on the Borg scale,[37] which correlates with a maximum functional capacity of 50–60%. Another option is the "Talk Test." The patient is instructed to exercise at an intensity where she can talk comfortably. If she encounters difficulty, the intensity should be reduced until she can once again carry on a conversation.

Exercise capabilities fluctuate during pregnancy. It is important to adjust exercise workloads to meet these changes and to alert the patient that they will occur. Changing to less-intense modes of exercise may have to occur during the final weeks if continued participation in exercise is desired.

Hypoglycemia

Hypoglycemia can be a consequence of exogenous insulin administration. If injections are involved in achieving blood-sugar control, strategies for preventing the occurrence of hypoglycemia during exercise need to be developed. The use of insulin dosage adjustments or preexercise snacks need to be assessed for their appropriateness, for each patient. Blood-sugar monitoring is instrumental in evaluating the glucose response to exercise and in establishing acceptable glucose ranges for pre- and postexercise.

There is a potential for the delayed onset of hypoglycemia, which can occur up to 24 hours after the exercise session. Once identified, specific strategies for insulin adjustment and snacking need to be developed and then utilized by the patient.

Timing of Exercise

Exercise should be scheduled at a consistent time in the day. This makes the glucose response more predictable and assists in the formation of strategies to prevent hypoglycemia. Usually, the optimal time to exercise is 30–60 minutes after a meal or 15 minutes after a snack. This helps to prevent hypoglycemia and blunt the rise in the glucose level that occurs after consuming food. If this is not possible, then definitive strategies must be designed to reduce the risk of hypoglycemia.

Terminating an Exercise Session

After an individualized exercise program is developed and a plan to prevent hypoglycemia is provided, the patient should be made aware of when to terminate an exercise session. She should know that pain, bleeding, dizziness, shortness of breath, palpitations, faintness, tachycardia, back pain, pubic pain, and difficulty in walking are signs and symptoms that should prompt her to stop exercising. In addition, her physician should be contacted immediately and be made aware of these occurrences and any other exercise-related events that cause her concern.[38]

REFERENCES

1. Summary and Recommendations of the Second International Workshop–Conference on Gestational Diabetes Mellitus. Diabetes 40 (suppl 2):175–185, 1991.
2. American College of Obstetricians and Gynecologists: Exercise during pregnancy and the postpartum period. ACOG Technical Bulletin 189. Washington, DC: ACOG, 1994.
3. Wolfe LA, Ohtake PJ, Mottola MF, McGrath MJ: Physiological interactions between pregnancy and aerobic exercise. Exerc Sport Sci Rev 17:295–351, 1989.
4. Clapp JF III: Maternal heart rate in pregnancy. Am J Obstet Gynecol 152:659–660, 1985.
5. Mashini IS, Albazzaz SJ, Fadel HE, et al: Serial noninvasive evaluation of cardiovascular hemodynamics during pregnancy. Am J Obstet Gynecol 156:1208–1213, 1987.
6. Capeless EL, Clapp JF: Cardiovascular changes in early phase of pregnancy. Am J Obstet Gynecol 161:1449–1452, 1989.
7. Hytten FE, Paintin DB: Increase in plasma volume during normal pregnancy. J Obstet Gynaecol Br Commonw 75:1193–1197, 1968.
8. Sullivan JM, Ramanathan KB: Management of medical problems in pregnancy—Severe cardiac disease. N Engl J Med 313:304–309, 1985.
9. Morton MJ, Paul NS, Compos GR, Hartz MV, Metcalfe J: Exercise dynamics in late gestation: Effects of physical training. Am J Obstet Gynecol 152:91–97, 1985.
10. Pivarnik JM, Lee W, Clark SL, Cotton DB, Spillman HT, Miller JF: Cardiac output responses of primigravid women during exercise determined by the direct Fick technique. Obstet Gynecol 75:954–959, 1990.
11. Wiswell RA, Artal R, Romem Y, Kammula R, Dorey, FJ: Hormonal and metabolic response to exercise in pregnancy (abstract). Med Sci Sports Exerc 17:206, 1985.
12. McMurray RG, Hackney AC, Katz VL, Gall M, Watson WJ: Pregnancy-induced changes in the maximal physiological responses during swimming. J Appl Physiol 71:1454–1459, 1991.

13. Sady M, Haydon B, Sady S, Carpenter M, Coustan D, Thompson P: Maximal exercise during pregnancy and postpartum (abstract). Med Sci Sports Exerc 20:511, 1988.
14. Alaily AB, Carroll KB: Pulmonary ventilation in pregnancy. Br J Obstet Gynecol 85:518–524, 1978.
15. Artal R, Wiswell R, Romem Y, Dorey F: Pulmonary responses to exercise in pregnancy. Am J Obstet Gynecol 154:378–383, 1986.
16. Clapp JF III: Oxygen consumption during treadmill exercise before, during and after pregnancy. Am J Obstet Gynecol 161:1458–1464, 1989.
17. Edwards MJ: Hyperthermia as teratogen: A review of experimental studies and their clinical significance. Teratogenesis Carcinog Mutagen 6:563–582, 1986.
18. Milunsky A, Ulcickas M, Rothman KJ, Willett W, Jick SS, Jick H: Maternal heat exposure and neural tube defects. JAMA 268:882–885, 1992.
19. Clapp JF III: The changing thermal response to endurance exercise during pregnancy. Am J Obstet Gynecol 165:1684–1689, 1991.
20. National Research Council: "Recommended Dietary Allowances," 10th ed. Washington, DC: National Academy Press, 1989.
21. Blackburn MW, Calloway DH: Energy expenditure and consumption of mature, pregnant and lactating women. J Am Diet Assoc 69:24–28, 1976.
22. Artal R, Friedman MJ, McNitt-Gray JL: Orthopedic problems in pregnancy. Physician and Sports Medicine 18(9):93–105, 1990.
23. Calguneri M, Bird HA, Wright V: Changes in joint laxity occurring during pregnancy. Ann Rheum Dis 41:126–128, 1982.
24. Rauramo I, Forss M: Effects of exercise on placental blood flow in pregnancies complicated by hypertension, diabetes orintrahepatic cholestasis. Acta Obstet Gynecol Scand 67:115–120, 1988.
25. Hay WW, Sparks JW: Placental, fetal and neonatal carbohydrate metabolism. Clin Obstet Gynaecol 28:473–483, 1985.
26. Artal R, Wiswell R, Romem Y: Hormonal responses to exercise in diabetic and nondiabetic pregnant patients. Diabetes 34 (suppl 2):78–80, 1985.
27. Clapp JF III: The effects of maternal exercise in early pregnancy outcome. Am J Obstet Gynecol 161:1453–1457, 1989.
28. Jovanovic-Peterson L, Durak EP, Peterson C: Randomized trial of diet versus cardiovascular conditioning on glucose levels in gestational diabetes. Am J Obstet Gynecol 161:415–419, 1989.
29. Philipson EH, Super DM: Gestational diabetes mellitus: Does it recur in subsequent pregnancy? Am J Obstet Gynecol 160:1324–1331, 1989.
30. Gaudier FI, Hauth JC, Poist M, deLacee C, Cliver SP: Recurrence of gestational diabetes. Obstet Gynecol 80:755–758, 1992.
31. Horton ES: Exercise in the treatment of NIDDM: Application for GDM? Diabetes 40 (suppl 2)175–178, 1991.
32. O'Sullivan JB: Diabetes mellitus after GDM. Diabetes 40 (suppl 2):131–139, 1991.
33. Durak EP, Jovanovic-Peterson L, Peterson CM: Comparative evaluation of uterine response to exercise on five aerobic machines. Am J Obstet Gynecol 162:754–756, 1990.
34. Artal R, Masaki DI, Khodiguian N, Romem Y, Rutherford SE, Wiswell RA: Exercise prescription in pregnancy: Weight-bearing versus non-weight-bearing exercises. Am J Obstet Gynecol 161: 1464–1469, 1989.
35. Collings CA, Curet LB, Mullin JP: Maternal and fetal responses to a maternal aerobic exercise program. Am J Obstet Gynecol 145:702–707, 1983.
36. American College of Sports Medicine: "Guidelines for Exercise Testing and Prescription," 4th ed. Philadelphia: Lea & Febiger, 1991.

37. Borg G, Linderholm H: Perceived exertion and pulse rate during graded exercise in various age groups. Acta Med Scand (Suppl) 472:194–206, 1967.
38. American College of Obstetricians and Gynecologists: "Exercise during Pregnancy and the Postnatal Period." ACOG Home Exercise Programs. Washington, DC: ACOG, 1985.

CHAPTER 7

Diabetic Retinopathy in Pregnancy

Timothy J. Murtha, MD

Many physicians warn of the progression of diabetic retinopathy during pregnancies in patients with diabetes mellitus. While it appears that pregnancy may be a risk factor for the progression of diabetic retinopathy, this general warning requires elaboration and qualification since there is a significant body of literature questioning its broad application.

Our understanding of the natural history of diabetic retinopathy makes it clear that pregnancy alone does not alter the course of diabetic retinopathy. Pregnancy, however, may accelerate the rate of progression of retinopathy, but this effect does not occur in isolation. Rather, pregnancy must be considered in the context of recognized clinical risk factors that impact on the natural history of diabetic retinopathy. Among known clinical risk factors that contribute to the progression of diabetic retinopathy in the nonpregnant patient are:

- Duration of diabetes
- Retinopathy level
- Glucose control
- Hypertension
- Renal disease

To understand the role of pregnancy in the progression of diabetic retinopathy, each of these variables must be considered. Unfortunately, much of the literature examining the effect of pregnancy on diabetic retinopathy is difficult to interpret because of the failure to address adequately or document the exacerbating effect of the clinical risk factors listed above. In addition, many of the pregnancy studies suffer from small sample sizes, absent or inadequate control groups, a retrospective format

Diabetes Complicating Pregnancy: The Joslin Clinic Method, Edited by Florence M. Brown, MD and John W. Hare, MD.
ISBN 0-471-11031-0 © 1995 John Wiley & Sons, Inc.

or lack of a standardized retinopathy grading scale. In spite of these shortcomings, it is instructional to review this literature in order to evaluate the interaction of known risk factors with pregnancy and to consider pregnancy's role in the progression of diabetic retinopathy.

DURATION OF DIABETES MELLITUS

The duration of diabetes is a significant predictor of the presence or severity of diabetic eye disease. Klein[1] reported that 98% of nonpregnant diabetic persons will have some form of diabetic retinopathy by 15 years duration. Similarly, Aiello et al[2] demonstrated that the duration (in years) of diabetes mellitus is a significant factor for predicting the presence or severity of diabetic retinopathy in pregnancy (See Table I). Other authors have also documented this relationship.[3–5] However, Moloney and Drury's data indicate that pregnant women with diabetes of similar duration demonstrate greater progression of diabetic retinopathy than a nonpregnant diabetic control group, thus implicating pregnancy as an additional risk factor.[4] Therefore, it seems reasonable to expect fewer ophthalmic complications in pregnant diabetic women with shorter duration of diabetes

TABLE I. Retinopathy Status of 80 Pregnant Diabetics, According to Age and Duration of Diabetes

Status of retinopathy	Number of patients	Age	(S.E.)	Duration	(S.E.)
No retinopathy	18	25.9	(1.74)	6.6	(1.0)
Background*	48	27.3	(0.66)	11.7	(0.95)
Preproliferative**	12	26.2	(0.95)	17.7	(1.18)
Proliferative***	2	27.5	(5.5)	15.5	(4.5)
	80				

*Background retinopathy consists of microaneurysms and hemorrhages without the preproliferative characteristics defined by the ETDRS Manual of Operations.
**Pre-proliferative retinopathy includes groupings of the following lesions: moderate to severe hemorrhages and microaneurysms, soft exudates, venous beading, and intraretinal microvascular abnormalities.
***Proliferative retinopathy indicates the presence of definite neovascularization.
From Aiello LM, Rand LI, Sebestyen JG, Weiss JN, Bradbury MJ, Wafai MZ, Briones JC: The eyes and diabetes. In Marble A, Krall LP, Bradley RF, Christlieb AR, Soeldner JS (eds): "Joslin's Diabetes Mellitus," 12th ed. Philadelphia: Lea and Febiger, 1985; 621. Reprinted with permission.

mellitus. Diabetic women may be counseled that earlier pregnancies may be advantageous in preserving ocular health.

BASELINE LEVEL OF DIABETIC RETINOPATHY

A significant predictor for the progression of diabetic retinopathy in pregnancy is the baseline level of retinopathy at the outset of pregnancy. The Early Treatment of Diabetic Retinopathy Study (ETDRS)[5] provides a substantial data base and framework for grading and categorizing levels of diabetic retinopathy. Employing this reproducible and defined grading system, we can more accurately predict the progression of diabetic retinopathy. For example, mild nonproliferative diabetic retinopathy (ETDRS level 20 and 35) carries a less than 5% risk of progressing to proliferative diabetic retinopathy within one year; however, severe nonproliferative retinopathy (level 53) carries a greater than 50% risk of progressing to proliferative diabetic retinopathy within one year.[5] Unfortunately, similar statistics of ETDRS quality are not available regarding the progression of diabetic retinopathy in pregnancy as a function of baseline retinopathy level. Consequently, quantitative comparisons of the pregnant versus nonpregnant state are difficult. However, it is possible to qualitatively assess progression of diabetic retinopathy in pregnancy.

Mild Nonproliferative Diabetic Retinopathy

For those women with no retinopathy or only mild retinopathy at the outset of pregnancy, progression to proliferative disease has been rare[6–8] and prior experience is consistent with the predictions of the ETDRS for nonpregnant patients. However, each of these pregnancy studies did acknowledge mild progression of diabetic retinopathy in some of the patients over the course of the pregnancy. In no instance were these changes visually significant. A return to baseline levels of retinopathy postpartum is the rule. Therefore, it appears that any effect exerted by pregnancy on diabetic retinopathy at this level is mild and transient.

Moderate to Moderately Severe Nonproliferative Diabetic Retinopathy (NPDR)

In pregnant women with diabetes, progression to proliferative diabetic retinopathy has been somewhat more common in those who meet ETDRS classification equivalents of moderate to severe NPDR. Dibble et al[3] reported that 16% (3/19) of patients with this level of retinopathy progressed to proliferative diabetic retinopathy during pregnancy. This finding has been confirmed in additional studies,[9,10] while others have reported very low rates of progression.[4,6,7,11] The ETDRS data predict progression rates to proliferative disease of 12–26% for moderate to moderately severe retinopathy over the course of one year in nonpregnant diabetic persons.[5] Therefore, many of the studies evaluating progression to proliferative diabetic retinopathy in pregnancy report lower rates of progression than would be expected. This discrepancy most likely reflects the inaccuracies of retinopathy grading systems prior to the ETDRS, selection bias, and inadequate sample sizes. Although progression to proliferative disease in pregnant diabetic women of this group was unusual, there was a pronounced predilection for some advance in the retinopathy grading score, often exceeding nonpregnant control groups and ETDRS expectations. Similarly, pospartum regression of diabetic retinopathy was almost uniform. These observations suggest that pregnancy may exacerbate the disease process. For those nonpregnant patients with severe or very severe nonproliferative diabetic retinopathy, the ETDRS reports have suggested consideration of early panretinal photocoagulation. In the setting of a diabetic pregnancy, severe or very severe NPDR prior to conception or in the first trimester are particularly worrisome. It has been our policy to immediately undertake panretinal photocoagulation in these patients.

Proliferative Diabetic Retinopathy

In those diabetic patients with proliferative diabetic retinopathy at the onset of pregnancy, the risk of progression to more severe levels of proliferative disease is quite high. Beetham,[6] Johnston,[12] and Dibble et al[3] all report rates of progression that approach or exceed those predicted in the ETDRS. Fortunately, our experience and studies suggest favorable outcomes for preserving useful vision with laser surgery in pregnant diabetic women. For those patients who enter pregnancy with either spontaneous or laser-induced remission of proliferative disease, the risk of reactivation or progression is quite low.[12–14] For those patients who develop proliferative disease during the course of pregnancy, laser treatment at or prior to the development of Diabetic Retinopathy Study (DRS) high-risk characteristics induces a favorable response similar to that in the nonpregnant diabetic patient.[15] Ultimately, proliferative disease may result in vitreous hemorrhage, fibrovascular tissue, or traction retinal detachment and a concomitant loss of vision. Modern vitrectomy techniques have provided a safe and effective treatment for these vision-threatening sequelae. Today, given timely and effective vitrectomy and laser surgery, diabetic eye disease is rarely a long-term contraindication to pregnancy or an indication for termination of pregnancy.

GLUCOSE CONTROL

Clearly, there appears to be some acceleration of diabetic retinopathy during diabetic pregnancies, albeit mild and transient in most instances. Previously, it had been assumed that pregnancy was the offending insult in diabetic retinopathy progression. Further investigation suggests that the intense glucose control requirements of the pregnant state are a contributing factor for mild progression of diabetic retinopathy. The role of glucose control has been linked to the onset and progression of diabetic retinopathy.[16] In particular, the role of blood-glucose regulation has been implicated as a third variable that may impact on progression of diabetic retinopathy in pregnancy. The Kroc study,[17] Oslo study,[18] and the Diabetes Control and Complication Trial[16] have demonstrated transient retinopathy progression with rapid and acute normalization of glycemic control in the nonpregnant diabetic population. The primary goal of current obstetrical diabetic management is imposition of strict and abrupt glycemic control for improved fetal outcomes. As a result of this management, progression of diabetic retinopathy in pregnancy may be a necessary and unavoidable complication. Phelps et al[9] and O'Hare et al[19] have attempted to assess glucose control as a predictor of diabetic retinopathy progression in pregnancy. Both studies have concluded that pregnant diabetic women who have the greatest fall in glucose values[9] or hemoglobin A_1c[19] levels also experience the greatest progression of characteristic NPDR lesions. In both studies, progression to proliferative diabetic retinopathy was rare. Given that progression of diabetic retinopathy as the result of improved glucose control is both mild and transient, ophthalmic considerations should not be invoked as an excuse to manage blood glucose less than aggressively. By eliminating the need to introduce strict and abrupt glycemic control in the setting of a diabetic pregnancy, presumably one less aggravating factor is eliminated. In this regard, preconception counseling, with the goal of gradual strict diabetic glucose control prior to pregnancy, may represent the safest therapy.

HYPERTENSION AND RENAL COMPLICATIONS

Hypertension has been implicated as an aggravating factor in the progression of diabetic retinopathy in the nonpregnant population.[20,21] Similarly, progression of diabetic retinopathy in pregnancy may be a function of both chronic and pregnancy-induced hypertension,[22,23] although other authors[4,11] have not confirmed this association. Such discrepancies once again underline the difficulties of isolating the impact of one clinical factor from multiple variables.

Diabetic renal complications are a recognized risk factor for progression of diabetic retinopathy in the nonpregnant population, but have not been well studied in the setting of pregnancy. It is reasonable to expect that renal disease will create similar, if not more pronounced, progression of diabetic retinopathy during pregnancy. Therefore, it follows that ideal management of diabetic retinopathy requires optimal management of blood pressure and renal dysfunction prior to and throughout pregnancy.

PREGNANCY

The progression of diabetic retinopathy in pregnancy may occur in the presence of many interacting clinical risk factors, but our understanding of the influence of pregnancy alone on diabetic retinopathy remains unclear. In an attempt to clarify the influence of pregnancy as a sole factor on the progression of diabetic retinopathy, Klein et al[23] conducted a prospective, controlled clinical study. In this study, the variables of diabetes duration, blood-glucose control, baseline retinopathy, and blood-pressure control were taken into account. The study shows that pregnancy is associated with progression of retinopathy ($p < 0.005$). By controlling for all of the confounding variables, this study confirms the general belief that pregnancy is an independent risk factor for the progression of diabetic retinopathy.

DIABETIC MACULAR EDEMA IN PREGNANCY

A second form of vision-threatening diabetic retinopathy is diabetic macular edema. While its natural history and positive response to focal laser therapy have been well documented in the ETDRS,[24,25] its incidence and course in pregnancy are less well defined than proliferative disease.[26] Our experience is that diabetic macular edema in pregnancy, usually characterized by retinal thickening only, is a transient phenomenon that resolves postpartum. Our policy has been to observe this condition throughout pregnancy. If this condition persists at 3–4 months postpartum, intervention with focal laser therapy may be beneficial. As with proliferative disease, macular edema is aggravated by systemic factors such as hypertension, elevated cholesterol, and poor glucose control. In particular, toxemia of pregnancy may act as a catalyst for development or progression of retinal thickening, including macular edema. With fastidious attention to control of these systemic factors, diabetic macular edema can be managed effectively during the pregnancy.

GUIDELINES

Detailed retinal examinations through dilated pupils by an ophthalmologist experienced in the management of diabetic eye disease and appropriate counseling prior to conception will provide optimal eye care. For those patients who are found to have no, minimal, or moderate retinopathy, the effects of pregnancy are minimal, but a follow-up eye exam early in the second trimester is advisable. In those patients with moderate to moderately severe NPDR, a more guarded prognosis requires close follow-up throughout the pregnancy and a low threshold for intervention with panretinal photocoagulation therapy. If severe NPDR or early proliferative disease is detected prior to conception, deferral of pregnancy and early laser surgery are appropriate. The goal of therapy is to induce remission prior to pregnancy. This approach may require a few months to as much as 1–2 years to attain adequate quiescence. Active high-risk proliferative disease with hemorrhage and fibrovascular tissue requires panretinal photocoagulation prior to pregnancy and, possibly, vitrectomy. In all instances, pregnant diabetic women should have an ophthalmic exam early in the first trimester with follow-up as dictated by the situation.

SUMMARY

Pregnancy is an independent risk factor for progression of diabetic retinopathy. In addition, variables including duration of diabetes mellitus, degree of diabetic control, elevated blood pressure, baseline level of retinopathy, and the presence of renal disease contribute to the progression of diabetic retinopathy and must be considered in evaluating retinopathy in pregnancy. Although the impact of pregnancy on diabetic retinopathy may be mild and transient in most instances, close follow-up and timely laser surgery are important in reducing the risk of severe visual loss to less than 5% for those who may reach high risk levels of retinopathy. It is our policy and the recommendation of the American Academy of Ophthalmology that "Diabetic women contemplating pregnancy should have a complete eye examination before they conceive. Pregnant women with diabetes should have their eyes examined early in each trimester of their pregnancy or more frequently, as indicated by level of retinopathy, and 3 to 6 months after delivery. Since pregnancy may exacerbate existing retinopathy and be associated with hypertension, careful medical and ocular observation is crucial during pregnancy. In women with proliferative retinopathy, cesarean delivery may be preferable to vaginal delivery to reduce the risk of vitreous hemorrhage. Close communication among the various members of the health-care team is essential."[27]

ACKNOWLEDGMENT

I would like to thank Lloyd M. Aiello, MD and Jerry Cavallerano, OD, PhD for their thoughtful review and editorial assistance with this manuscript. I would also like to thank Marlene B. Messina for her gracious secretarial skills in the preparation of this manuscript.

REFERENCES

1. Klein R: The epidemiology of diabetic retinopathy: Findings from the Wisconsin Epidemiologic Study of Diabetic Retinopathy. Int Ophthalmol Clin 27:230–238, 1987.
2. Aiello LM, Rand LI, Sebestyen JG, Weiss JN, Bradbury MJ, Wafai MZ, Briones JC: The eyes and diabetes. In Marble A, Krall LP, Bradley RF, Christlieb AR, Soeldner JS (eds): "Joslin's Diabetes Mellitus," 12th ed. Philadelphia: Lea and Febiger, 1985, p. 621.
3. Dibble CM, Kochenour NK, Worley J et al: Effect of pregnancy on diabetic retinopathy. Obstetrics and Gynecology 59:699–704, 1982.
4. Moloney JBM, Drury MJ: The effect of pregnancy on the natural course of diabetic retinopathy. American Journal of Ophthalmology 93:745–756, 1982.
5. ETDRS Study Group #12: Fundus photographic risk factors for progression of diabetic retinopathy. May, (supplement): 98:823–833, 1991.
6. Beetham WP: Diabetic retinopathy in pregnancy. Trans Am Ophthalm Soc 48:205, 1950.
7. Horvat M, Maclean H, Godberg L, Crock GW: Diabetic retinopathy in pregnancy: A 12 year prospective survey. British Journal of Ophthalmology 64:398–403, 1980.
8. Jervell J, Moe N, Skjaeraasen J et al: Diabetes mellitus and pregnancy—Management and results at Riks Hospitalet, Oslo 1970-1977. Diabetologica 16:151–155, 1979.
9. Phelps RL, Sakol P, Metzger BE, Jampol LM et al: Changes in diabetic retinopathy during pregnancy correlations with regulation of hyperglycemia. Archives of Ophthalmology 104:1806–1810, 1986.
10. Price JH, Hadden DR, Archer DB et al: Diabetic retinopathy in pregnancy. British Journal of Obstetrics and Gynecology 91:11–17, 1984.
11. Ohrt V: The influence of pregnancy on diabetic retinopathy with special regard to the reversible changes shown in 100 pregnancies. Acta Ophthalmologica 62:603–616, 1984.
12. Johnston GP: Pregnancy and diabetic retinopathy. American Journal of Ophthalmology 90:519–524, 1980.
13. Aiello LM, Rand LI, Briones JC et al: Nonocular clinical risk factors in the progression of diabetic retinopathy. In Little HL, Jack RL, Patz A et al (eds): "Diabetic Retinopathy" New York: Thieme-Stratton, pp. 21–32, 1983.
14. Singerman LJ: Diabetic retinopathy in juvenile-onset diabetics: 1. Laser therapy in high risk proliferative 2. Effects of pregnancy. In Fine SL, Owens SL (eds): "Management of Retina Vascular and Macular Disorders." Baltimore: Williams & Wilkins, 1983, pp 43–46.

15. Hercules BL, Wozencroft M, Gayed II: Peripheral retinal ablation in the treatment of proliferative diabetic retinopathy during pregnancy. British Journal of Ophthalmology 64:87–93, 1980.
16. Diabetes Control and Complication Trial Research Group: The effect of intensive treatment of diabetes on the development and progression of long-term complications in insulin-dependent diabetes mellitus. New England Journal of Medicine 329:977–986, 1993.
17. The Kroc Collaborative Study Group: Blood glucose and the evolution of diabetic retinopathy and albuminuria. New England Journal of Medicine 311:365–372, 1984.
18. Dahl-Jorgensen K, Brinchmann-Hansen O, Hanssen KF, Sanduik L, Aagenaes O, Aker Diabetes Group: Rapid tightening of blood glucose control leads to transient deterioration of retinopathy in insulin dependent diabetes mellitus: The Oslo study. British Medicine Journal 290:811–815, 1985.
19. O'Hare J, Rand LI, Krolewski AS: Progression of background diabetic retinopathy in pregnancy. Personal communication of unpublished data.
20. Klein R, Klein BEK, Moss SE, Davis MD, DeMets DL: Is blood pressure a predictor of the incidence of progression of diabetic retinopathy? Journal of the Am Med Assoc 260:2864, 1988.
21. Knowler WC, Bennett PH, Ballentine EJ: Increased incidence of retinopathy in diabetics with elevated blood pressure. New England Journal of Medicine 302:645–650, 1980.
22. Rosenn B, Miodovnik M et al: Progression of diabetic retinopathy in pregnancy: Association with hypertension in pregnancy. American Journal of Obstetrics and Gynecology 166:1214–1218, 1992.
23. Klein BEK, Moss SE, Klein R: Effect of pregnancy on progression of diabetic retinopathy. Diabetes Care 33:34–40, 1990.
24. Early Treatment Diabetic Retinopathy Study Research Group: Photocoagulation for diabetic macular edema. ETDRS Report No. 1. Arch Ophthalmol 103:1796–1806, 1985.
25. Early Treatment Diabetic Retinopathy Study Research Group: Treatment techniques and clinical guidelines for photocoagulation of diabetic macular edema. ETDRS Report No. 2. Ophthalmology 94(7):761–774, 1987.
26. Sinclair SH, Nesler C, Foxman B et al: Macular edema and pregnancy in insulin-dependent diabetes. American Journal of Ophthalmology 97:154–167, 1984.
27. Aiello LM, Cavallerano JD: Ocular complications of diabetes mellitus. In Kahn CR, Weir GC (eds): "Joslin's Diabetes Mellitus," 13th ed. Philadelphia: Lea and Febiger, 1994, pp. 771–793.

CHAPTER 8

Maternal Complications: Nephropathy, Neuropathy, and Coronary Artery Disease

Florence M. Brown, MD and John W. Hare, MD

For most women with insulin-dependent diabetes mellitus (IDDM), pregnancy is associated with minimal maternal risk and good neonatal outcome. However, for women whose diabetes is complicated by nephropathy, neuropathy, retinopathy, or coronary artery disease, risk to the mother and infant is increased and may be substantial. Coronary artery disease, severe gastroparesis, and active proliferative retinopathy (see Chapter 7) are contraindications to pregnancy due to maternal risk. Diabetic nephropathy with prepregnancy creatinine greater than 2 mg/dl is usually associated with a uniformly poor fetal prognosis. Overall, the risk to the mother and infant must be individualized depending on the severity of the preexisting maternal diabetic complications.

DIABETIC NEPHROPATHY

Diabetic nephropathy is defined as persistent albuminuria of greater than 300 mg/24 hours. One-third of patients with IDDM will develop diabetic nephropathy in their lifetime.[1] Approximately 15% of pregnant patients with IDDM who are followed at the Joslin Diabetes Center have diabetic nephropathy (Class F diabetes). These complicated pregnancies present special problems to the obstetricians, diabetologists, and neonatologists who care for the affected mother and her child during the gestation and/or postpartum. The risk of Class F diabetes on pregnancy outcome is presented in Chapters 10 and 11 and summarized below.

Diabetes Complicating Pregnancy: The Joslin Clinic Method, Edited by Florence M. Brown, MD and John W. Hare, MD.
ISBN 0-471-11031-0 © 1995 John Wiley & Sons, Inc.

Perinatal mortality in Class F diabetes is 6–11%, compared with 3% in patients with Class B, C, D, or R diabetes.[2,3] This higher perinatal mortality rate is due to the higher incidence of preterm deliveries among patients with Class F diabetes.[2] Fifty percent of Class F pregnancies are premature (<37 weeks gestation), compared with 20% of Class B and C pregnancies. Furthermore, preeclampsia is the major cause of these premature deliveries, developing in 25% of Class F pregnancies compared with 5% of Class B and C pregnancies[4] and, consequently, is a common cause of respiratory distress syndrome in infants of Class F mothers. Recent studies suggest that microalbuminuria also may be associated with increased risk for preeclampsia[5] and small-for-gestational-age infants.[6]

The risk of Class F pregnancy on short- and long-term maternal kidney function is also of concern. Elucidation of the pathophysiology of diabetic nephropathy has helped define treatment strategies both pre- and postpartum. Diabetic nephropathy, in its early phases, is a disorder characterized by hyperfiltration with an increase in glomerular filtration rates above normal. The microscopic lesion is glomerular hypertrophy.[7] Kidney size is increased in patients with increased glomerular filtration rate (GFR).[8,9] Incipient diabetic nephropathy may be heralded by the detection of persistent microalbuminuria (30–300 mg/24 hours), which cannot be identified by urine dipstick testing. Several studies have established that microalbuminuria is a strong predictor of overt diabetic nephropathy.[10–13] As the pathogenic process continues, hyperfiltration leads to an increase in the glomerular transcapillary hydraulic pressure, increasing filtration of protein and the individual nephron glomerular filtration rate.[14] These changes lead to an expansion of the mesangium, and finally, glomerulosclerosis. Surviving glomeruli, then, have an added compensatory hyperfiltration causing a further increase in the surviving single-nephron glomerular filtration rate, more mesangial expansion, more glomerulosclerosis, and hence a vicious cycle.[15] When overt diabetic nephropathy is established, GFR begins to fall at a linear rate. A significant negative correlation exists between decreasing GFR and increasing protein excretion.[16]

Efforts to slow the progression of renal disease with antihypertensive agents have been successful. ACE inhibitors, in particular, have been shown to decrease albumin excretion and slow the fall in GFR over time.[17,18] While reductions in proteinuria, with the use of other antihypertensive agents, are probably directly related to the lowering of systemic blood pressure, ACE inhibitors decrease proteinuria and preserve GFR independent of changes in systemic blood pressure.[19] Animal models suggest that ACE inhibitors protect the kidney by reducing intraglomerular capillary pressure without reducing GFR.[20]

Studies have also demonstrated that initiation of ACE inhibitor therapy in normotensive patients with persistent microalbuminuria reduces microalbumin excretion and delays progression to overt diabetic nephropathy.[21,22] Nonpregnant patients with IDDM at the Joslin Clinic are screened yearly for microalbuminuria. Patients with an elevated random urine albumin/creatinine are screened three months later. If persistent elevation of albumin/creatinine 100 μg/mg or greater is demonstrated, patients are treated with ACE inhibitors. Women of child-bearing age are advised to stop ACE inhibitors when pregnancy has been diagnosed. While ACE inhibitors do not appear to cause teratogenesis during the first trimester, they have been associated with fetal skeletal abnormalities due to oligohydramnios and with transient acute renal failure in the neonate and, therefore, should not be used in the second or third trimester.[23]

Since pregnancy is associated normally with an increase in glomerular filtration rate, one can speculate that it could aggravate preexisting renal disease. Additionally, urinary albumin excretion increases during the third trimester as a normal phenomenon.[24–25] Women with IDDM who have normal albumin excretion rates early in pregnancy likewise have minimal variation during the first and second trimesters. However, by 36 weeks, these women demonstrate an exaggerated rise in albumin excretion compared with nondiabetic control subjects. By six weeks postpartum urinary albumin excretion returns to normal in both groups.[24] Two studies involving women with Class F diabetes have demonstrated marked increases in urinary protein excretion.[2,3] Nephrotic range proteinuria developed in a majority of these patients. Nevertheless, postpartum urinary protein excretion returned almost to baseline early pregnancy levels. Creatinine clearance in these patients does not rise as it does in the nondiabetic population. For individual patients, creatinine clearance may rise, fall or stay the same during pregnancy, though overall there is a slight decrease in creatinine clearance. For most Class F patients, this likely represents the natural course of diabetic nephropathy. Therefore, pregnancy does not seem to adversely affect the rate of decline of kidney function in the long run.

There is one other major philosophical issue that needs to be addressed. Because diabetic nephropathy proceeds inexorably, if it is established at the time a woman is pregnant, she faces the possibility of renal failure, dialysis, and possible transplantation in the next ten years. It is not our policy to volunteer this information to a woman who is determined to be pregnant and does not inquire about the future. If she does, and the physician senses that she wishes to use this information to help her decide whether or not to become pregnant or to continue a pregnancy, the prognosis is revealed to her. Some women will wish to have a child despite the presence of renal disease. If this is the case, the sooner the better, because as discussed above, if her renal disease is mild, the chance for a successful outcome is relatively high.

Treatment

Women who have hypertension that predates pregnancy usually continue medical treatment, albeit with drugs that are safe for use in pregnancy. Selective beta-adrenergic blocking agents are our drugs of choice for the treatment of hypertension. Their safety during pregnancy is well established.[26] Methyldopa may be used but it is less effective than beta adrenergic blocking agents and produces somnolence. Hydralazine may be given in combination with a beta-adrenergic blocking agent if hypertension is not well controlled with a single agent. Diuretics are rarely used in patients who had been taking them as part of combination therapy for severe hypertension prior to pregnancy. Angiotensin-converting enzyme inhibitors are not used during pregnancy.

Guidelines for when to initiate or continue treatment for elevated blood pressure during diabetic pregnancy are not well established in the medical or obstetrical literature. The National Institutes of Health report of the Working Group on High Blood Pressure in Pregnancy recommends initiating antihypertensive therapy for diastolic blood pressures greater than 100 mm Hg.[27,28] These guidelines are based on the findings that treatment with antihypertensive medication may not reduce the incidence of preeclampsia in women with mild to moderate hypertension. Nevertheless, it has been well established that even mild hypertension in patients with diabetes is a risk factor for progression of retinopathy as well as kidney disease. We, therefore, suggest using antihypertensive therapy at lower diastolic blood pressures, i.e., above 85–90 mm Hg in the second trimester and 90–95 mm Hg in the third trimester until further risk/benefit studies are available for the hypertensive diabetic population. Women who have microalbuminuria without preexisting hypertension are taken off their ACE inhibitor without substituting other antihypertensive therapy.

In mid- to late pregnancy, it is often helpful to have the mother spend an hour or two each morning and each afternoon recumbent, particularly in the left lateral position. This reduces the accumulation of edema and reduces the mother's blood pressure and increases uteroplacental flow. This prescription is also incompatible with most forms of employment. Thus, women with renal disease need to be told at the beginning of their pregnancy that it is unlikely that they will be able to work late in the pregnancy. It is possible that they may have to cease working in mid-pregnancy and quite often that they will have to cease working by the beginning of the third trimester. If they already have small children at home, it may be necessary to arrange for child care. This all needs to be made clear at the outset so that the mother has ample time to make preparations for a difficult pregnancy.

Postpartum, ACE inhibitors may be resumed in women who choose to bottle feed their infants. Women who choose to breast feed their infants for less than three or four months may continue the antihypertensive agent used during their pregnancy. For women who choose to nurse their infants for longer periods of time, a decision must be made whether or not to resume the ACE inhibitors. Preservation of renal function in the mother may outweigh the risk to the infant. While the drug companies that manufacture ACE inhibitors caution against their use during lactation, available data for Captopril and Enalapril reveal that drug levels in breast milk are less than 1% of maternal serum levels and are considered safe for use during lactation by the American Academy of Pediatrics.[23,29]

If the serum creatinine is elevated and the clearance diminished at the beginning of pregnancy, the likelihood of a successful outcome is markedly diminished. Although it is not our policy to recommend termination of pregnancy, we view these pregnancies with great trepidation and make our views known to those mothers who choose to embark upon this course. As a general guideline, a serum creatinine level of greater than 3.0 mg/dl is incompatible with fetal life, so that if the serum creatinine at the outset is already 2.0 mg/dl or higher, it is quite possible that the pregnancy will be terminated by the natural history of the disease. Unfortunately, this tends to occur after fetal viability has been reached, so that the psychological magnitude of the loss is greater than if it had occurred in the first trimester.

Transplantation

Several case reports and series have reported on successful pregnancies following renal transplantation.[30–32] These pregnancies are complicated by prematurity in nearly 100%, and preeclampsia and hypertension in two-thirds. Immunosuppressive drugs such as azathioprine and prednisone have little direct deleterious effect on the fetus. Prednisone is the steroid of choice because the fetoplacental unit lacks the capability to convert it to its active metabolite prednisolone. Nevertheless steroid therapy may increase insulin resistance. Alternate-day steroids may render good glucose control difficult. If possible, daily prednisone, with unchanging dosages, is preferred in order to achieve consistency of insulin requirements. Stress-dose steroid coverage should be given during labor and delivery in order to prevent Addisonian crisis.

DIABETIC NEUROPATHY

Although clinical studies of diabetic neuropathy abound in the literature, very few report on this complication in pregnancy. While the Diabetes Control and Complications Trial (DCCT) has demonstrated that excellent diabetes control reduces the risk of neuropathy in nonpregnant individuals,[33] it is not known whether this applies to pregnancy as well. It is also unclear whether pregnancy itself influences the short-term or long-term complications of neuropathy. While the presence of autonomic neuropathy may have serious potential impact on the diabetic pregnancy, other forms of neuropathy (i.e., peripheral and cranial) are less common and of less clinical significance.

AUTONOMIC NEUROPATHY

Autonomic neuropathy refers to dysfunction of the nerves that innervate the stomach, bladder, bowel, heart, blood vessels, and sweat glands. In the setting of pregnancy, gastroparesis has been reported as a cause of significant maternal and fetal morbidity and mortality. First trimester "morning sickness" may exacerbate preexisting symptoms of gastroparesis, such as early satiety, nausea, and postprandial vomiting. Mechanical compression of the stomach, by an enlarging uterus, late in pregnancy can result in more pronounced delays in gastric emptying. Gastroparesis may undermine blood sugar management, resulting in either severe maternal hypoglycemia due to delayed absorption of food or profound hyperglycemia when food is finally absorbed and there is an inadequate amount of insulin available to metabolize the glucose. It is our belief that metoclopramide improves metabolic stability in these patients without significant risk to the fetus and should be instituted when symptoms of gastroparesis are present. In the worst cases, intractable vomiting has resulted in severe malnutrition and dehydration and the need for hyperalimentation during pregnancy.[34,35] Women with symptoms of gastroparesis prior to pregnancy should be aware that exacerbations are likely to occur during pregnancy and that there is a potential for significant maternal or fetal morbidity.

Incomplete bladder emptying secondary to bladder neuropathy may predispose to urinary tract infections. Monthly routine urine screening, for culture and antibiotic sensitivities, is performed and positive urine cultures are treated with appropriate antibiotics. Lower bowel neuropathy may result in embarrassing symptoms of nocturnal diarrhea and fecal incontinence alternating with constipation. Infectious causes of diarrhea should be ruled out before treating with loperamide (Food and Drug Administration pregnancy Category B). Constipation, whether it occurs as a result of bowel neuropathy, supplementation with iron, or as a direct result of pregnancy may be treated with sugar-free bulking agents and increased per oral water intake.

Orthostatic hypotension is defined as a 20–30 mm Hg fall in systolic blood pressure or a 10–15 mm Hg fall in diastolic blood pressure, when changing from a supine to standing blood pressure. Failure of the heart rate to increase with standing distinguishes orthostatic hypotension from hypovolemia. Symptoms include postural light-headedness or near syncope. Reports of orthostatic hypotension complicated diabetic pregnancies are rare. One interesting case report notes amelioration of severe orthostatic hypotension during pregnancy, possibly as a result of the volume expansion of the pregnant state.[36]

Prospective controlled studies from Finland have demonstrated that women with IDDM who have asymptomatic autonomic neuropathy, as defined by an abnormality of either expiratory to inspiratory ratio (E:I ratio) or heart rate response to standing (30:15 ratio), have double the risk of aggregated pregnancy-related complications when compared with IDDM women who have normal autonomic function tests. Data comparing the risk of specific complications between the two groups, such as maternal ketoacidosis, severe maternal hypoglycemia, congenital malformations, spontaneous abortion, preeclampsia, respiratory distress syndrome, and perinatal mortality were not significant, possibly because the study group was too small to evaluate these low-frequency complications independently.[37] In addition, cross-sectional studies demonstrated that increasing parity was not associated with a higher incidence of abnormal autonomic function tests. Thus, it appears that pregnancy itself does not lead to deterioration of autonomic neuropathy.[38]

We do not routinely screen asymptomatic women with IDDM for autonomic neuropathy since management decisions have not been altered with this information. We do advise women with symptomatic gastroparesis prior to pregnancy that exacerbations may occur during pregnancy and that there is a potential for significant maternal and fetal morbidity. Metoclopramide may help nutritional status, blood-sugar control, and comfort level in women who have symptomatic gastroparesis during pregnancy. In cases of severe gastroparesis, total parenteral nutrition should be instituted early when malnutrition threatens the pregnancy.

PERIPHERAL NEUROPATHY

While peripheral neuropathy is a common complication of both IDDM and NIDDM, it rarely complicates the diabetic pregnancy. The longest nerves of the body, innervating feet, hand, and thoracoabdominal area are affected initially. Patients complain of pain, burning, tingling, and numbness. The physical examination reveals loss of vibration, pinprick, light touch, proprioception, and temperature sensations. Patients with peripheral neuropathy should be instructed to avoid exposure to extreme temperatures, avoid walking barefoot, wear properly fitting shoes, and visually inspect the feet twice daily for evidence of unrecognized injury.

Peripheral neuropathy involving the hand may be clinically difficult to distinguish from carpal tunnel syndrome. Nerve conduction velocities reveal pronounced slowing at the wrist in patients with carpal tunnel syndrome compared with gradual slowing of nerve conduction in patients with peripheral neuropathy. Conservative management of carpal tunnel syndrome, i.e., the use of wrist splints, is advised because carpal tunnel syndrome usually improves postpartum.

CRANIAL NEUROPATHIES

The 3rd, 6th, and 7th (Bell's Palsy) cranial nerves (CN) may be involved in diabetic patients. Similarly, Bell's Palsy is more common in pregnancy. Patients may present with diplopia (CNs III and VI) or ipsilateral facial weakness, including the forehead (CN VII). Absence of other neurologic findings distinguish these cranial neuropathies from a more serious central nervous system process, such as a stroke or space-occupying lesion. Imaging studies are unnecessary and the palsy usually resolves completely over several weeks to months.

CORONARY ARTERY DISEASE (CLASS H DIABETES)

In the general population, myocardial infarction is infrequent in women of childbearing age, occurring in approximately 1 in 10,000 pregnancies.[39,40] Data from the Framingham Heart Study demonstrates a low cumulative mortality rate of 4% for women up to the age of 55 years, which is half the risk of men of similar age.[41] The incidence of coronary disease in the general population is 2 per 10,000 persons-years in 35–45 year old women and negligible for women less than 35 years of age. In contrast, women with IDDM have an eight-fold higher cumulative mortality rate from coronary artery disease (35%) by age 55 years. This cumulative mortality rate in women does not differ from that of men of similar ages, indicating that the protective effect of female gender is eliminated in premenopausal women with IDDM.[42]

Additionally, diabetic nephropathy is a powerful risk factor for coronary artery disease in patients with IDDM. The yearly incidence of death from coronary artery disease for IDDM women ages 25–35 is 1 per 1000 for those without nephropathy and 3–4 per 1000 for those with nephropathy.[42] For women ages 35–45 years, the yearly incidence of death from coronary artery disease is 7 per 1000 for those without nephropathy and 30 per 1000 for those with nephropathy. Deaths from coronary artery disease in both the IDDM and Framingham cohorts do not seem to occur before the latter part of the 3rd decade.[42] However, for women with IDDM who delay their childbearing until the fourth and sometimes fifth decades, there is an associated increased risk of coronary artery disease just on the basis of age.

While there have been occasional case reports of coronary artery disease occurring during the pregnancies of women with IDDM, the incidence during these pregnancies has not been reported.[35,43–51] Our experience from 1978 through 1993 has included four cases of Class H diabetes in approximately 1400 pregnancies. Of note, three of four women had ages greater than 35 years during their pregnancies. All women had IDDM of greater than 20 years duration. All had at least one additional risk factor other than IDDM, such as smoking, family history of coronary artery disease, or hypertension, and all women had renal involvement; one had microalbuminuria noted prior to pregnancy and three had diabetic nephropathy.

It seems prudent that women with IDDM who seek preconception counseling be provided with an assessment of coronary artery disease risk. Women who are of age greater than 30–35 years and who have other risk factors for coronary artery disease, including diabetic nephropathy, should probably perform exercise-tolerance testing prior to pregnancy. Women with established coronary artery disease should be counseled against pregnancy. While there have been case reports of successful pregnancies following coronary artery bypass surgery, the high maternal mortality rate associated with symptomatic coronary artery disease and the lack of experience following these women through pregnancy precludes encouraging pregnancy in this situation.

A very difficult management issue arises when symptoms suggestive of coronary artery disease occur for the first time during pregnancy. Establishing a definitive diagnosis is difficult since angiographic and nuclear medicine studies are contraindicated during pregnancy and exercise-tolerance testing is usually nondiagnostic. If the symptoms are mild and resolve spontaneously, watchful waiting with the assistance of a cardiologist may be employed. If symptoms recur or worsen, it becomes necessary to establish definitively whether or not the woman has coronary artery disease. Early delivery or termination (if fetal viability has not been reached) may be necessary for those women with coronary artery disease.

In summary, for women of child bearing age, coronary artery disease is more prevalent in those with IDDM compared with the general population. Our experience suggests that coronary artery disease may be more common in the diabetic gravida as well. In particular, older age at the time of pregnancy and the presence of diabetic nephropathy are substantial risk factors for coronary artery disease.

REFERENCES

1. Krolewski AS, Warram JH, Christlieb AR, Busick EJ, Kahn CR: The changing natural history of nephropathy in Type I diabetes. Am J Med 78:785–794, 1985.
2. Kitzmiller JL, Brown ER, Phillippe M, Stork AR, Acker D, Kaldany A, Singh S, Hare JW: Diabetic nephropathy and perinatal outcome. Am J Obstet Gynecol 141:741–751, 1981.
3. Reece EA, Coustan DR, Hayslett JP, Holford T, Coulehan J, O'Connor TZ, Hobbins JC: Diabetic nephropathy: Pregnancy performance and fetomaternal outcome. Am J Obstet Gynecol 159:56–66, 1988.
4. Green MF, Hare JW, Krache M, Phillippe M, Barrs VA, Saltzman DH, Nadel A, Younger MD, Heffner L, Sherl JE: Prematurity among insulin-requiring gravid women. Am J Obstet Gynecol 161:106–111, 1989.
5. Combs CA, Rosenn B, Kitzmiller JL, Khoury JC, Wheeler BC, Miodovnik M: Early-pregnancy proteinuria in diabetes related to preeclampsia. Obstet Gynecol 82:802–807, 1993.
6. Laffel LMB, Greene MF, Wilkins-Haug L: First trimester urinary albumin excretion predicts birth weight in diabetic pregnancies. Diabetes 41 (Suppl 1):133A, 1992.
7. Osterby R, Gundersen HJG: Glomerular size and structure in diabetes mellitus 1. Early abnormalities. Diabetologia 11:225–229, 1975.
8. Christiansen JS, Gammelgaard J, Frandsen M, Parving H-H: Increased kidney size, glomerular filtration rate and renal plasma flow in short-term insulin-dependent diabetics. Diabetologia 20:451–456, 1981.
9. Mogensen CE, Andersen MJF: Increased kidney size and glomerular filtration rate in early juvenile diabetes. Diabetes 22:706–712, 1973.
10. Viberti GC, Hill RD, Jarrett RJ, Argyropoulos A, Mahmud U, Keen H: Microalbuminuria as a predictor of clinical nephropathy in insulin dependent diabetes mellitus. Lancet 1:1430–1432, 1982.
11. Parving H-H, Øxenboll B, Svendsen PA, Christiansen JS, Andersen AR: Early detection of patients at risk of developing diabetic nephropathy. A longitudinal study of urinary microalbumin excretion. Acta Endocrinol (Copenhagen) 100:550–555, 1982.
12. Mathiesen ER, Øxenboll B, Johansen K, Svendsen PA, Deckert T: Incipient nephropathy in Type I insulin-dependent diabetes. Diabetologia 26:406–410, 1984.
13. Mogensen CE, Chistensen CK: Predicting diabetic nephropathy in insulin-dependent diabetic patients. N Engl J Med 311:89–93, 1984.
14. Zatz R, Meyer TW, Rennke HG, Brenner BM: Predominance of hemodynamic rather than

metabolic factors in the pathogenesis of diabetic glomerulopathy. Proc Natl Acad Sci USA 82:5963–5967, 1985.
15. Osterby R, Gundersen HJ, Nyberg G, Aurell M: Advanced diabetic glomerulopathy. Quantitative structural characterization of non-occluded glomeruli. Diabetes 36:612–619, 1987.
16. Viberti GC, Bilous RW, Mackintosh D, Keen H: Monitoring glomerular function in diabetic nephropathy: A prospective study. Am J Med 74:256–263, 1983.
17. Lewis EJ, Hunsicker LG, Bain RP, Ronde RD: The effect of angiotensin-converting-enzyme inhibition on diabetic nephropathy. N Engl J Med 329:1456–1462, 1993.
18. Parving H-H, Hammel E, Smidt UM: Protection of kidney function and decrease in albuminuria by captopril in insulin dependent diabetics with nephropathy. Br Med J 297:1086–1091, 1988.
19. Kasiske BL, Kalil RSN, Ma JZ, Liao M, Keane WF: Effect of antihypertensive therapy on the kidney in patients with diabetes: A meta-regression analysis. Ann Intern Med 118:129–138, 1993.
20. Zatz R, Dunn BR, Meyer TW et al: Prevention of diabetic glomerulopathy by pharmacologic amelioration of capillary hypertension. J Clin Invest 77:1925–1930, 1986.
21. Marre M, LeBlanc H, Suarez L, Guyenne T-T, Menard J, Passa P: Converting enzyme inhibition and kidney function in normotensive diabetic patients with persistent microalbuminuria. Br Med J 294:1148–1152, 1987.
22. Mathiesen ER, Hommel E, Giese J, Parving H-H: Efficacy of captopril in postponing nephropathy in normotensive insulin-dependent diabetic patients with microalbuminuria. Br Med J 303:81–87, 1991.
23. Briggs GG, Freeman RK, Yaffe SJ: "Drugs in Pregnancy and Lactation." Baltimore: Williams and Wilkins, 1994.
24. McCance DR, Traub AI, Harley JMG, Hadden DR, Kennedy L: Urinary albumin excretion in diabetic pregnancy. Diabetologia 32:236–239, 1989.
25. Konstantin-Hansen KF, Hesseldahl H, Pedersen SM: Microalbuminuria as a predictor of preeclampsia. Acta Obstet Gynecol Scand 71:343–346, 1992.
26. Ferris TF: Pregnancy complicated by hypertension and renal disease. Adv Intern Med 35:269–288, 1990.
27. National High Blood Pressure Education Working Group: Report on High Blood Pressure in Pregnancy. Am J Obstet Gynecol 163:1689–1712, 1990.
28. Lindheimer MD, Cunningham FG: Hypertension and pregnancy: Impact of the Working Group report. Am J Kidney Diseases 21(5 Suppl 2):29–36, 1993.
29. Committee on Drugs, American Academy of Pediatrics: The transfer of drugs and other chemicals into human milk. Pediatrics 93:137–150, 1994.
30. Levine MG, Miodovnik M, Siddiqi TA, First MR, Knowles HC: A successful pregnancy in a juvenile diabetic with a renal transplant complicated by preeclampsia. Transplantation 8:498–499, 1983.
31. Vinicor C, Golichowski A, Filo R, Smith EJ, Maxwell D: Pregnancy following renal transplantation in a patient with insulin-dependent diabetes mellitus. Diabetes Care 7:280–284, 1984.
32. Ogburn PL, Kitzmiller JL, Hare JW, Phillippe M, Gabbe SG, Miodovnik M, Tagatz GE, Nagel TC, Williams PP, Goetz FC, Barbosa JJ, Sutherland DE: Pregnancy following renal transplantation in Class T diabetes mellitus. JAMA 255:911–915, 1986.
33. The DCCT Research Group: The effect of intensive treatment of diabetes on the development and progression of long-term complications in insulin-dependent diabetes mellitus. N Engl J Med 329:977–986, 1993.

34. Macleod AF, Smith SA, Sonksen PN, Lowy C: The problem of autonomic neuropathy in diabetic pregnancy. Diabetic Med 7:80–82, 1990.
35. Brown FM, Hare JW: Diabetic neuropathy and coronary artery disease. In: Reece EA and Coustan DR (eds): "Diabetes Mellitus in Pregnancy: Principles and Practice." New York: Churchill Livingstone, in press.
36. Scott AR, Tattersall RB, McPherson M: Improvement of postural hypotension and severe diabetic autonomic neuropathy during pregnancy. Diabetes Care 11:369–370, 1988.
37. Airaksinen KEJ, Anttila LM, LinnaCuoto MK, Jouppila PI, Takkunen JT, Salmela PI: Autonomic influence on pregnancy outcome in IDDM. Diabetes Care 13:756–761, 1990.
38. Airaksinen KEJ, Salmela PI: Pregnancy is not a risk factor for a deterioration of autonomic nervous function in diabetic women. Diabetic Med 10:540–542, 1993.
39. Fletcher E, Knox EW, Morton P: Acute myocardial infarction in pregnancy. B Med J 3:586–588, 1967.
40. Sullivan JM, Ramanathan KB: Management of medical problems in pregnancy—Severe cardiac disease. N Engl J Med 313:304–309, 1985.
41. Lerner DJ, Kannel WB: Patterns of coronary heart disease morbidity and mortality in the sexes: A 26 year follow-up of the Framingham population. Am Heart J 111: 383–390, 1986.
42. Krolewski AS, Kosinski EJ, Warram JH, Leland OS, Busick EJ, Asmal AC, Rand LI, Christlieb AR, Bradley RF, Kahn CR: Magnitude and determinants of coronary artery disease in juvenile-onset, insulin-dependent diabetes mellitus. Am J Cardiol 59:750–755, 1987.
43. Brock HJ, Russel NG, Randall CL: Myocardial infarction in pregnancy: Report of a case with normal spontaneous vaginal delivery seven months later. JAMA 152:1030–1031, 1953.
44. Siegler AM, Hoffman J, Bloom O: Myocardial infarction complicating pregnancy. Obstet Gynecol 7:306–311, 1956.
45. Delaney JJ, Ptacek J: Three decades of experience with diabetic pregnancies. Am J Obstet Gynecol 106:550–556, 1970.
46. White P: Life cycle of diabetes in youth. JAMWA 27:293–313, 1972.
47. Hibbard LT: Maternal mortality due to cardiac disease. Clin Obstet Gynecol 18:27–36, 1975.
48. Hare JW, White P: Pregnancy in diabetes complicated by vascular disease. Diabetes 26:953–955, 1977.
49. Silfen SL, Wapner RJ, Gabbe SG: Maternal outcome in Class H diabetes mellitus. Obstet Gynecol 55:749–751, 1980.
50. Reece EA, Egan JFY, Coustan DR, Tamborlane W, Bates SE, O'Neil TM, Fitzpatrick JG: Coronary artery disease in diabetic pregnancies. Am J Obstet Gynecol 154:150–151, 1986.
51. Hare JW: Complicated diabetes complicating pregnancy. In Oats JN (ed): Clinical Obstetrics and Gynecology, 5, 1991, pp. 349–366.

SECTION III

OBSTETRICAL CONSIDERATIONS

CHAPTER 9

Obstetrical Management

Robert N. Blatman, MD and Vanessa A. Barss, MD

INTRODUCTION

In 1898, Dr. Elliot P. Joslin cared for the first diabetic gravida at what was to become the Joslin Clinic. At that time, a quarter century before the introduction of insulin, maternal mortality was 20% and perinatal mortality was 60% in pregnant diabetics.[1] Currently, most diabetic women can look forward to a pregnancy outcome that is comparable to that of the general population (Table I). This reduction in perinatal and maternal mortality over the past century can be attributed to the introduction of insulin and sophisticated technologies for monitoring glycemic control and fetal well-being. It can also be attributed to intensive medical, obstetrical, and neonatal management of the diabetic gravida and her infant by specialized teams of physicians interested and experienced in caring for the pregnancy complicated by diabetes.[2]

In this chapter, the obstetrical management of women with diabetes is described with respect to the antepartum care, fetal surveillance, delivery, and postpartum care of the uncomplicated patient. Although most diabetic patients can expect a pregnancy outcome as favorable as their nondiabetic counterparts, this success is achieved at a price. These patients have to commit themselves to a management program that requires frequent prenatal visits, strict adherence to diet, compulsive self-monitoring of blood sugars, and intensive fetal surveillance.

FIRST TRIMESTER

First Prenatal Visit

An obstetrician uses the first prenatal visit to obtain basic historical, physical and laboratory information about the patient and to educate her

Diabetes Complicating Pregnancy: The Joslin Clinic Method, Edited by Florence M. Brown, MD and John W. Hare, MD.
ISBN 0-471-11031-0 © 1995 John Wiley & Sons, Inc.

TABLE I. Perinatal Survival at the Joslin Clinic

Time period	Perinatal survival (%)
1898–1917	40
1924–1938	54
1938–1958	86
1958–1975	90
1975–1994	97

regarding the management and potential complications of diabetes in pregnancy. A thorough medical history is obtained and the patient is examined. Every effort is made to establish an accurate estimated date of confinement. If the last menstrual period is unreliable or if the uterine size is not appropriate for dates, an ultrasound examination is obtained. The obstetrician describes the entire management program for the diabetic gravida, emphasizing the importance of good glycemic control to reduce perinatal mortality and morbidity (Chapter 3). The patient is given forms on which to record her home glucose monitoring results during the next week (Chapter 4). This surveillance can be achieved using one of the many home glucose monitoring systems currently available. The general goals of therapy are to keep the fasting glucose levels below 100 mg/dl and the postprandial levels below 120 without having periods of hypoglycemia.

The patient is seen by a nutritionist, a diabetic educator and a social worker, if appropriate. An appointment may be scheduled for an ophthalmologist.

In addition to the routine prenatal laboratory examination, baseline renal function is assessed with either an early morning urine microalbumin or a 24-hour urine collection for total protein excretion and creatinine clearance. A glycosylated hemoglobin level is obtained for purposes of counseling regarding the risks of miscarriage and congenital malformations.

Patients who are in poor metabolic control at the first prenatal visit, or at any other time, are admitted to the hospital for adjustment of insulin and diet; otherwise, care is provided in an outpatient setting. Both an obstetrician and a diabetologist are continuously on call to answer questions and make insulin adjustments by telephone. This availability is crucial in order for outpatient management to work.

Second Prenatal Visit

At the second prenatal visit, the results of the laboratory tests and physical examination are discussed with the patient. Special emphasis is placed on any new evidence of nephropathy or retinopathy, and the previous week's blood sugar values are reviewed. The main focus of this visit, however, is the glycosylated hemoglobin result. Data from the Joslin Clinic have confirmed an increasing risk of spontaneous abortion and major congenital malformations associated with increasing first trimester glycosylated hemoglobin values (see Chapter 12). Each patient is told her glycohemoglobin result and its significance. If the glycohemoglobin indicates a high risk for a congenital anomaly, options include: (1) immediate termination of the pregnancy, (2) continuing the pregnancy and then dealing with any neonatal problems that arise, or (3) delaying the decision until 18 weeks gestation when the findings from a sonographic survey and maternal serum analytes (alpha-fetoprotein panel) are available. It has been our experience that ultrasound examination performed by experienced personnel can pick up the vast majority of major malformations. In one study including pregestational diabetic gravidas from the Joslin Clinic and the Brigham and Women's Hospital, the negative predictive value of ultrasound for the diagnosis of anomalies was 97%.[4] Therefore, a normal ultrasound can be quite reassuring. The disadvantage of this approach is the necessity of waiting until 18 weeks gestation to obtain an adequate fetal survey, with the resulting need, in some cases, for a late, second trimester termination.

After the first two prenatal visits, which are scheduled one week apart, patients are seen by the obstetrician every four weeks through the 30th week of gestation and then weekly until delivery. However, patients continue to come to the clinic each week to be seen by the diabetologist for review of their blood sugar sheets and adjustment of insulin dose. The internist–diabetologist and obstetrician work side by side in the same clinical area to facilitate the flow of clinical information regarding each patient. At the end of each clinical session, the diabetologists, obstetricians, nurses, social worker, nutritionist, and clerical staff meet to review each patient's visit, progress, and management plans in detail.

SECOND TRIMESTER

Congenital-disease screening is a particular concern for the second trimester. The "triple panel" of serum analytes is drawn, consisting of maternal serum alfa-fetoprotein (aFP), beta-subunit of human chorionic gonadotropin, and unconjugated estriol. An elevated aFP can be associated with an open neural tube defect. Traditionally, an elevated maternal serum aFP has been followed up with an amniocentesis after ultrasound confirmation of gestational age and singleton pregnancy. More recently, Nadal et al. demonstrated that a normal, high-resolution ultrasound examination can detect neural-tube defects with close to 100% accuracy.[5] At the Joslin Clinic, we offer these patients amniocentesis, but counsel that a normal ultrasound examination may be as predictive with no risk of pregnancy loss.

These serum analytes can also be used to help determine a woman's risk of carrying a chromosomally abnormal fetus. The results are typically reported as a risk ratio. We offer invasive prenatal diagnosis to women whose risk of a chromosomally abnormal fetus is approximately that of a procedure-related loss.

A thorough fetal anatomic survey is performed between 18 and 20 weeks gestation. A full discussion of the prevention and diagnosis of congenital anomalies in diabetic pregnancies is presented in Chapter 12.

THIRD TRIMESTER

The major hazards of the third trimester are the risks of (1) intrauterine fetal demise, (2) obstetrical or medical complications necessitating premature delivery, and (3) potential fetal–maternal trauma during delivery because of fetal macrosomia. Therefore, obstetrical management during the final weeks of pregnancy is primarily concerned with the assessment of continued fetal well-being. Obstetrical surveillance is directed toward electronic and sonographic fetal monitoring, maintenance of good glycemic control, estimation of fetal size, and determination of fetal pulmonary maturity. Potential obstetrical complications that may develop during the period, such as preeclampsia, premature rupture of membranes, premature labor, and hydramnios, are discussed in Chapter 10.

Fetal Surveillance

Antepartum fetal heart rate testing utilizing the nonstress test (NST) or the oxytocin challenge test (OCT) was introduced in the United States in the 1970s. In a large, prospective, multiinstitutional study of these tests, the neonatal death rate was 3.2 per thousand after a reactive nonstress test and 0.4 per thousand after a negative oxytocin challenge test (OCT).[6] Two relatively large series, in well-controlled, insulin-requiring diabetics employing a combination of the NST and the OCT, have shown excellent results. In Golde's series of 107 patients followed with biweekly NSTs, three stillbirths occurred, two of which were associated with congenital anomalies incompatible with life, and one with maternal diabetic ketoacidosis in a noncompliant, untested patient of 24 weeks who stopped taking insulin.[7] In Ray's series of 170 diabetic pregnancies followed with the OCT, there were no stillbirths.[8] It has not been clearly resolved whether the NST or the OCT should be the primary method of antepartum fetal surveillance in high-risk pregnancies. Although Freeman's multiinstitutional study concluded that monitoring with the OCT improved antenatal survival eight-fold over NST surveillance, the groups studied were not appropriately matched, the criteria for NSTs varied from hospital to hospital, and the management of the pregnancies was not standardized.[6] Because the risk of antenatal death within seven days of a reactive NST was very low in that study (3.2 per thousand) and in our own experience (2.7 per thousand), we think that the NST is an adequate method of antepartum fetal surveillance.[9] Evertson and associates found a reactive NST to be a better predictor of fetal well-being than a negative OCT.[10] The clear advantages of the NST are (1) it does not require intravenous medications, (2) it takes less time, (3) it is easier to interpret, and (4) it costs less.

The role of the biophysical profile, first introduced in 1980 by Manning et al,[11] is still unclear. Golde et al. performed 459 fetal biophysical profiles in 107 diabetic patients semiweekly and found that a reactive NST was as predictive of fetal well-being in the diabetic population as a fetal biophysical profile score of eight.[7] However, they did not feel that the fetal biophysical profile improved the predictive value of fetal surveillance if the NST was reactive. There were not enough patients in the study to conclude whether or not the biophysical profile or the OCT was a better back-up test for a nonreactive NST. When performed in a careful, standardized manner, it may be an appropriate follow-up test for a nonreactive NST.

It is important to keep in mind the limitations of all methods of antepartum surveillance and not to expect the impossible of them. No antepartum test of fetal well-being can identify the fetus at risk from sudden environmental changes such as severe acute hyperglycemia.

Our general scheme for antepartum surveillance is to begin weekly NST at 32 weeks gestation, increasing the frequency of testing to two times per week at 36 weeks gestation. However, this scheme must be individualized. In complicated patients with intrauterine growth restriction, hypertension, oligohydramnios, preeclampsia, or poorly controlled blood sugars, testing may start as early as 26 weeks gestation and may be performed more frequently. The OCT is probably reliable this early in gestation.[12] Although a reactive NST is probably a reliable indicator of fetal well-being between 26 and 32 weeks, there is a high frequency of false positive results before 30 weeks, and thus does not justify the routine use of the NST for fetal surveillance before this time.[13–15] Thus, if testing needs to be started before 32 weeks of gestation an OCT will often be required to confirm fetal well-being.

If the NST is nonreactive, we further evaluate fetal status with an OCT. Subsequent obstetrical management then depends on the results of the

OCT, gestational age of the fetus, indices of lung maturity, maternal condition and, in selected cases, the results of the sonographic biophysical profile score. If an ominous pattern (nonreactive NST, positive OCT) is related to a potentially reversible problem such as ketoacidosis, it is advisable to resuscitate the fetus in utero. Often, pathologic fetal heart rate patterns will revert to normal when the mother's metabolic status is corrected. In nonreversible situations, the degree of prematurity strongly influences our choices. In premature infants, consideration should be given to delaying delivery, at least long enough to treat with corticosteroids in an effort to accelerate fetal lung maturation. This can be done while monitoring the fetus continuously. Obviously, the degree of compromise indicated by fetal surveillance will dictate how comfortable the obstetrician can be with a delay in delivery.

Ultrasound

The ultrasound examination is repeated at 28 weeks to assess fetal growth and repeat the fetal survey. If there is evidence of intrauterine growth restriction, the pregnancy is followed more carefully with earlier and more frequent tests of fetal well-being.

Hospitalization versus Outpatient Care

The most important aspect for insuring a good outcome in a diabetic pregnancy is good glycemic control. Although previously this was achieved by prolonged maternal hospitalization, equally good outcomes have been noted with outpatient care.[16,17] This depends on a total commitment by the patient to adhering to her diet, frequently checking her blood sugars, and constantly adjusting her insulin in consultation with the diabetologist. Unfortunately, there are some brittle diabetics who cannot be satisfactorily managed as an outpatient, even with great dedication.

Patients are admitted antepartum for the usual obstetric indications, i.e., preeclampsia, premature rupture of membranes, premature labor, etc. If there is poor glycemic control at any time during pregnancy, patients are admitted to the antepartum unit to evaluate their diet, adjust their insulin and to look for potential underlying problems such as infection. As long as glycemic control is good, and there are reassuring tests of fetal well-being, no evidence of preeclampsia or hypertension, and normal fetal growth, most patients can expect to remain at home until their delivery. Many patients with vascular complications of diabetes will not meet these strict criteria and often require admission before term.

DELIVERY

At term, a number of issues arise concerning the assessment of fetal maturity, timing of delivery, and route of delivery.

Fetal Pulmonary Maturity

In the past, early delivery of the infant of the diabetic mother was advocated to prevent fetal death in late gestation.[18–20] This seemed reasonable since, in one series before 1950, 50% of stillbirths occurred after the 38th week of gestation.[21] The hazards of this approach related to morbidity and mortality from prematurity. Robert reported that respiratory distress syndrome (RDS) was 5.6 times more likely to develop in the infants of diabetic mothers delivered early than in the infants of nondiabetic mothers, and that the risk did not become equal in the two groups until after 38.5 weeks of gestation.[22] Among neonatal deaths of infants of diabetic mothers, respiratory distress syndrome was the most frequently lethal process, occurring in 52% of deaths.[23] For this reason, the development of a test to estimate fetal lung maturity was a significant contribution to the management of diabetic pregnancies.

We employ the saturated phosphatidylcholine (SPC) in amniotic fluid to determine fetal pulmonary maturity.[24] We require an SPC ≥1000, before electively delivering a diabetic patient prior to 39 completed weeks of gestation or even after 39 weeks if dating of the pregnancy is in question. We have not seen respiratory distress syndrome in any infants delivered at or beyond 39 weeks gestation.

The inclusion of phosphatidylglycerol (PG) may also be helpful in assessing fetal lung maturation.[25,26] We do not routinely measure PG levels and cannot correlate neonatal outcome in infants of diabetic mothers with amniotic fluid PG levels.

Timing of Delivery

It is unclear whether or not the well-controlled diabetic woman with reassuring antepartum surveillance has an increased risk of an intrauterine demise. Girz et al. report three fetal deaths occurring within 72 hours of reassuring fetal testing in gravidas with gestational diabetes, despite maternal euglycemia.[27] Our experience has been more fortunate, but we still see little benefit in continuing a pregnancy beyond 38 weeks if fetal pulmonary maturity can be demonstrated and the cervix is favorable. Generally, if the cervix is unfavorable, induction can be safely delayed until 39 to 40 weeks in patients with excellent glycemic control, no vascular disease or preeclampsia, and normal fetal growth. If these criteria for continued pregnancy are not met, and induction is indicated before the cervix is favorable, cervical ripening agents can be employed safely.[28]

Route of Delivery

Diabetes by itself is not an indication for cesarean section. It should be performed only for the usual obstetric indications and for fetal macrosomia. The risk of shoulder dystocia was reported by Benedetti and Gabbe to be 0.07% in vaginal deliveries of infants weighing less than 4000 g, 1.2% in vaginal deliveries of infants weighing >4000 g, and 23% in infants weighing >4000 g with a prolonged second stage and midpelvic delivery.[29] Morbidity from shoulder dystocia has been reported to be as high as 11–30%.[30–32] In comparing the risk of shoulder dystocia in infants of diabetic mothers >4000 g with that in infants of nondiabetic mothers of similar weight, the risks were >23% and 10%, respectively.[30] Furthermore, the associated morbidity average was 18.2% and 5.5%, respectively. It has been suggested that neonates with shoulder dystocia have greater shoulder and chest to head disproportion than macrosomic infants without this complication.[33,34] In particular, macrosomic infants of diabetic mothers are more likely to exhibit this disproportion than infants of nondiabetic mothers of comparable weight.[32] For these reasons, we advise most insulin-requiring diabetics with fetuses whose estimated weight is >4000 g to have an elective cesarean section. This is clearly a guideline, and recommendations must be individualized, taking into account past obstetric history and pelvic adequacy. It is also important to recognize the limitations of ultrasound. Using this guideline, we occasionally perform an elective cesarean section for ultrasonographically detected macrosomia, only to find that the neonate is not actually macrosomic. This is a trade-off that we are willing to make in order to avoid the significant morbidity associated with shoulder dystocia.

Delivery Day

Every effort is made to schedule inductions or cesarean sections early in the morning, as this facilitates following and controlling maternal blood sugars. It is important to maintain euglycemia during this period as well (see Chapter 3). The patient should not take anything by mouth after midnight the evening before the planned delivery. She may be admitted the morning of the induction or surgery. Patients who are induced receive either no morning insulin, or only a small dose of an intermediate-acting insulin. On the labor and delivery floor, the patient is continuously monitored both for fetal heart rate and uterine contractions, as these patients are at increased risk for abnormal heart rate patterns.[35] An intravenous line is placed for administering oxytocin and fluids, generally 5% dextrose and half-normal saline at 125 ml per hour delivered by a controlled pump. A liter of normal saline is "piggy-backed" into the IV line to be continuously available for giving fluid boluses, if necessary. It is important not to give any parturient, especially the diabetic, boluses of glucose-containing solutions. An excess infusion of glucose, even over a short period, can raise maternal blood sugars and increase the risk of neonatal hypoglycemia, fetal hypoxia, and fetal and neonatal acidosis.[36–40] Maternal capillary blood sugars are checked every hour with a glucometer and charted on the flow sheet by the labor nurse. If the blood glucose values rise above 120mg/dl, intravenous insulin infusion is begun and adjusted with a sliding scale. A sample method of infusion would consist of 15 units of regular insulin in 150 ml of normal saline administered at 1–2 units per hour. It is not necessary to add albumin to the solution, but several milliliters of solution should be run through the line before beginning the infusion, to avoid the problem of insulin absorbing to the tubing surface.[42,43] Because there appears to be a decreased insulin requirement during labor, some patients do not require any intravenous insulin to maintain normal glucose levels. When insulin is needed, good glycemic control is readily achieved using the constant-infusion pump. Before elective cesarean section, approximately one-third of the patient's prepregnancy insulin dose is given as an intermediate-acting insulin on the morning of surgery.

There are no contraindications in the diabetic patient to natural childbirth, epidural anesthesia, or general anesthesia. Maternal hypotension, more commonly associated with spinal than epidural anesthesia, may be associated with lower pH and less base excess in the neonate.[44]

The diabetic woman can expect to have a normal postpartum course and hospital stay. Insulin requirements for the first two days postpartum usually are less than antepartum levels, and are often less than prepregnancy needs, but return to baseline rapidly in most patients. It is better to relax glycemic control during this time to avoid symptomatic hypoglycemia from too much insulin. There is no contraindication to breast-feeding in diabetic mothers, and it may be encouraged.

Obstetrical Management of Gestational Diabetes

Gestational diabetics who can maintain normal blood sugars (fasting <105 mg/dl and two-hour postprandial <120 mg/dl) on a diabetic diet do not appear to be at an increased risk for stillbirth over the normal pregnant population and do not require fetal surveillance before 40 weeks.[45] They

TABLE II. Summary of Management of the Diabetic Gravida

Prepregnancy	Achieve euglycemia
First Visit	Glycohemoglobin Thyroid function studies Baseline renal function Nutritional instruction Ophthalmologic status
Second trimester	
15 weeks	MS-aFP, triple panel
18 weeks	Ultrasound
Third trimester	
28 weeks	Ultrasound
32 weeks	NSTs weekly
36 weeks	NSTs biweekly
38 weeks	Estimation of fetal weight, cervical favorability, possible amniocentesis, pulmonary maturity
38–40 weeks	Delivery
Postpartum	Contraceptive counseling Reevaluation of insulin needs

should be followed with weekly blood sugars until delivery, since approximately 10–15% will develop hyperglycemia and require insulin.[45] Gestational diabetics who (1) develop an insulin requirement, (2) required insulin in a previous pregnancy, (3) have a history of prior stillbirth, or (4) develop preeclampsia, should undergo the same antepartum fetal surveillance and glucose monitoring as women whose diabetes antedated pregnancy, as they are at increased risk of an adverse outcome. Management of their diabetes before, during, and after delivery is discussed in Chapter 2.

CONTRACEPTION

Contraception affords a means of intentionally avoiding pregnancy. It enhances a woman's control of her body, her family, and, to a large extent, her socioeconomic condition. Because reproductive risk is associated with the degree of glycemic control in diabetics, contraception can reduce the incidence of poor reproductive outcome, by allowing diabetic women to postpone conception until good metabolic control is achieved. In patients suffering from some of the long-term sequelae of diabetes, pregnancy may increase maternal risk. Thus, contraception may impact significantly on a woman's survival.

Natural Family Planning

The basis of natural family planning is to try to determine when ovulation occurs and to avoid intercourse during the periovulatory part of the menstrual cycle. It is safe and without significant cost; however, the typical user failure rate is 20%.[46] To be effective, it requires a great deal of motivation on the part of the couple to abstain from intercourse during the fertile portion of the cycle, keep a basal body temperature chart, check cervical mucous, and maintain a constant awareness of the cyclic signs of fertility. It is an unsatisfactory method for women with irregular cycles.

Barrier Methods

Barrier methods of contraception, i.e., diaphragm and condom, are also safe and relatively inexpensive techniques. Used with a spermicide, the lowest reported failure rates are 2 to 4%, respectively. The typical user failure rates are 18 and 12%.[46] To be effective, barrier methods of contraception must be used during each coital experience, and therefore should be used by highly motivated couples.

Intrauterine Contraceptive Devices

Because the intrauterine contraceptive device has emerged as a major "litogen" (a cause of litigation), its use has decreased substantially over the last decade and a half. Only over the last few years is the IUD making a comeback as a popular form of contraception in selected women. The main benefits of the IUD include a high rate of effectiveness, the lack of need for multiple acts of willful use, and a lack of systemic metabolic side effects. The IUD has a continuation rate second only to subdermal progestational inserts.

A careful analysis of available data was published by the Center for Disease Control evaluating various risk factors for developing pelvic inflammatory disease (PID), such as the frequency of intercourse and the number of sexual partners among IUD users and users of no contraception.[47] In a group of married or cohabitating women who used the IUD, the relative risk of developing PID was not significantly higher than for those using no method of contraception. The IUD is probably safe in this group of patients.

For the diabetic woman who has a consistent single partner, particularly if she has completed her child bearing, the IUD is an attractive choice. Concern has been voiced in the past that since diabetic women are generally more prone to infection, they may be more prone to complications associated with the IUD. This has not been realized by clinical experience.[48]

Hormonal Contraception

Combined oral contraceptives (OCPs) are the most effective reversible method of contraception presently available, with failure rates as low as 0.5% and a typical user failure rate of 2%.[46] They do not require much motivation, at least as compared to barrier methods, and they do not restrict sexual spontaneity.

The absolute contraindications to the use of oral contraceptives, such as estrogen-dependent neoplasia, thromboembolic disorders, coronary artery disease, cerebrovascular disease, and severe liver dysfunction are only rarely altered significantly by diabetes. Little data is available comparing the risks of OCPs in diabetic women to those in nondiabetics. In a poorly controlled, retrospective study of 120 women with diabetes mellitus, who had taken or were taking OCPs, Steel et al. described three episodes of cerebral ischemia, one case of myocardial infarction, and one instance of axillary vein thrombosis. In a control group of 150 diabetics who had never taken the pill, there was only one myocardial infarction.[49] Further studies are needed. There are no prospective, well-controlled trials that show an increase in adverse cardiovascular or cerebrovascular events in diabetics using OCPs.

The effect of exogenous sex steroids on lipid metabolism varies with the dose and ratio of steroids. In general, the use of oral contraceptives is associated with increased levels of low density lipoproteins, very low density lipoproteins, cholesterol, and triglycerides.[50] However, the long-term meaning of this and any incremental risk for diabetics have not yet been elucidated.

Another area of great concern for the use of OCPs in diabetic women is the potential adverse effects on carbohydrate metabolism. Women on OCPs have increased peripheral resistance to insulin, possibly owing to a decrease in the concentration of insulin receptors.[51] In practice, only a few diabetic women who start OCPs experience a clinically significant alteration in carbohydrate metabolism. Steel and Duncan noted in their series of 88 patients that 81% did not require a change in insulin, 17% increased the daily insulin requirement by 8–20 units, and 2% required more than 20 additional units of insulin.[49] Any tendency for higher blood glucose values can easily be treated by increasing the exogenous insulin dose.

In short, we feel quite comfortable giving OCPs to diabetic women, but recommend particular attention to possible changes in insulin requirements that may ensue.

Subdermal Implants: Norplant®

Norplant® is the patented name of a contraceptive method consisting of silastic capsules containing levo-norgestrel that are placed under the skin of the upper arm. The capsules release a slow, continuous dose of the drug. This is a very well tolerated, safe and effective form of contraception. The typical user failure rate is 0.04%, which is even lower than tubal ligation.[46] Although our experience with using this form of contraception in diabetics is limited, our initial patients have generally been quite satisfied. They have not experienced any significant metabolic disturbances. Larger studies are required to further evaluate the safety of this form of contraception in diabetic women.

CONCLUSIONS

At the present time, virtually all diabetic women can undergo pregnancy with the expectation of a good maternal and fetal outcome. This is being achieved because of (1) commitment by the patient and physician to strict glycemic control, (2) accurate determination of gestational age, (3) careful fetal surveillance, (4) ability to assess fetal pulmonary maturity, (5) liberal use of cesarean section to avoid dystocia and difficult vaginal delivery, and (6) improved understanding of the pathophysiology of diabetes in pregnancy. Furthermore, careful obstetrical management has resulted in shorter maternal and neonatal hospital stays. Major challenges remain in preventing congenital anomalies and macrosomia. The solution appears to be to bring the metabolic milieu of the diabetic gravida as close to normal as possible. With improved methods of monitoring and treating the metabolic changes in diabetes complicated by pregnancy, attaining this goal is a realistic possibility.

REFERENCES

1. White P: Classification of obstetric diabetes. Am J Obstet Gynecol 130:228, 1976.
2. Gabbe S: Medical complications of pregnancy, management of diabetes in pregnancy: Six decades of experience. In Pitkin RM, Zlatnik FJ (eds): "Yearbook of Obstetrics and Gynecology. Part I. Obstetrics." Chicago: Yearbook, 1980, pp 37–49.
3. Greene MF, Hare JW, Cloherty JP, Benacerraf BR, Soeldner JS: First-trimester hemoglobin A_1 and risk for major malformation and spontaneous abortion in diabetic pregnancy. Teratology 39:225–231, 1989.
4. Greene MF, Benacerraf BR: Prenatal diagnosis in diabetic gravidas: Utility of ultrasound and maternal serum alpha-fetoprotein screening. Obstet Gynecol 77:520–524, 1991.
5. Nadal AS, Green NK, Holmes LB et al: Absence of need for amniocentesis in patients with elevated levels of maternal serum alpha-fetoprotein and normal ultrasonographic examinations. N Engl J Med 323:557, 1990

6. Freeman RK, Anderson G, Dorchester W: A prospective multi-institutional study of antepartum fetal heart rate monitoring. II. Contraction stress test versus nonstress test for primary surveillance. Am J Obstet Gynecol 143:778, 1982.
7. Golde SH, Montoro M, Good-Anderson B, Broussard P, Jacobs N, Loesser C, Trujillo M, Walla C, Phelan J, Platt LD: The role of nonstress tests, fetal biophysical profile and contraction stress tests in the outpatient management of insulin-requiring diabetic pregnancies. Am J Obstet Gynecol 148:269, 1984.
8. Ray DA, Yeast JF, Freeman RK: The current role of daily serum estriol monitoring in the insulin-dependent pregnant diabetic woman. Am J Obstet Gynecol 154:1257, 1986.
9. Barss VA, Frigoletto FD, Diamond F: Stillbirth after nonstress testing. Obstet Gynecol 65:541, 1985.
10. Evertson LR, Gauthier RJ, Collea JV: Fetal demise following negative contraction stress tests. Obstet Gynecol 51:671, 1978.
11. Manning FA, Platt LD, Sipos L: Antepartum fetal evaluation: Development of a fetal biophysical profile. Am J Obstet Gynecol 136:788, 1980.
12. Gabbe SG, Freeman RD, Goebelsmann U: Evaluation the contraction stress test before 33 weeks gestation. Obstet Gynecol 52:649, 1978.
13. Lavin JP, Miodovnik M, Barden TP: Relationship of nonstress test reactivity and gestational age. Obstet Gynecol 63:338, 1984.
14. Bishop EH: Fetal acceleration test. Am J Obstet Gynecol 141:905, 1981.
15. Devoe LD: Antepartum fetal heart rate testing in preterm pregnancy. Obstet Gynecol 60:431, 1982.
16. Gabbe SG: Management of diabetes mellitus in pregnancy. Am J Obstet Gynecol 153:829, 1985.
17. Schneider JM, Curet LB, Olson RW, et al: Ambulatory care of the pregnant diabetic. Obstet Gynecol 56:144, 1980.
18. Lawrence RD, Oakley W: Pregnancy and diabetes. Quart J Med 11:45, 1942.
19. Driscoll JJ, Gillespie L: Obstetrical considerations in diabetes in pregnancy. Med Clin North Am 49:1025, 1965.
20. Hagbard L: Pregnancy and diabetes mellitus; clinical study. Obstet Gynecol Scand (Suppl) 35:1, 1956.
21. Pedowitz P, Shlevin EL: Review of management of pregnancy complicated by diabetes and altered carbohydrate metabolism. Obstet Gynecol 23:716, 1964.
22. Robert MF, Neff RK, Hubbell JP, Taeusch HW, Avery ME: Association between maternal diabetes and the respiratory-distress syndrome in the newborn. N Engl J Med 294:357, 1976.
23. Driscoll SG, Benirschke K, Curtis GW: Neonatal deaths among infants of diabetic mothers. Am J Dis Child 100:818, 1960.
24. Torday J, Carson L, Lawson EE: Saturated phosphatidylcholine in amniotic fluid and prediction of the respiratory distress syndrome. N Engl J Med 301:1013, 1979.
25. Cunningham MD, Desai NS, Thompson SA, Greene JM: Amniotic fluid phosphatidylglycerol in diabetic pregnancies. Am J Obstet Gynecol 131:719, 1978.
26. Tsai MY, Shultz EK, Nelson JA: Amniotic fluid phosphatidylglycerol in diabetic and control pregnant patients at different gestational lengths. Am J Obstet Gynecol 149:388, 1984.
27. Girz BA, Divon MY, Merkatz IR: Sudden fetal death in women with well-controlled, intensively monitored gestational diabetes. J. Perinatol 12(3):229, 1992.
28. Rayburn WF: Prostaglandin E_2 gel for cervical ripening and induction of labor: A critical analysis. Am J Obstet Gynecol 160:529, 1989.
29. Benedetti TJ, Gabbe SG: Shoulder dystocia: A complication of fetal macrosomia

and prolonged second stage of labor with midpelvic delivery. Obstet Gynecol 5:526, 1978.

30. McCall JO: Shoulder dystocia: A study of after effects. Am J Obstet Gynecol 83; 1486, 1962.
31. Acker DB, Sachs BP, Friedman EA: Risk factors for shoulder dystocia. Obstet Gynecol 66:762, 1985.
32. Golditch IM, Kirkman K: The large fetus. Management and outcome. Obstet Gynecol 52:26, 1978.
33. Modanlou HD, Komatsu G, Dorchester W, Freeman RK, Bosu SK: Large-for-gestational age neonates: Anthropometric reasons for shoulder dystocia. Obstet Gynecol 60:417, 1982.
34. Wladimiroff JW, Boemsma CA, Wallenburg HCS: Ultrasonic diagnosis of the large-for-dates infant. Obstet Gynecol 52:285, 1978.
35. Gabbe SG, Mestman JH, Freeman RK, Goebelsmann UT, Lowensohn RI, Nochimson D, Cetrulo C, Quilligan EJ: Management and outcome of pregnancy in diabetes mellitus, classes B to R. Am J Obstet Gynecol 129:723, 1977.
36. Grylack LJ, Chu SS, Scanlon JW: Use of intravenous fluids before cesarean section: Effects on perinatal glucose, insulin and sodium homeostasis. Obstet Gynecol 63:654, 1984.
37. Kitzmiller JL, Phillippe M, von Oeyen P et al: Hyperglycemia, hypoxia and fetal acidosis in rhesus monkeys. Society for Gynecologic Investigation, Abstract 169, p 98, March, 1981.
38. Madsen H, Ditzel J: Changes in red blood cell oxygen transport in diabetic pregnancy. Am J Obstet Gynecol 143:421, 1982.
39. Robillard JE, Sessions C, Kennedy RL, Smith FG: Metabolic effects of constant hypertonic glucose infusion in well-oxygenated fetuses. Am J Obstet Gynecol 130:199, 1978.
40. Kenepp NB, Kumar S, Shelley WC, Stanley CA, Gabbe SG, Gutsche BB: Fetal and neonatal hazards of maternal hydration with 5% dextrose before caesarean section. Lancet 1:1150, 1982.
41. Peterson L, Caldwell, Hoffman J: Insulin absorbence to polyvinylchloride surfaces with implications for constant infusion therapy. Diabetes 25:72, 1976.
42. Jovanovic L, Peterson CM: Insulin and glucose requirements during the first stage of labor in insulin-dependent diabetic women. Am J Med 75:607, 1983.
43. Golde SH, Good-Anderson B, Montoro M, Artal R: Insulin requirements during labor: A reappraisal. Am J Obstet Gynecol 144:556, 1982.
44. Datta S, Brown WU: Acid-base status in diabetic mothers and their infants following general or spinal anesthesia for caesarean section. Anesthesiology 47:272, 1977.
45. Gabbe SG, Mestman JG, Freeman RK, Anderson GV, Lowensohn RI: Management and outcome of class A diabetes mellitus. Am J Obstet Gynecol 127:465, 1977.
46. Trussell J, Hatcher RA, Cates W Jr, Stewart FH, Kost K: Contraceptive failure in the United States: An update. Stud Fam Plann 21:51, 1990.
47. Lee NC and Rubin GL: The intrauterine device and pelvic inflammatory disease revisited: New results from the women's health study. Obstet Gynecol 72:1, 1988.
48. Skouby SO, Molsted-Pedersen L, Kosonen A: Consequences of intrauterine contraception in diabetic women. Fertil Steril 42:568, 1984.
49. Steel JM, Duncan LJP: Contraception for the insulin-dependent diabetic woman: The view from one clinic. Diabetes Care 3:557, 1980.
50. Powell MG, Hedlin AM, Cerskus I, Kakis G, Prudham D, Rosenrot P: Effects of oral contraceptives on lipoprotein lipids: A prospective study. Obstet Gynecol 63:764, 1984.
51. De Pirro R, Forte F, Bertoli A, Greco AV, Lauro R: Changes in insulin receptors during oral contraception. J Clin Endocrinol Metab 52:29, 1981.

CHAPTER 10

Obstetrical Complications

David B. Acker, MD and Vanessa A. Barss, MD

INTRODUCTION

The diabetic gravida is at risk for increased obstetrical complications. Quantification of the risks is difficult, as many reports predate or overlap the current era of tertiary care management and often do not distinguish between gestational and preexisting diabetes or among White classes. Cousins[1] searched 1,054 possible references but found only 24 suitable reviews. Table I aggregates his findings and Table II displays data collated from an additional eight reports. The tabulated items: hypertension, infection, prematurity, excessive fetal and uterine size, and operative delivery serve as the framework for this chapter. Data from recent publications and our experience at the Joslin Clinic are utilized to expand upon the above lists. This should help the clinician anticipate problems while caring for women who, in spite of serious illness, choose to conceive and continue their pregnancies, a choice we believe should not be discouraged.

HYPERTENSIVE COMPLICATIONS

The diagnosis of pregnancy-induced hypertension, occurring in patients with longstanding diabetes, is difficult to determine, due to the often confounding presence of secondary hypertension and coexisting proteinuria. It is equally difficult to be sure if increasing hypertension and proteinuria are due to worsening preeclampsia superimposed on chronic hypertension or to intensification of diabetic nephropathy secondary to physiologic renal changes from pregnancy (see Chapter 8). Table I displays rates of hypertensive complications, as does Table III, adapted from Greene's review of similar complications at the Joslin Clinic.[10] Diagnostic dilemmas notwithstanding, both found similiar rates. We concur with the

Diabetes Complicating Pregnancy: The Joslin Clinic Method, Edited by Florence M. Brown, MD and John W. Hare, MD.
ISBN 0-471-11031-0 © 1995 John Wiley & Sons, Inc.

TABLE I. Incidence of Complications by White Class

	Classes				
	B and C (No. and %)		D,F,R (No. and %)		Nondiabetic
Hypertension, pregnancy-induced	729	8.0	350	15.7*	3.8–10.0
Hypertension, chronic	411	8.0+	118	16.9*	N.R.
Pyelonephritis	356	2.2	264	4.9	N.R.
Hydramnios	199	17.6	167	18.6*	0.9
Preterm labor	183	7.7	86	4.7*	3.9–4.0
Cesarean section, primary	359	44.0	97	56.7*	N.R.
Cesarean section, repeat	359	13.4	97	19.6*	N.R.
Cesarean section, total	554	41.9(A)	175	58.3*	9.6–13.9

Adapted from Cousins, L: Obstet-Gynecol Survey 42:140–149, 1987.

N.R.—Not recorded in the control population.

*Differences between Classes B and C and D, F, and R achieved statistical significance.

A—Ceserean deliveries are aggregated from different sources and are *not* simply totalled.

+—Note that chronic hypertension is an inclusion criterion for Class D but Cousins includes them in Classes B and C, based on age and duration criteria only.

evidence that pregestational diabetes is associated with an increased risk of hypertension.[11–13] In anticipation of these difficulties, we obtain baseline blood pressure, serum creatinine, BUN, and morning urine microalbumin or a 24-hour urine for protein and creatinine clearance in the first trimester or at the first visit. Our surveillance includes weekly blood pressure readings and monthly 24-hour quantification of urine protein for those patients who measure one plus or greater on urine dipstick. We do not offer low-dose aspirin to patients based solely upon the presence of insulin-requiring diabetes. We are however, utilizing this medication for patients who, in addition to diabetes, have a prior history of severe preeclampsia or chronic hypertension. We recognize that data confirming the effectiveness of aspirin to prevent/alleviate preeclampsia is controversial[14–17] and, for those with diabetes, the published data is insufficient for a firmly grounded recommendation.

TABLE II. Obstetrical Complications*

Author/Reference	Interval	Geographical area	N	PIH (%)	Macrosomia (%)	Preterm delivery (%)	Cesarean birth (%)
Diamond et al[2]	1977–1983	Nashville, TN	177	23.2	16.9	35.6	NR
Roberts et al[3]	1986–1989	Belfast, Northern Ireland	135	28.1	12.0	28.9	51.9
Lang and Kimzel[4]	1982–1986	Hesse, Germany	446	9.2	NR	13.8	44.9
Neilson and Neilson[5]	1976–1990	Jutland, Denmark	328	NR	28.0	NR	NR
Mittal et al[6]	1976–1982	New Delhi, India	98	21.6	13.5	38.3	NR
French Study Group[7]	1986–1988	France	232	14	32	42.0	61.0
Johnstone et al[8]	1984–1986	Kuwait	161	NR	10.6	NR	NR
Kjos et al[9]	1987–1991	Los Angeles, CA	100	NR	23.0	NR	31.0
Total			1516	16.0	17.5	27.4	48.5

*PIH = Pregnancy-induced hypertension; N = number of patients; NR = not reported.

TABLE III. Incidence of Hypertensive Complications, Joslin Clinic 1983–1987

White class	*N* (% of Total)	Number of hypertensive complications (% of total)
B	103 (24.5)	18 (14.4)
C	121 (28.8)	28 (22.4)
D	101 (24.0)	31 (24.8)
F	59 (14.0)	39 (31.2)
R	36 (8.6)	9 (7.2)
Total	420 (100.0)	125 (100.0)

Adapted from Greene MF, Hare JW, Krache M: Am J Obstet Gynecol 161:106, 1989.

Hypertension is treated during pregnancy when the diastolic blood pressure remains greater than 100 mm Hg. In the setting of diabetes, where the potential for end-organ damage is greater, treatment with antihypertensive agents at lower diastolic blood pressure may be warranted (see Chapter 8). Methyldopa, beta-adrenergic blocking agents, and calcium-channel blocking agents are used; diuretics and angiotensinase inhibiting agents are avoided.[18,19] Patients who develop hypertension and proteinuria at greater than 24 weeks' gestation are admitted to the hospital for maternal/fetal surveillance. In-hospital management includes: (1) frequent blood pressure monitoring, (2) sonograms to assess fetal growth, (3) antihypertensive drugs, if indicated by persistent diastolic hypertension ≥100 mm of Hg, (4) nonstress tests at gestational ages ≥28 weeks, (5) laboratory evaluation that includes BUN, creatinine, platelet count, liver function tests, 24-hour urinalysis for protein and creatinine clearance, (6) daily weight measurements, and (7) bedrest. In patients with poorly controlled hypertension, signs of severe preeclampsia, intrauterine growth retardation (IUGR), or sonographic evidence of reversed diastolic flow through the umbilical artery, consideration is given to amniocentesis, betamethasone administration, and delivery.

In those patients with hypertension preceding pregnancy or diagnosed in the first trimester that is stable, and whose proteinuria is believed to be secondary to diabetic nephropathy, outpatient care is acceptable, provided the patient can be seen one to two times per week. A small or gradual worsening of hypertension or proteinuria in the third trimester may be attributed to physiologic changes of pregnancy but any sudden or marked worsening should be considered superimposed preeclampsia.

INFECTIOUS COMPLICATIONS

These occur more frequently in the diabetic gravida and some may be associated with severe sequelae.

Genito-Urinary

The urine should be cultured at the first prenatal visit and monthly thereafter.[20] During pregnancy, asymptomatic bacteriuria is frequently followed by pyelonephritis. Infections of the upper urinary tract are associated with an increased risk for preterm delivery and deterioration of glycemic control. Therefore, the primary purpose for treating asymptomatic or symptomatic bacteriuria is the prevention of pyelonephritis.[21,22]

Therapy for asymptomatic bacteriuria should consist of a seven-day course of an appropriate antibiotic, followed by a urine culture after treatment. We believe that a single dose or even a three-day course of therapy is less effective during pregnancy. All pregnant women diagnosed with pyelonephritis should be hospitalized for parenteral antibiotic therapy until afebrile for at least 24 hours and then treated with oral antibiotics for a 10–14-day total course. If bacteriuria/pyelonephritis recurs, suppressive antibiotic therapy should be instituted and continued until delivery is achieved.

Postoperative

Diabetic gravidas may be at an increased risk for postcesarean-section infection, compared to nondiabetic women. Diamond et al. studied 83 pregnant diabetic women undergoing cesarean section and noted an increased incidence of postoperative endometritis and wound infection, after controlling for duration of labor, ruptured membranes, and obesity.[23] Prophylactic antibiotics may be efficacious in reducing such postcesarean section infections in insulin-requiring diabetics. The treatment of endometritis and wound infection is the same as in the nondiabetic patient.

Necrotizing Fascitis

Although rare, necrotizing fascitis involving the vulva is a potentially fatal complication of vulvar infection. The early signs of this disorder include induration, edema, violaceous discoloration, tenderness, and crepitation.[24,25] The diagnosis is confirmed if the following criteria are met: (1) extensive necrosis of the superficial fascia with widespread undermining of skin; (2) moderate to severe systemic toxic reaction; (3) absence of muscle involvement; (4) absence of clostridia in wound and blood cultures; (5) absence of major vascular occlusion; (6) intensive leukocyte infiltration, necrosis of subcutaneous tissue, and microvascular thrombosis on pathologic examination of debrided tissue.[26] The treatment is early, aggressive surgical debridement to the level of healthy tissue.

Vaginitis

Monilial vulvovaginitis, although benign, may cause significant maternal discomfort. Both pregnancy and poorly controlled diabetes can increase the frequency and severity of attacks. Monilial vaginitis is treated with mycostatin suppositories in the first trimester and miconazole or clotrimazole vaginal cream or suppositories in the second or third trimester.

PREMATURITY

Greene and coworkers evaluated complications of prematurity in insulin-requiring diabetics at the Joslin Clinic between 1983 and 1987.[10] The distribution of premature deliveries, by White Class, is displayed in Table IV. Among the 420 neonates emanating from one triplet, six twin, and 413 singleton gestations that progressed beyond 20 gestational weeks, 110 (26.6%) delivered prior to the 37th gestational week. This included six of the seven multiple gestations and 104 (25.2%) of the singleton pregnancies. Preeclampsia was the most frequent cause of prematurity (Table V), and of

TABLE IV. Incidence of Prematurity—Joslin Clinic, 1983–1987

White class	*N*	% of total	Number premature deliveries*[a]	% of total
B	103	24.5%	21	19.1%
C	121	28.8%	21	19.1%
D	101	24.0%	26	23.6%
F	59	14.0%	31	28.2%
R	36	8.6%	11	10.0%
Total	420		110	26.6%

*Adapted from Greene MF, Hare JW, Krache M: Am J Obstet Gynecol 161:106, 1989.
[a]Delivery at ≤ completion of 37th gestational week.

TABLE V. Causes of Prematurity—Joslin Clinic, 1983–1987*

Indication for delivery	Singleton (N)	% of singleton total	Multiple gestation (N)	% of Multiple gestation total
Preeclampsia	34	32.7%	2	33.3%
Spontaneous rupture of membranes	26	25.0%	1	16.7%
Fetal distress	13	12.5%	2	33.3%
Idiopathic premature labor	14	13.5%	0	0.0%
Hemorrhage	4	3.8%	1	16.7%
Fetal demise[a]	4	3.8%	0	0.0%
Hydramnios/maternal discomfort	4	3.8%	0	0.0%
Other[b]	5	4.8%	0	0.0%
Total	104		6	

*Adapted from Greene MF, Hare J, Krach M: Am J Obstet-Gynecol 161:106, 1989.
[a]Fetal demise: 22 weeks—severe hypertension; 30 weeks—chorioamnionitis/sepsis after amniocentesis; 33 weeks—chronic alcoholism, pancreatitis, renal failure, disseminated intravascular coagulation, diabetic ketoacidosis; 35 weeks—poor glycemic control, otherwise normal.
[b]Other: 22 weeks—induced abortion for congenital defects; 34 weeks—spontaneous ruptured uterus (c/s × 4); 35 weeks—nephrogenic diabetic insipidis; 35 weeks—preeclampsia with hypoglycemic seizure; 35 weeks—intractable headache.

36 such cases, 9 were superimposed upon chronic hypertension. Although hydramnios was counted separately from spontaneous rupture of the membranes, the extent that excessive fluid contributed to ruptured membranes could not be calculated. Longstanding diabetes, especially when associated with peripheral vascular disease and hypertensive complications, contributed disproportionately to prematurity among patients with diabetic nephropathy. Coombs and Kitzmiller found a 56% incidence of preterm births prior to 37 gestational weeks and a 23% incidence of birth before 34 gestational weeks.[27] Greene found no relationship between prematurity and maternal age, number of previous pregnancies, previous term births, number of living children, a history of previous perinatal mortality, or previous spontaneous or induced abortions.[10]

The success of pharmacological treatment of premature labor remains controversial.[28] Especially for insulin-requiring diabetics, potential efficacy must be balanced by the potential for complications generally associated with their use: transient elevations in serum insulin and glucose; tremulousness; palpitations; anginal symptoms; pulmonary edema; and fetal and maternal tachycardia, as well as those not usually seen in the nondiabetic population: severe ketoacidosis, significant hyperglycemia, and fetal demise.[29–36]

Miodovnik et al evaluated the safety and efficacy of beta-sympathomimetic agents in diabetic gravidas.[37] On average, tocolytic therapy initiated at 31.5 weeks delayed delivery 30.5 days, resulting in a mean gestational age at delivery of 35.8 weeks. Adjuvant glucose and insulin infusion were administered to control blood sugars as follows: if serum glucose was less than 70 mg/dl, 5% dextrose in water was administered at a rate of 125 cc/hr; if serum glucose was 70–100 mg/dl, an infusion of Ringer's lactate was administered; and if the initial glucose was greater than 100 mg/dl, Ringer's lactate was administered in conjunction with a continuous intravenous infusion of regular insulin starting at a rate of 1 U/hr, given by piggyback infusion. In three cases in which glucocorticoid treatment was simultaneously given, glucose control was "difficult, but . . . adequate. . . ." Blood glucose started to rise one hour after initiation of continuous intravenous beta-sympathomimetic administration. Insulin increases followed in a couple of hours, reflecting the lag time during which the changes in glucose concentration were noted and adjustments in insulin made. Maternal and fetal heart rates increased within one hour and by six hours, respectively. Mean arterial pressure did not vary significantly. The authors concluded that this class of agents may be used under strictly controlled clinical settings. We concur.

Magnesium sulfate therapy, as an alternative to beta-sympathomimetic agents, has been evaluated by many investigators.[38–41] The tocolytic loading dose of 4–6 gm, followed by a continuous infusion of 2–3 gm per hour to achieve tocolysis, was found to be safe and effective; however, the data are from small and not well controlled studies. Calcium channel blockers are a recent addition to the tocolytic armamentarium. Initial experience indicates that they may be more effective than the beta-sympathomimetics, with fewer maternal metabolic and hemodynamic side effects.[42] Antiprostaglandin drugs have not achieved widespread acceptance because of the risk of premature closure of the fetal ductus arteriosus leading to in-utero heart failure or neonatal pulmonary hypertension.[43]

We use magnesium sulfate or nifedipine for tocolysis, before employing beta-sympathomimetic drugs in patients who have demonstrated cervical change with uterine contractions. All such tocolytic therapy is administered under strict controls in a well-supervised labor and delivery unit.

Currently, there are insufficient data to confirm or deny the efficacy of glucocorticoids to enhance lung maturity in fetuses of insulin-requiring diabetic gravidas.[44] Nonetheless, we treat gravidas at high risk for preterm delivery with 12 mg of betamethasone, given to the mother by intramuscular injection twice, twenty-four hours apart. If the pregnancy is less than 34 gestational weeks, fetal lung maturity is unlikely, and we give the steroids empirically. After 34 weeks, we perform an amniocentesis and offer steroids for confirmed lung immaturity (L/S ratio <2 or SPC <500). Steroids are not used for intermediate lung immaturity (L/S >2 but <3.5 or SPC >500 but <1000).

The decision to treat the diabetic gravida, with either corticosteroids, beta-sympathomimetic agents or both, should be made only for well-documented indications, and the metabolic status of the patient should be followed very carefully. Diabetic patients who are receiving steroids or beta-sympathomimetics (IV or SC) are monitored with capillary blood sugars, at one to two hour intervals for 48 hours, or as long as blood sugars are unstable. The steroid effect on blood sugars begins approximately 12 hours after the first dose and may last up to 5 days. When hyperglycemia occurs, it is vigorously treated by continuous, intravenous insulin infusion, with close maternal/fetal monitoring, on the labor and delivery floor. We have found that patients may require anywhere from 2 to 30 units of regular insulin per hour. Other investigators have had a similar experience.[37,45]

Maternal tachycardia and mild hypotension regularly occur. Fluid overload, sustained tachycardia greater than 140 beats per minute, undiagnosed cardiopulmonary disease, or infection in association with beta-sympathomimetic drug administration can lead to pulmonary edema.[46] Cerebral ischemia and angina pectoris have also been reported.[34,35] Therefore, the cardiopulmonary status of patients, especially those with peripheral vascular disease or nephropathy, should be carefully monitored with particular attention to fluid balance. Therapy should only be undertaken in centers where continuous, experienced maternal/fetal supervision is possible. After labor is arrested with parenteral therapy, oral therapy is begun. Athough metabolic derangements produced by oral therapy are less dramatic than those with parenteral therapy, they are associated, nevertheless, with some deterioration of control and a higher insulin requirement.[36,47]

MACROSOMIA

The distribution curve of birth weights of infants of diabetic mothers (IDM) is shifted to the right of infants of nondiabetic population, so that the former neonates tend to be relatively heavier than the latter, after adjustment for gestational age. This finding suggests that, irrespective of the actual birth weight, all infants of diabetic mothers exceed their genetic potential for growth.[48] As an absolute, a birth weight over 4,000 g is described as macrosomic.

Macrosomia, a probable shoulder dystocia and an intrauterine fetal demise were described in what may be the first recorded case of a diabetic pregnancy.[49] In 1824, a 22 year old Berlin housewife was delivered by Dr. H. G. Bennewitz, who described the sudden and unexpected arrival of the head of the fetus. Then the shoulders became "... stuck in the womb exit ... in the end, [the baby] ... was born dead, but not without a great struggle. The child, whom you would have thought Hercules would have begotten ... weighed twelve pounds. His shoulders were of such a width that I could not span their circumference with my fingers spread out." Despite advances in the care of the diabetic gravida, macrosomia remains a common complication.

The macrosomic fetus of a diabetic gravida is susceptible to all birth complications found in fetuses delivered of nondiabetic parturients. Such morbidity includes: asphyxia, meconium aspiration, fractures, facial palsy, and central nervous system trauma. However, shoulder dystocia and its attendant palsy occur more frequently in the diabetic gravida's fetus.[50,51]

In general, the risk of shoulder dystocia has been reported by Benedetti and Gabbe to be 1.2% in vaginal deliveries of all infants weighing greater than 4,000 g, and 23% in infants weighing greater than 4,000 g whose second stage of labor required a midpelvic delivery.[52] Acker evaluated 14,721 gravidas delivering, per vagina, infants of birth weight >2,500 g.[51] This series included 144 diabetic patients, more than half of whom were treated with diet only. Table VI displays the incidence of shoulder dystocia by birth weight category, comparing nondiabetic and diabetic patients. Infants of diabetic gravidas experienced shoulder dystocia five times more frequently than those of nondiabetic women. Nearly one-quarter (23.1%) of the IDM's weighing 4,000–4,500 g had a shoulder dystocia and, of those weighing >4,500 g, half experienced the complication.

The diabetic population was examined to determine if labor patterns and delivery method might serve as clinical indicators of shoulder dystocia. Among 144 diabetic gravidas, 36 experienced a vaginal delivery of an infant with a birth weight >4,000 g. Table VII displays the labor patterns and the delivery methods. Shoulder dystocia occurred in 11 (30.6%) cases. Normal labors were complicated by shoulder dystocia in 24% of cases, and three of four precipitate labors also had this problem. Spontaneous deliveries were associated with a 29% rate. Of particular concern, infants of diabetic gravidas sustained a disproportionate incidence of an immediate Erb-Duchenne palsy as a complication of shoulder dystocia.[53]

TABLE VI. Shoulder Dystocia by Birth Weight in Diabetic and Nondiabetic Gravidas Who Delivered Vaginally*

Birth weight (g)	Nondiabetic			Diabetic			Rate ratio
	Number	ShD[a]	%	Number	ShD[a]	%	
4500 +	208	47	22.6	10	5	50.0	2.21
4000–4499	1074	107	10.0	26	6	23.1	2.31
3500–3999	4249	94	2.2	43	4	9.3	4.23
3000–3499	6252	40	0.6	47	0	0.0	0.00
2500–2999	2794	6	0.2	18	0	0.0	0.00
Total	14577	294	2.0	144	15	10.4	5.20

*Adapted from Acker DB, Sachs BP, Friedman EA: Obstet Gynecol 66:762, 1985.
[a]ShD = shoulder dystocia.

TABLE VII. Shoulder Dystocia in Diabetic Gravidas Delivering large (4000+ g) Infants by Labor Pattern and Delivery Method*

	Number	ShD[a]	%
Labor pattern[b]			
Normal	25	6	24.0
Prolonged latent phase	1	0	0.0
Protraction disorder	3	2	66.7
Arrest disorder	4	1	25.0
Precipitate labor	4	3	75.0
Delivery method			
Spontaneous	31	9	29.0
Low forceps	4	2	50.0
Midforceps	1	0	0.0
Total gravidas	36	11	30.6

*Adapted from Acker DB, Sachs BP, Friedman EA: Obstet Gynecol 66:762, 1985.
[a]ShD = shoulder dystocia.
[b]The total number of labor patterns is greater than the total number of patients because any given patient can have more than one labor abnormality.

We therefore advise all insulin-requiring diabetic women with fetuses whose estimated weight is greater than 4,000 g to have a cesarean section, especially if there has been no previous uncomplicated vaginal delivery of a macrosomia infant. We offer this advice despite the realization that the ultrasonographic estimation of fetal weight greater than 4,000 g may be erroneous. Largely because of the high incidence of macrosomia in our population, the primary cesarean section rate in our patients is approximately 47%.[11]

HYDRAMNIOS

Hydramnios, or increased amniotic fluid volume, has been reported in 1.5–66% of diabetic pregnancies.[54] The large variance in incidence is probably due both to nonrandom selection of patients and the qualitative assessment of amniotic fluid volume. The mechanism for the increase in amniotic fluid volume has not been clearly defined but may be due to fetal polyuria secondary to hyperglycemia, to macrosomia, or to an imbalance in water movement between the fetal and maternal compartments.[54,55] Mild hydramnios does not usually cause problems; however, with increasingly severe hydramnios, premature rupture of membranes (PROM), premature labor, cord prolapse or abruption may occur. Severe polyhydramnios leading to maternal discomfort or respiratory embarrassment is uncommon.

SUMMARY

Although obstetrical complications are more frequent and potentially more severe in the diabetic pregnancy, careful surveillance and management can reduce the morbid consequences of these problems. During prenatal care, the physician should (1) assess fetal growth and well-being with ultrasound; (2) diligently look for infection and vigorously treat it when it occurs; (3) see the patient frequently to monitor blood pressure, glucose control, and maternal and fetal well-being; (4) scrupulously follow blood sugars, particularly during hyperglycemic stress from drugs or infection; and (5) liberally employ hospitalization or surgery to prevent serious maternal or fetal complications.

ACKNOWLEDGMENT

The authors respectfully acknowledge the commitment and service rendered to countless diabetic gravidas by the obstetric faculty, fellows and residents of the Boston Lying-In Hospital and the Brigham & Women's

Hospital and especially wish to note the efforts of Drs. Luke Gillespie, John Kitzmiller, Mark Phillippe, and Michael Greene.

REFERENCES

1. Cousins L: Pregnancy complications among diabetic women: Review 1965-1985. Obstet Gynecol Survey 42:140–149, 1987.
2. Diamond MP, Shah DM, Hester RA, et al: Complication of insulin-dependent pregnancies by preeclampsia and/or chronic hypertension: Analysis of outcome. Am J Perinat 2:263–266, 1985.
3. Roberts RN, Moohan JM, Foo RLK, et al: Fetal outcome in mothers with impaired glucose tolerance in pregnancy. Diabetic Med 10:438–443, 1993.
4. Lang U, Kunzel E: Diabetes mellitus in pregnancy. Management and outcome of diabetic pregnancies in the state of Hesse, F.R.G.: A five-year survey. Europ J Obstet Gynecol Repro Endo 33:115–129, 1989.
5. Nielson GL, Nielson PH: Outcome of 328 pregnancies in 205 women with insulin-dependent diabetes in the county of Northern Jutland from 1976 to 1990. Europ J Obstet Gynecol Repro Endo 50:33–38, 1993.
6. Mittal S, Agarwal N, Buckshee K: The diabetic pregnancy: Review of management and results over seven year period. Asia Oceania J Obstet Gynecol 13:277–281, 1987.
7. Gestation and Diabetes in France Study Group: Multicenter survey of diabetic pregnancy in France. Diabetes Care 14:994–1000, 1991.
8. Johnstone FD, Nasrat AA, Prescott RJ: The effect of established and gestational diabetes on pregnancy outcome. British J Obstet Gynecol 97:1009–1015, 1990.
9. Kjos SL, Henry OA, Montoro M, et al: Insulin-requiring diabetes in pregnancy: A randomized trial of active induction of labor and expectant management. Am J Obstet Gynecol 169:611–615, 1993.
10. Greene MF, Hare JW, Krache M, Phillipe M, Barss VA, Saltzman DH, Nadel A, Younger MD, Heffner L, Scherl JE: Prematurity among insulin-requiring diabetic gravidas. Am J Obstet Gynecol 161:106–111, 1989.
11. Gabbe SG, Mestman JH, Freeman RK et al: Management and outcome of pregnancy in diabetes mellitus, Classes B to R. Am J Obstet Gynecol 129:723–732, 1977.
12. Kitzmiller JL, Cloherty JP, Younger MD et al: Diabetic pregnancy and perinatal morbidity. Am J Obstet Gynecol 131:560–580, 1978.
13. Leveno KJ, Hauth JC, Gilstrap LC et al: Appraisal of "rigid" blood glucose control during pregnancy in the overtly diabetic woman. Am J Obstet Gynecol 135:853–859, 1979.
14. Sibai BM, Caritis SN, Thom E, Klebanoff M, McNellis D, Rocco L, Paul RH, Romero R, Whitter F, Rosen M, et al: Prevention of preeclampsia with low-dose aspirin in healthy nulliparous pregnant women. The National Institute of Child Health and Human Development Network of Maternal-Fetal Medicine Units. N. Engl J Med 329 (17):1213–1218, 1993.
15. Dekker GA, Sibai BM: Low-dose aspirin in the prevention of preeclampsia and fetal growth retardation: Rationale, mechanisms and clinical trials. Am J Obstet Gynecol 168:214–227, 1993.
16. Imperiale TF, Petrulis AS: A meta-analysis of low-dose aspirin for the prevention of pregnancy induced hypertensive disease. JAMA 266:260–264, 1991.
17. Clasp. A randomised trial of low-dose aspirin for the prevention and treatment of preeclampsia among 9364 pregnant women. Lancet 343:619–629, 1994.

18. Sibai BM, Grossman RA, Grossman HG: Effects of diuretics on plasma volume in pregnancies with hypertension. Am J Obstet Gynecol 150: 831, 1984.
19. Fiocchi R, Ligmen P, Fagard R et al: Captopril during pregnancy. Lancet 2:1153, 1984.
20. Vejlsgaard R: Studies on urinary infection in diabetes III. Significant bacteriuria in pregnant diabetics and matched controls. Acta Med Scand 193:377, 1973.
21. Ayromlooi J, Mann LI, Weiss RR et al: Modern management of the diabetic pregnancy. Obstet Gynecol 49:137, 1977.
22. Pederson J: "The Pregnant Diabetic and Her Newborn. Problems and Management," 2nd ed. Baltimore: Williams and Wilkins, 1977, p 46.
23. Diamond MP, Entmann SS, Salyer SL et al: Increased risk of endometritis and wound infection after cesarean section in insulin-dependent diabetic women. Am J Obstet Gynecol 155:297, 1986.
24. Addison WA, Livengood CH, Hill GB et al: Necrotizing fasciitis of vulvar origin in diabetic patients. Obstet Gynecol 63:473, 1984.
25. Roberts DB: Necrotizing fasciitis of the vulva. Am J Obstet Gynecol 157:568, 1987.
26. Fisher JR, Conway MJ, Takeshita RT et al: Necrotizing fasciitis. Importance of roentgenographic studies for soft-tissue gas. JAMA 241:803, 1979.
27. Combs CA, Kitzmiller JL: Diabetic nephropathy in pregnancy. Clin Obstet Gynecol 34:505–515, 1991.
28. Canadian Preterm Labor Investigators Group: Treatment of preterm labor with beta-adrenergic agonist ritodrine. N Eng J Med 327:308–312, 1992.
29. Thiagarajah S, Harbert GM, Bourgeois FJ: Magnesium sulfate and ritodrine hydrochloride: Systemic and uterine hemodynamic effects. Am J Obstet Gynecol 153:666, 1985.
30. Mordes D, Kreutner K, Metzger W et al: Dangers of intravenous ritodrine in diabetic patients. JAMA 248:973, 1982.
31. Desin D, Coevorden AV, Kirkpatrick C et al: Ritodrine-induced acidosis in pregnancy. Br Med J 1:1194, 1978.
32. Thomas DJ, Gill B: Salbutamol-induced diabetic ketoacidosis. Br Med J 2:438, 1977.
33. Schilthuis MS, Aaronoudse JG: Fetal death associated with severe ritodrine induced ketoacidosis. Lancet 1:11:45, 1980.
34. Rosene KA, Featherstone HJ, Beneddetti TJ: Cerebral ischemia associated with parenteral terbutaline use in pregnant migraine patients. Am J Obstet Gynecol 143:405, 1982.
35. Ying Y, Tejani NA: Angina pectoris as a complication of ritodrine hydrochloride therapy in premature labor. Obstet Gynecol 60:385, 1982.
36. Main EK Main DM, Gabbe SG: Chronic oral terbutaline tocolytic therapy is associated with maternal glucose intolerance. Am J Obstet Gynecol 157:644, 1987.
37. Miodovnik M, Peros N, Holroyde JC et al: Treatment of premature labor in insulin dependent diabetic women. Obstet Gynecol 65:621, 1985.
38. Elliott JP: Magnesium sulfate as a tocolytic agent. Am J Obstet Gynecol 147:277, 1983.
39. Spisso KR, Harbart GM, Thiagarajah S: The use of magnesium sulfate as the primary tocolytic agent to prevent premature delivery. Am J Obstet Gynecol 142:840, 1982.
40. Beall MH, Edgar BW, Paul RH et al: A comparison of ritodrine, terbutaline and magnesium sulfate for the suppression of preterm labor. Am J Obstet Gynecol 153:854, 1985.
41. Holander DI, Nagey DA, Pupkin MJ: Magnesium sulfate and ritodrine hydrochloride: A randomized comparison. Am J Obstet Gynecol 156:631, 1987.
42. Read MD, Wellby DE: The use of a calcium antagonist (nifedipine) to suppress preterm labor. Br J Obstet Gynaecol 93:933, 1986.
43. Manchester D, Margolis HS, Sheldon RE: Possible association between maternal indomethacin therapy and primary hypertension of the newborn. Am J Obstet Gynecol 126:467, 1976.

44. NIH Consensus Development Conference on Effect of Corticosteriods for Fetal Maturation on Perinatal Outcome. Feb 28–March 2, 1994.
45. Barnett AH, Stubbs SM, Mander AM: Management of premature labor in diabetic pregnancy. Diabetologia 18:365, 1980.
46. Souney PF, Kaul A, Osathanondh R: Pharmacotherapy of preterm labor. Clin Pharmacy 2:29, 1983.
47. Steel JM, Parboosingh J: Insulin requirements in pregnant diabetics with premature labor controlled by ritodrine. Br Med J 1:880, 1977.
48. Bradley RJ, Nicolaides KH, Brudenell JM: Are all infants of diabetic mothers "macrosomic"? BMT 297:1583–1584, 1988.
49. Neiger R: Fetal macrosomia in the diabetic patient. Clin Obstet Gynecol 35:138–150, 1992.
50. McCall JO: Shoulder dystocia: A study of after effects. Am J Obstet Gynecol 83:1486. 1962.
51. Acker DB, Sachs BP, Friedman EA: Risk factors for shoulder dystocia. Obstet Gynecol 66:762, 1985.
52. Benedetti TJ, Gabbe SG: Shoulder dystocia: A complication of fetal macrosomia and prolonged second stage of labor with midpelvic delivery. Obstet Gynecol 5:526, 1978.
53. Acker DB, Gregory KD, Sachs BP et al: Risk factors for Erb-Duchenne Palsy. Obstet Gynecol 71:389–392, 1988.
54. Wallenberg HC, Wladimiroff JW: The amniotic fluid II. Polyhydramnios and oligohydramnios. J Perinat Med 6:233, 1977.
55. Seeds AE: Current concepts of amniotic fluid dynamics. Am J Obstet Gynecol 138:575, 1980.

SECTION IV

FETAL CONSIDERATIONS

CHAPTER 11

Neonatal Management

John P. Cloherty, MD

INTRODUCTION

The recent reduction in perinatal mortality and morbidity in infants of diabetic mothers (IDMs) has been due to improvements in medical and obstetric care of the mothers and advances in the care of the newborn.[1–3] Two of the major causes of this improvement have been the prolongation of pregnancy and the ability to assess pulmonary maturity in the fetus, thus reducing the incidence of respiratory distress syndrome (RDS) in the IDM. Infants of mothers with severe renal and vascular disease are often delivered early because of maternal problems (hypertension, renal failure) or fetal distress. These infants are more likely to have complications, such as poor fetal growth, prematurity, asphyxia, respiratory distress syndrome, jaundice, and poor feeding.

Before the delivery of the IDM, there should be clear communication between specialists in medicine, obstetrics, and pediatrics, so that problems can be anticipated. Areas that should be discussed are (1) outcome of previous pregnancies, (2) gestational age and fetal assessment, (3) control of diabetes during pregnancy, (4) present maternal diabetic and medical state, (5) maternal HbA1 levels in pregnancy, (6) results of fetal monitoring for malformations or distress, (7) fetal size, (8) evidence for pulmonary maturity, and (9) monitoring during labor.

DELIVERY ROOM MANAGEMENT

If pulmonary maturity has not been assured prenatally, amniotic fluid can be obtained by aspiration of the amniotic sac, before it is opened at cesarean section. Fluid may be evaluated by gram stain, culture, shake test,

Diabetes Complicating Pregnancy: The Joslin Clinic Method, Edited by Florence M. Brown, MD and John W. Hare, MD.
ISBN 0-471-11031-0 © 1995 John Wiley & Sons, Inc.

lecithin/sphingomyelin (L/S) ratio, or saturated phosphatidylcholine (SPC) content, if indicated.

After the baby is born, an assessment is made on the basis of the Apgar score to determine the need for any resuscitative efforts. The infant should be dried well and placed under a heat source. The airway is cleared of mucous with bulb suction, but the stomach is not aspirated at this point, because of the risk of reflex bradycardia and apnea with pharyngeal stimulation in the first five minutes of life. A screening physical exam for the presence of major congenital anomalies should be performed. The placenta should be examined. A glucose level and pH should be determined on cord blood. The general approach to resuscitation of the newborn in the delivery room has been discussed by Ringer.[3]

NURSERY EVALUATION AND MANAGEMENT

The initial care involves the simultaneous provision of what is needed to support the baby while making continuous evaluation. This includes providing warmth, suction, and oxygen as needed, while checking vital signs (heart rate, temperature, respiratory rate, perfusion, color, and blood pressure). The presence of cyanosis may indicate cardiac disease, respiratory distress syndrome (RDS), transient tachypnea of the newborn, or polycythemia. A careful exam should be performed for the presence of anomalies because of the 6–9% incidence of major congenital anomalies in IDMs.[5,6] Blood glucose levels are checked at 1, 2, 3, 6, 12, 24, 36, and 48 hours of age. Hematocrit levels are checked at 1 and 24 hours of age. Calcium and bilirubin levels are checked if the baby is jittery or appears jaundiced. The baby is given glucose orally or intravenously by one hour of age (see Hypoglycemia, below). Every effort is made to involve the parents in the care of the baby as soon as possible.

Specific Problems

Respiratory Distress Syndrome. Robert et al showed a six-fold increased risk of RDS in infants of diabetic mothers compared to infants of nondiabetic mothers of the same gestational age.[7] With changes in the management of pregnant diabetics resulting in longer gestations and more vaginal deliveries, the incidence of RDS in IDMs has fallen from 28% in 1950–1960,[8] to 8% in 1975–1976,[9] to 5.7% in 1983–1984,[10] and to 4% in 1990.[10] The major difference in the incidence of RDS, between diabetics and nondiabetics, occurs in infants born before 37 weeks of gestation. Therefore, the longer gestations, resulting from better in utero surveillance and the more accurate prediction of pulmonary maturity, have had a marked influence on the reduction of RDS in the IDM (see Chapter 9). Causes of respiratory distress, besides RDS, that must be considered in IDMs are (1) cardiac or pulmonary anomalies, (2) hypertrophic cardiomyopathy, (3) transient tachypnea of the newborn, (4) pneumonia, (5) pneumothorax, (6) meconium aspiration, (7) diaphragmatic hernia, and (8) polycythemia.

The management of RDS is complex but includes maintenance of adequate oxygenation and metabolic support until the disease resolves.[11] Oxygen is given in amounts necessary to maintain a PaO_2 of 50–80 mm Hg. If the provision of ambient oxygen in the range of 40–50% FiO_2 is not adequate to provide a PaO_2 in a safe range, continuous distending airway pressure is used along with oxygen. Nasal prongs, a nasopharyngeal tube, or an endotracheal tube may be used for this purpose. If there is evidence of inadequate ventilation ($PaCO_2$ over 50 mm Hg, PaO_2 less than 50 mm Hg with an FiO_2 of 0.6, or apnea), mechanical ventilation is required. Infants with RDS, who do not suffer any complications, may be weaned from the ventilator in three to four days. Problems that prolong therapy are pneumothorax, intracranial hemorrhage, infection, extreme prematurity, and bronchopulmonary dysplasia.

Surfactant replacement therapy, early in the treatment of infants with RDS, decreases morbidity and mortality and now is routine in their care. Important areas to be managed in infants with RDS are as follows:

1. Temperature control. The infants should be placed in a neutral thermal environment to minimize oxygen demand and conserve calories for growth. Neutral thermal environment is defined as the thermal condition at which heat production (as measured by oxygen consumption) is minimum yet core temperature is within the normal range.
2. Fluid balance, metabolic balance, nutrition, provision of fluids, electrolytes, and calories must be carefully monitored to provide maintenance requirements yet not overload the circulation. Water loss may be increased by the need to use an open bed under phototherapy or decreased by providing humidified air through a nasotracheal tube.
3. Circulation. This is assessed by monitoring pulse, blood pressure, and peripheral perfusion. Blood, plasma, or pressors are often needed to maintain circulation. Frequent transfusions of packed red cells are used to keep the hematocrit ≥45%. The major source of blood loss is the frequent blood sampling needed to monitor blood gases, hematocrit, electrolyte balance, and glucose.

4. Infection. It is often difficult to distinguish between RDS and pneumonia. Because of this, most infants with RDS are treated with antibiotics after cultures are obtained. If the cultures are negative at 72 hours, antibiotics are usually stopped.

The major complications of respiratory distress syndrome are as follows:

1. Air Leak. Pneumothorax, pneumomediastinum, pneumopericardium, or pulmonary interstitial emphysema occur in 5–10% of infants with RDS.
2. Infection. In addition to the initial risk of infection from maternal sources, infants with RDS are susceptible to nosocomial infection. The use of endotracheal tubes, indwelling catheters, and chest tubes, in these infants puts them at great risk for infection.
3. Intraventricular hemorrhage. Bleeding into the lateral ventricles of the brain may occur in up to 40% of infants with birth weight under 1,500 g. The incidence is higher in infants who are mechanically ventilated.
4. Patent ductus arteriosus (PDA). A PDA, with left-to-right shunt and congestive heart failure, is seen in 30–50% of patients with RDS. Medical management includes fluid restriction and diuretics. Pharmacologic (indomethacin) or surgical treatment is usually required.

Long-term complications of RDS and its therapy are as follows:

1. Bronchopulmonary dysplasia (BPD). Chronic lung disease in the form of BPD occurs in 5–30% of survivors of neonatal respiratory therapy for RDS. This often necessitates prolonged treatment with oxygen and the respirator.
2. Retinopathy of prematurity (ROP). Previously called retrolental fibroplasia, ROP occurs in about 10% of infants ventilated for RDS. The smaller the infant the greater the risk for ROP. In most infants, ROP spontaneously resolves and there are no long-term sequelae.
3. Neurologic impairment. Ten to fifteen percent of the survivors of respirator therapy for RDS have neurologic impairment including cerebral palsy, mental retardation, or seizures.

Hypoglycemia. Blood glucose concentrations, measured serially on the first day of life in IDMs, reveal that 30% will have hypoglycemia, defined as a blood glucose of <30 mg/dl. The fall in blood glucose in IDMs is more rapid, more severe, and more prolonged than in babies born to nondiabetic mothers.[12] However, in most IDMs, provision of glucose, via oral feeding or parenteral glucose infusion, results in a rapid and sustained correction to a euglycemic state.

The hypoglycemia of IDMs results from the stimulation of the fetal pancreas by the abnormally elevated levels of glucose in maternal blood during pregnancy. The elevated maternal blood glucose levels result in elevated fetal blood glucose levels. The fetal pancreatic islet cells, which are normally relatively unresponsive to glucose, respond to this chronic hyperstimulation by hyperplasia and hypertrophy of the beta cells. As a result, the serum insulin levels in IDMs are inappropriately elevated for the blood glucose concentrations. Also, the IDM responds to a glucose load with an exaggerated insulin secretion. In addition, the hormones glucagon and epinephrine, that normally are released to hold and reverse the usual fall in blood glucose after birth, are present in diminished concentrations in the serum of IDMs. As a result, the usual balance between glycogenolysis and glycogenesis is tipped toward the latter, and hypoglycemia is a common finding in these babies.[13] The risk of hypoglycemia appears to correlate with the presence of macrosomia, elevated maternal blood glucose at delivery, and elevated cord blood C-peptide or immunoreactive insulin levels.

Hypoglycemia is usually asymptomatic in IDMs. When signs or symptoms are present, they most frequently are irritability, jitteriness, lethargy or hypotonia, respiratory distress, cyanosis or apnea, and, occasionally, seizures. Although the low frequency of symptoms argues for an alternate energy source for central nervous system metabolism, we have been aggressive in trying to prevent hypoglycemia and treating it when present.

The best prevention is to ensure good maternal control during the last trimester and euglycemia during delivery. Asymptomatic babies are fed 10% dextrose and formula orally or by gavage, within the first 30–60 minutes after birth, and Dextrostix® and blood glucose levels are measured hourly for three hours. If two consecutive blood glucose levels are <40 mg% despite oral feeding, or if symptoms occur at any time, parenteral glucose is administered as a minibolus and continuous infusion.[14,15] Administration of 200 mg/kg of glucose (2 ml/kg of 10% dextrose) over two to three minutes, followed by 10% dextrose at 80–120 ml/kg/day, provides 6–8 mg/kg/min of glucose, the usual rate to achieve and maintain euglycemia in newborn infants. Administration of a large amount of dextrose, as is advised in the older literature (500 mg/kg over several minutes), can cause a rapid elevation of blood glucose and result in an outpouring of insulin and a return of hypoglycemia.

If there is a delay in achieving vascular access in a macrosomic infant, glucagon may be administered intramuscularly or subcutaneously in a dose of 300 μg/kg (maximum dose 1.0 mg). Blood glucose will rise 20–40 mg% within 10–20 minutes. Glucagon is ineffective in premature infants or those small for gestational age. In unusual cases, vascular access can only be achieved by an umbilical venous catheter placed in the inferior vena cava.

Most IDMs can achieve euglycemia on a normal feeding schedule (either breast or bottle) by 24–48 hours of age.

Hypocalcemia. Calcium levels begin to decline immediately upon cord clamping. As with glucose, the decrease in serum calcium is greater and more prolonged in the IDM. The nadir in calcium levels occurs between 24 and 72 hours, and between 30% and 50% of IDMs will become hypocalcemic (defined as a serum total calcium level under 7 mg/dl). Most of these babies are asymptomatic. Occasional infants manifest lethargy or jitteriness, and the differential diagnosis includes hypocalcemia and hypoglycemia, as well as central nervous system trauma, malformations, or infection.

Infants who have symptoms that remain after adequate treatment of hypoglycemia should be evaluated for hypocalcemia. Most IDMs show a spontaneous rise in serum calcium on day 2 or 3 after delivery. When symptoms coexist with a low serum calcium level, calcium is added as the chloride or gluconate salt to a parenteral glucose infusion or to oral feedings. The dose is 200 mg/kg of 10% calcium gluconate intravenously over 10–20 minutes in symptomatic infants or 400–500 mg/kg/day as an infusion for asymptomatic infants who are not feeding adequately.

Neonatal hypomagnesemia may impair parathyroid response and blunt end-organ response to parathyroid hormone. If, after adequate treatment of hypocalcemia and hypoglycemia, the infant remains symptomatic, treatment for hypomagnesemia with 0.1–0.3 ml/kg of 50% magnesium sulfate should be considered. We have not had to do this in years. Management of hypocalcemia is discussed in reference 15.

Polycythemia. Polycythemia (a peripheral venous hematocrit over 65%) is common in IDMs. In infants who are small for gestational age, due to maternal vascular disease and placental insufficiency, polycythemia may be caused by chronic fetal hypoxia and increased fetal erythropoiesis. Polycythemia may also be caused by reduced oxygen delivery to fetal tissue because of elevated glycosylated hemoglobin in maternal blood. In cases of fetal distress, there may be shifts of blood from the placenta to the fetus. Other mechanisms, such as altered prostaglandin metabolism, may explain the association of polycythemia and IDM. Most infants with polycythemia are asymptomatic but some have respiratory distress, cyanosis, congestive heart failure, lethargy, poor feeding, convulsions, hypoglycemia, jaundice, priapism, renal vein thrombosis, cerebral vein thrombosis, necrotizing enterocolitis, or testicular infarcts. Infants with any of the above symptoms, who have a venous hematocrit over 65%, should have a partial exchange transfusion with 5% albumin, plasma, or plasmanate.

There is controversy about the need to perform exchange transfusion on asymptomatic infants with a venous hematocrit between 65% and 70%. Most neonatologists would perform a partial exchange transfusion in the absence of symptom if the venous hematocrit is over 70% because of concern about silent thrombi in the central nervous system. The general approach to neonatal polycythemia has been described by Goorin.[16]

Jaundice. Hyperbilirubinemia (over 15 mg/dl) is seen with increased frequency in IDMs. Kitzmiller reported that bulirubin levels over 16 mg/dl were seen in 19% of the IDMs at the Brigham and Women's Hospital.[9] When carboxyhemoglobin production is used as an indication of increased heme turnover, IDMs are found to have increased heme turnover.[17] The etiology of this increased heme turnover may be hemolysis, ineffective erythropoiesis, or catabolism of nonhemoglobin hemes. Infants with polycythemia may have increased red cell destruction. Other factors that may account for increased jaundice are prematurity, impairment of the hepatic conjugation of the bilirubin, and an increased enterohepatic circulation of bilirubin due to poor feeding.

Jaundice in IDMs is treated, as in other infants, with adequate fluid intake, phototherapy, or exchange transfusion.[18]

Congenital Anomalies. In a series of 147 IDMs from the Boston Hospital for Women in 1976–1977, 9% had major malformations, and malformations accounted for 50% of the perinatal mortality.[9] As mortality from other causes such as prematurity, stillbirth, asphyxia, and RDS falls, malformations become the major cause of perinatal mortality in IDMs. Most studies show a 6–9% incidence of major anomalies in IDMs.[2,19,20] This is three-to-five-fold greater than the rate of major congenital malformations in the general population.[21] The type of anomalies seen are central nervous system (anencephaly, meningocele syndrome) cardiac, vertebral, skeletal, renal, and caudal regression syndrome (sacral agenesis). The central nervous system and cardiac anomalies make up two-thirds of the malformations occurring in IDMs. Although there is a general increase in the anomaly rate in IDMs, no anomaly is specific for IDMs. However, half of all cases of caudal regression syndrome are seen in IDMs. There have been several studies correlating poor metabolic control of diabetes, as measured by maternal glycohemoglobin values in early pregnancy, with increased incidence of anomalies in offspring.[22,24]

The study by Miller et al showed 3.4% major malformation in the best controlled group of mothers versus a 22.4% incidence in the group with poor control.[4] The study by Ylinen et al[24] showed 3.1% incidence of malformations in patients with good control and 23.5% incidence in patients with poor control. In the Diabetes in Early Pregnancy Study (DIEP) there were 2.4% malformations in the nondiabetic state and 4.9% malformations in the IDMs whose mothers entered the study before pregnancy or in early pregnancy.[25] Diabetic patients who entered the study late (after the first trimester) had a malformation rate of 9%. This study failed to show a correlation between hyperglycemia, elevated glycosylated hemoglobin levels, and malformations in women who prospectively opted for rigorous control of diabetes. The authors felt that some, but not all malformations, can be prevented by good control of blood sugar and that other etiologies must be sought to identify the teratogenic mechanisms in IDMs. However, only a few diabetic women in the full participant group had glycosylated hemoglobin levels as high as those seen in references 4 and 24. Thus, most women in this group had good control of diabetes in pregnancy, with glycohemoglobin levels below the threshold for the appearance of malformations.

A second study performed by the Joslin Clinic again showed a relationship between elevated hemoglobin A1 (HBA1) in the first trimester and major anomalies in IDMs[20] (see Chapter 12). The data are consistent with the hypothesis that poor metabolic control of maternal diabetes in the first trimester is associated with an increased risk for major congenital malformations in IDMs.

Because of the high incidence of malformations in IDMs, an ultrasound should be performed in early pregnancy. Maternal alpha feroprotein (AFP) should also be measured (Chapter 11). The newborn should have a careful physical exam to diagnose any anomalies that were missed by interuterine surveillance.

Feeding. Poor feeding is a major problem in IDMs. It occurred in 37% of 150 IDMs at the Boston Hospital for Women.[9] Sometimes poor feeding is related to prematurity, respiratory distress, or other problems; however, it is often present in the absence of other problems. In our more recent experience, it was found in 17% of IDMs of Classes B–D mothers and in 31% of Class F. Infants born to Class F diabetic women are usually premature (average gestation age is 34 weeks). There was no difference in the incidence of poor feeding in large-for-gestational-age (LGA) infants versus appropriate-for-gestational-age (AGA) infants and no relation to polyhydramnios. Poor feeding is a major reason for prolongation of hospital stay and parent–infant separation.

Macrosomia. Macrosomia is defined as birth weight over the 90th percentile, i.e., over 4,000 g, and is common in IDMs. It was found in 28% of IDMs at the Brigham and Women's Hospital in 1983–1984.[10] IDMs born to mothers without vascular or renal disease have an increased incidence of macrosomia. The obstetrical management of the macrosomic infant is discussed in Chapters 9 and 10. The macrosomic infant should be carefully examined for complications of shoulder dystocia, such as Erbs palsy, Klumpkes paralysis, fractured clavicle, or phrenic-nerve palsy.

Myocardial Dysfunction. Transient hypertrophic subaortic stenosis resulting from ventricular septal hypertrophy in IDMs has been frequently reported.[26,27,28,29] The infants may present with congestive heart failure, poor cardiac output, and cardiomegaly. This cardiomyopathy may complicate the management of other illnesses such as RDS. The diagnosis, made by echocardiography, shows hypertrophy of the ventricular septum, the right ventricular anterior wall, and the left ventricular posterior wall in the absence of chamber dilation.[26] Cardiac output decreases with increasing septal thickness.[28]

Most symptoms resolve by two weeks of age. The septal hypertrophy resolves by four months of age. In the series by Walther, 18/42 (43%) of IDMs had hypertrophic cardiomyopathy; 7 of the 18 were symptomatic. Most infants respond to supportive care. Digitalis and other inotropic drugs are contraindicated, unless myocardial dysfunction is seen on echocardiography. Propanolol is the most useful drug.[29]

The differential diagnosis of myocardial dysfunction owing to diabetic cardiomyopathy of the newborn includes: (1) postasphyxial cardiomyopathy, (2) myocarditis, (3) endocardial fibroelastosis, (4) glycogen storage disease of the heart, and (5) aberrant left coronary artery coming off the pulmonary artery. There is some evidence that good control of diabetes in pregnancy may reduce the severity of hypertrophic cardiomyopathy.[30]

Other Problems in IDMs. These include renal vein thrombosis and small left colon syndrome. Renal vein thrombosis may occur in utero or postpartum. Intrauterine diagnosis may be made by ultrasound. Postnatal signs may include hematuria, flank mass, hypertension, or embolic phenomena. Most renal vein thrombosis can be managed conservatively, with preservation of renal tissue.[31]

Small left colon syndrome presents as generalized abdominal distention, because of the inability to pass meconium. Meconium is removed by passage of a rectal catheter. An enema, with meglumine diatrizoate (Gastrograffin®), is used to make the diagnosis and often results in evacuation of the colon. The infant should be well hydrated before Gastrograffin® is used. The infant may have some problems with passage of stool in the first week of life, but this usually resolves after treatment with half-normal saline enemas (5 ml/kg) and glycerine suppositories.[31]

Genetics. The parents of IDMs are often concerned about the eventual development of diabetes in their new offspring. There are conflicting data on the incidence of insulin dependent diabetes in IDMs.[32–35] Although there is an increased risk, the absolute magnitude is at present uncertain.

Perinatal Survival. Despite all these problems, the diabetic woman has a 95% chance of having a healthy child, if she is willing to participate in a program of pregnancy management and surveillance in a modern perinatal center. During 1976–1977, the perinatal mortality rate was 34/1,000 at the Boston Hospital for Women, based on a group of 147 IDMs who were over 24 weeks gestation when born to mothers who required insulin.[32–35] Between 1977 and 1980, at the same center, the perinatal mortality of infants born to women with Class B, C, D, H, or R diabetes was 20/1,000 (unpublished). In the earlier series, 24 infants born to Class F diabetic women had a perinatal mortality of 125/1,000.[36]

In a series of 215 IDMs at the Brigham and Women's Hospital from 1983 to 1984, the total perinatal mortality, from 24 weeks gestation to 28 days postpartum, was 28/1,000. There was one intrauterine demise of a singleton near term.[9]

Thus, perinatal survival is encouragingly good as a result of advances in medical, obstetrical, and neonatal treatment. More infants are born healthy than ever before, and if ill, more survive.

REFERENCES

1. Gabbe SG: Management of diabetes mellitus in pregnancy. Am J Obstet 153:824–828, 1985.
2. Freinkel N, Dooley SL, Metzger BE: Care of the pregnant woman with insulin-dependent diabetes mellitus. N Engl J Med 313:96–101, 1985.
3. Ringer S: Resuscitation in the delivery room. In Cloherty JP, Stark AR (eds): "Manual of Neonatal Care of the Joint Program in Neonatology," chapter 17. Boston: Little, Brown 1995.

4. Miller EM, Hare JW, Cloherty JP, Dunn PJ, Gleason RE, Soeldner JS, and Kitzmiller JL: Elevated maternal hemoglobin AIC in early pregnancy and major anomalies in infants of diabetic mothers. N Engl J Med 304:1331–1334, 1981.
5. Kitzmiller JL, Gavin LA, Gin GD, Javanovic-Peterson L, Main EK, Zigrand WD: Preconception care of diabetes: Glycemic control prevents congenital anomalies. JAMA 265:731, 1991.
6. Steel JM, Johnstone FD, Hepburn DA, Smith AF: Can prepregnancy care of diabetic women reduce the risks of abnormal babies? Br Med J 301:1070, 1990.
7. Robert MF, Neff RK, Hubbell JP, Taeusch HW, Avery ME: Association between maternal diabetes and the respiratory distress syndrome in newborn. N Engl J Med 294:357–360, 1976.
8. Hubbell JP, Muirhead DM, Drobough JE: The newborn infant of the diabetic mother. Med Clin North Am 49:1035–1052, 1965.
9. Kitzmiller JL, Cloherty JP, Younger MD, Tabatubaii A, Rothchild SB, Sosenko I, Epstein MF, Singh S, Neff RK: Diabetic pregnancy and perinatal mortality. Am J Obstet Gynecol 131:560–580, 1978.
10. Greene MF: personal communication.
11. Liley H and Stark AR: Respiratory disorders—Hyaline membrane disease. In Cloherty JP, Stark AR (eds): "Manual of Neonatal Care, Joint Program in Neonatology," 3rd ed, chapter 25. Boston: Little, Brown, 1995.
12. Cornblath M, Schwartz R: "Disorders of Carbohydrate Metabolism in Infancy." Philadelphia: Saunders, 1976, pp. 115–154.
13. Cowett RM: Metabolism in the fetus and infant of the diabetic mother. In "Infant of the Diabetic Mother." Report of the 93rd Ross Conference on Pediatric Research. Columbus: Ross Laboratories, 1987.
14. Lillien LD, Pildes RS, Srinivasan G, Voora S, Yeh TF: Treatment of the neonatal hypoglycemia with minibolus and intravenous glucose infusion. J Pediatr 97:295–298, 1980.
15. Huttner K: Hypocalcemia, Hypercalcemia, and Hypermagnesemia. In Cloherty JP, Stark AR (eds): "Manual of Neonatal Care of the Joint Program in Neonatology," chapter 30. Boston: Little, Brown, 1995.
16. Goorin AM: Polycythemia. In Cloherty JP, Stark AR (eds): "Manual of Neonatal Care, Joint Program in Neonatology," chapter 27. Boston: Little, Brown, 1994.
17. Peevy KJ, Landow SA, Gross SJ: Hyperbilirubinemia in infants of diabetic mothers. Pediatrics 66:417–419, 1980.
18. Hyperbilirubinemia. In Freeman RK, Poland RL (eds): "Guidelines for Perinatal Care." American Academy of Pediatrics and American College of Obstetrics and Gynecologists. Evanston, IL: American Academy of Pediatrics, 1992, pp 204–210.
19. Gabbe SG, Mostman JH, Freeman RK, Goebelsmann UT, Lowensohn RI, Nichimson D, Cetrulo C, Quilligan EG: Management and outcome of pregnancy in diabetes mellitus classes B to R. Am J Obstet Gynecol 129:723–732, 1977.
20. Greene MF, Hare JW, Cloherty JP, Benacerraf BR, Soeldner JS: First-trimester hemoglobin A1, and risk for major malformation and spontaneous abortion in diabetic pregnancy. Teratology 39:225–231, 1989.
21. Holmes LB: Congenital malformations. In Cloherty JP, Stark AR (eds): "Manual of Newborn Care, Joint Program in Neonatology," chapter 12. Boston: Little, Brown, 1985.
22. Greene MF: Prevention and diagnosis of congenital anomalies in diabetic pregnancies. In Landon MB (ed): "Clinics in Perinatology Diabetes in Pregnancy." Philadelphia: W.B. Saunders, 1993, pp 533–547.
23. Reid M, Hadden D, Hanley JMG, Halliday HL, McClure BG: Fetal malformations in

diabetics with high hemoglobin A1C values in early pregnancy. Br Med J [Clin Res] 289:1001, 1984.
24. Ylinen K, Aula P, Stenman UH, Kesaniemi-Kuokkanen T, Teramo K: Risk of minor and major malformations in diabetics with high hemoglobin A1C values in early pregnancy. Br Med J [Clin Res] 289:345–346, 1984.
25. Mills JL, Knopp RH, Simpson JL, Jovanovic-Peterson L, Metzger BE, Holmes LB, Aarons JH, Brown Z, Reed GF, Bieber FR, Van Allen M, Holzman I, Ober C, Peterson CM, Withiam MJ, Duckles A, Mueller-Heubach E, Polk BF, and the National Institute of Child Health and Human Development: Diabetes in Early Pregnancy Study: Lack of relation of increased malformation rates in infants of diabetic mothers to glycemic control during organogenesis. N Engl J Med 318:671–676, 1988.
26. Mace S, Hirschfeld SS, Riggs T, Franaroff AA, Merkatz IR: Echocardiographic abnormalities in infants of diabetic mothers. J Pediatr 95:1013–1019, 1979.
27. Gutgesell HP, Speer ME, Rosenberg HS: Characterization of the cardiomyopathy in infants of diabetic mothers. Circulation 61:441–450, 1980.
28. Walther FJ, Siassi B, King J, Wu PY: Cardiac output in infants of insulin dependent diabetic mothers. J Pediatr 107:109–114, 1985.
29. Way GI, Wolfe RR, Eskaghpour E, Bender RL, Jaffe RB, Ruttenberg HP: The natural history of hypertrophic cardiomyopathy in IDM's. J Pediatr 95:1020–1025, 1979.
30. Reller MD, Tsang RC, Meyer RA, Braun CP: Relationship of prospective diabetes control in pregnancy to neonatal cardiorespiratory function. J Pediatr 106:86–90, 1985.
31. Ringer S: Surgical emergencies in the newborn. In Cloherty JP, Stark RS (eds): "Manual of Neonatal Care," chapter 34. Boston: Little, Brown, 1995.
32. Warrem JH, Krolewski AS, Gottlieb MS, Kahn CR: Differences in risk of insulin–dependent diabetes in offspring of diabetic mothers and diabetic fathers. N Engl J Med 311:149–152, 1984.
33. Hod M, Diamant YZ: The offspring of a diabetic mother—short- and long-range implications. Isr J Med Sci 28:81–86, 1992.
34. Martin AO, Simpson JL, Ober C, Freinkel N: Frequency of diabetes mellitus in mothers of probands with GDM. Possible maternal influence on the predisposition to gestational diabetes. Am J Obstet Gynecol 151:971–975, 1985.
35. McFarland KF, Edwards JG, Strickland AL, Lampert R: Incidence of diabetes mellitus in parents and grandparents of diabetic children. Cleve Clin J Med 55:217–219, 1988.
36. Kitzmiller J, Brown ER, Phillipe M, Stark AR, Acker D, Kaldany A, Singh S, Hare JW: Diabetic nephropathy and perinatal outcome. Am J Obstet Gynecol 141:741–751, 1981.

CHAPTER 12

Congenital Malformations

Michael F. Greene, MD and Florence M. Brown, MD

INTRODUCTION

Historical Perspective

Dr. Elliott Joslin's initial publication concerning diabetes and pregnancy appeared in 1915, seven years before the discovery of insulin. In that lengthy communication in the Boston Medical and Surgical Journal[1] he described ten pregnancies among seven women with four maternal mortalities and three living children. Twenty years after the introduction of insulin, Lawrence and Oakley[2] published their results from Kings College Hospital and reviewed the existing literature. It was striking that although the maternal mortality rate had fallen to 2–5% following the introduction of insulin, the perinatal mortality of approximately 40% had not changed substantially. The sources of that mortality were ketoacidosis, congenital anomalies, late intrauterine demise, and prematurity. Dr. Priscilla White recognized that scrupulous diabetic control was the key to reducing losses from ketoacidosis and late intrauterine demise, but was frustrated when she conceded that congenital anomalies were "doubtless beyond our therapeutic control."[3] Over the next 30 years, improvements in the care of pregnancies complicated by diabetes reduced perinatal losses from other causes to the point that major congenital anomalies emerged as the single greatest cause of perinatal death.

Numerous reports from around the world spanning several decades documented the fact that the incidence of congenital anomalies among infants of diabetic mothers (IDMs) is higher than that among the non-diabetic population. Except for the results of several recent European studies, the actual incidence of major and minor anomalies among IDMs has been found to be 6–9%, which is two to three times greater than that

Diabetes Complicating Pregnancy: The Joslin Clinic Method, Edited by Florence M. Brown, MD and John W. Hare, MD.
ISBN 0-471-11031-0 © 1995 John Wiley & Sons, Inc.

for a nondiabetic population. Table I lists several representative studies of major malformations among IDMs. The incidence of major anomalies found in a general population depends upon the age at which the children are examined, definitions of malformation, and other factors. Generally, this incidence is 2–3%.

The anomalies found among IDMs span the range of the anomalies found in the nondiabetic population. Kucera compiled a series of 7,100 IDMs from the literature from nine countries spanning 30 years.[17] He compared the 340 anomalous fetuses among them to a control group of 7,100 anomalous fetuses from 431,000 nondiabetic women from a WHO database. He found 10 malformations whose frequencies were increased from 6- to 200-fold among the IDMs, which he considered "very probably" specific for diabetes. These anomalies and their incidence ratios are listed in Table II.

Although the incidence ratio of 212 for the caudal regression syndrome looks formidable, its absolute risk of occurrence is still only 1.3 per 1,000 among IDMs. In this series the risk of neural tube defects was 4.6 per 1,000. In a recent series from the Joslin Clinic, the risk of a neural tube defect was found to be 19.5/1,000, tenfold greater than in the general population.[18]

TABLE I. Incidence of Major Malformations among Infants of Diabetic Mothers*

Source	N	Percentage
Stockholm (Hanson et al, 1990)[4]	10/532	1.9
Nottingham (Gregory et al, 1992)[5]	3/139	2.2
France (Gestation and Diabetes Group, 1991)[6]	9/208	4.3
Paris (Tchobroutsky et al, 1991)[7]	22/389	5.5
Copenhagen (Pedersen et al, 1964)[8]	44/791	5.6
Dublin (Drury et al, 1977)[9]	34/558	6.1
Los Angeles (Gabbe et al, 1977)[10]	19/260	7.3
Boston (Greene and Benacerraf, 1991)[11]	32/432	7.4
Birmingham U.K. (Soler et al, 1976)[12]	44/585	7.5
Helsinki (Ylinen et al, 1984)[13]	11/142	7.7
Chicago (Simpson et al, 1983)[14]	9/106	8.5
Boston (Kitzmiller et al, 1978)[15]	13/137	9.5
Cincinnati (Ballard et al, 1984)[16]	19/196	9.7
Total	269/4475	6.0

*Reprinted with permission from Clinics in Perinatology 20:533–547, 1993. Philadelphia: W.B. Saunders.

TABLE II. Anomalies and Incidence Ratios among IDMs from Kucera's Study[17]*

Anomaly	Incidence ratio
Caudal regression syndrome	212
Situs inversus	42
Arthrogryposis	28
Spinal anomalies	23
Ureter duplex	23
Pseudohermaphroditism	11
Gross skeletal anomalies	10
Hydronephrosis	7
Gross skeletal and associated anomalies	6
Anencephalus	6

*Adapted with permission from the Journal of Reproductive Medicine 7:61–70, 1971.

Several years later, Mills[19] reviewed the anomalies cited by Kucera in light of what is known of the normal timetable for human development. He pointed out the fact that all of these malformations arise from perturbation of development before the seventh week of gestation. Table III lists the gestational age in postovulatory weeks when each of the anomalies cited by Kucera arises. From this analysis it can be seen that if these malforma-

TABLE III. Gestational Age at Which Anomalies Arose in Kucera''s Study According to Mills et al[19]*

Anomaly	Postovulatory weeks
Caudal regression syndrome	3
Neural tube defect	4
Cardiac anomalies	5-6
Anal/rectal atresia	6
Renal/ureteral anomalies	5
Situs inversus	4

*Adapted from Diabetes 28:292–293, 1979, with permission from the American Diabetes Association, Inc.

tions are preventable, then any effort to intervene must be made very early in pregnancy. This is so early in pregnancy that most women would not ordinarily have seen their obstetricians for the first time, or even have recognized their pregnancies.

The increased risk of malformation appears rather clearly to be limited to patients whose diabetes antedates their pregnancies. McCarter et al[20] have shown that it is not found among the nondiabetic pregnancies of women who develop diabetes in later life. Studying the data from the Collaborative Perinatal Project, Chung and Myrianthopoulos[21] found no increased risk of malformation among the offspring of women with gestational diabetes whose carbohydrate metabolism was normal during early pregnancy. Comess et al[22] found no increased risk for malformation among the children of men with diabetes. These facts seem to indicate that the teratogenic stimulus is a disturbance in the environment of the developing embryo rather than a genetic predisposition to major malformation among persons who also have a genetic predisposition to diabetes mellitus.

The first hint that malformations among IDMs might be related to Hb A_1 levels, and therefore metabolic control, came from Leslie et al.[23] They noted that three out of five diabetic women in poor metabolic control delivered babies with major congenital malformations. Miller et al at the Joslin Clinic provided the first reasonably large data set to suggest that this might be true. They examined the relationship between the concentration of Hb A_{1c} obtained before 14 weeks gestation and the risk for major congenital malformation. The results of that study are summarized in Table IV. Patients with reasonably good metabolic control in the first tri-

TABLE IV. Results of Study by Miller et al, 1981[24]*

Hb A_{1c} before 14th wk of gestation (%)	Major malformations	Number of malformations	Percent
≤6.9	0	19	3.4
7.0–8.5	2	37	
8.6–9.9	8	27	22.4
≥10.0	5	18	

*Reprinted with permission from the New England Journal of Medicine 304:1331–1334, 1981.

mester, defined as an Hb A_{1c} of less than or equal to 8.5%, had a risk for major malformation of 3.4%. Patients with poor metabolic control, defined as a Hb A_{1c} greater than 8.5%, had a 22.4% risk of major malformation. This difference was statistically highly significant. Three years later Ylinen et al[13] published a similar series that confirmed remarkably closely Miller's original findings. The risk for major malformation at lower levels of Hb A_{1c} was 3.2%, and 23.5% at very high Hb A_{1c} levels.

In the early 1980s the NICHHD developed a protocol for a multicenter study to examine the biochemical events in early pregnancy associated with malformations among IDMs.[25] The Diabetes in Early Pregnancy Study (DIEP) recruited both diabetic and nondiabetic women either before pregnancy or within 21 days of conception. Patients who volunteered for the study were followed through a rigorous protocol, which included two ultrasound examinations in the first trimester and weekly interviews and blood sampling for a wide variety of biochemical parameters.

Well into the study, it became obvious that the incidence of adverse outcomes among the recruited patients was going to be very low. To provide more adverse outcomes for study, the DIEP Study also enrolled "late entry" diabetic women whenever they presented for care. Unfortunately, the DIEP Study has no first trimester biochemical data for these late entrants. The incidence of major malformations for each group is listed in Table V.[26] Note that the incidence of major malformations in the early entry patients is lower than the average for all of the studies cited in Table I. The incidence of major malformations in the late entry patients seems much more typical for a diabetic patient population.

Contrary to the studies of Miller and Ylinen, the DIEP Study was unable to demonstrate a relationship between degree of glycemic control in the first trimester and risk for major malformation. Data from these apparently conflicting studies can be reconciled when glycohemoglobin values are expressed in terms of standard deviations above the mean for a nondiabetic population. This is necessary since methods of determining glycohemoglobin vary from one laboratory to another. Miller's Hb A_{1c} of 8.5%

TABLE V. Diabetes in Early Pregnancy Study: Major Malformations[26]

Patients	Number	Percent
Nondiabetics	8/389	2.1
Early entry diabetics	17/347	4.9
Late entry diabetics	25/279	9.0

proved to be approximately seven standard deviations above the non-diabetic mean for that assay. Among the DIEP early entrants, only 7% were above seven standard deviations above the mean, and thus "at risk" for major malformation as defined by Miller et al.

Stimulated by the findings of the DIEP Study, we have examined our recent experience at the Joslin Clinic regarding Hb A_1 in the first trimester and risk for congenital malformation and spontaneous abortion. All patients in this series had Hb A_1 determinations performed by the current technique at the Joslin Clinic before 12 weeks gestation. Where two or more determinations were available before 12 weeks, the earliest one was used. None of the patients in this series were included in the original series of Miller et al. Congenital malformations were ascertained by routine clinical examinations performed by six pediatricians by 72 hours of age. Babies with known malformations were followed for a minimum of 28 days.

There were 451 patients available for study with known Hb A_1 and pregnancy outcome status. The distribution of these patients with respect to Hb A_1 in the first trimester and outcome status is shown in Table VI.[27] The risk of major malformations among all pregnancies, progressing beyond the first trimester was 7.8%. Among women with excellent blood sugar control (less than six standard deviations [SD] above the mean), this risk was 3.1%. In contrast, the incidence of major congenital abnormalities for women with glycohemoglobin levels greater than 12 standard devia-

TABLE VI. Major Malformations According to First-Trimester Hb A_1 Level

SD above mean	Percentage†	Major malformations	No major malformations	Percentage‡	Risk ratio (95% confidence interval)
≤6	≤9.3	6	187	3.1	1.0
6.1–9.0	9.4–11.0	9	134	6.3	2.0 (0.7–5.4)
9.1–12.0	11.1–12.7	6	70	7.9	2.5 (0.9–7.4)
12.1–15.0	12.8–14.4	9	18	33.3	10.7 (4.8–23.8)
>15.0	>14.4	5	7	41.7	13.4 (5.5–32.5)

*Reprinted with permission from Clinics in Perinatology 20:533–547, 1993. Philadelphia: W.B. Saunders.

†Hb A_1 as a percentage of total hemoglobin.

‡Major malformations as a percentage of all pregnancies progressing beyond the first trimester.

tions above the mean was 36%. Similarly, deaths from malformations occurred in 6 of 412 (1.4%) infants of women with a first trimester glycohemoglobin less than or equal to 12 SD above the mean, compared to 8 of 39 (20%) infants whose mothers had a glycohemoglobin more than 12 SD above the mean.

The risk of spontaneous abortion relative to first trimester hemoglobin A_1 level is presented in Table VII. First trimester glycohemoglobin levels above 9 SD above the mean are associated with twice the risk of spontaneous abortions as seen in well-controlled diabetic patients. The risk of spontaneous abortion in women with well-controlled diabetes is similar to the background rate seen in the general nondiabetic population.

HUMAN STUDIES: CONCLUSIONS AND DILEMMA

It appears from the very carefully done DIEP Study (Table V) with its own nondiabetic concurrent controls that even well-controlled diabetic women have a greater incidence of major malformations than nondiabetic women. The risk of malformation does not vary over a broad range of glycemic control but rises sharply with very poor control.

What then causes the increased incidence of major malformations in well-controlled diabetic women? If the etiology is genetic, then one would expect to find an increased incidence of malformations among the offspring of men with diabetes and women who develop diabetes after their pregnancies. As noted above, this is not the case. If the etiology is en-

TABLE VII. Spontaneous Abortions According to the First Trimester Hb A_1 Levels*

SD above mean	Percentage†	Spontaneous abortions	Continuing pregnancies	Percentage	Risk ratio (95% confidence interval)
≤6	≤9.3	31	193	13.8	1.0
6.1–9.0	9.4–11.0	18	143	11.2	0.8 (0.5–1.4)
9.1–12.0	11.1–12.7	23	76	23.2	1.7 (1.03–2.7)
12.1–15.0	12.8–14.4	13	27	32.5	2.4 (1.3–4.2)
>15.0	>14.4	7	12	36.8	2.7 (1.3–5.5)

*Reprinted with permission from Clinics in Perinatology 20:533–547, 1993. Philadelphia: W.B. Saunders.

†Hb A_1 as a percentage of total hemoglobin.

vironmental, owing to the metabolic derangements of diabetes, then how can we explain this very unusual "dose–response" curve?

Since congenital abnormalities develop very early in pregnancy, recent studies have aimed at further reducing the incidence of congenital malformation by enrolling women in preconception counseling programs. These programs are designed to ensure that women conceive under good metabolic control. Results of these studies reveal that diabetic women who attend these clinics have less than a 2% incidence of malformations (Table VIII)[28–32] compared to nonattendees who have an incidence between 6 and 10%. Although small numbers of women have participated in these studies, initial data are encouraging. Nevertheless, interpretation of these studies is not straightforward. Randomization of women to preconception versus postconception care groups has not been done for ethical reasons. Therefore, women who choose to participate in preconception programs represent a self-selected motivated group invested in meticulous care of their diabetes.[33] Despite intensive recruiting efforts, many women still fail to plan their pregnancies and present postconception with poor metabolic control. Approximately half of pregnancies in the United States are unplanned.[34] Addressing this statistic in women with diabetes is an important goal in reducing the risk of congenital abnormalities, spontaneous abortions, and, ultimately, perinatal mortality.

MECHANISM

The mechanism of the diabetic embryopathy is still incompletely understood. Observations in humans were confused by the inability to separate

TABLE VIII. Trials of Preconception Care for Women with Diabetes Mellitus: Incidence of Major Malformations*

Study	Attenders (%)	Nonattenders (%)
Fuhrmann et al (1983)[28]	1/128 (0.8)	22/292 (7.5)
Damm et al (1989)[29]	2/193 (1.0)	5/61 (8.2)
Steel et al (1990)[30]	2/143 (1.4)	10/96 (10.4)
Kitzmiller et al (1991)[31]	1/84 (1.2)	12/110 (10.9)
Willhoite et al (1993)[31]	1/62 (1.6)	8/123 (6.5)

*Reprinted with permission from Clinics in Perinatology 20:533–547, 1993. Philadelphia: W.B. Saunders.

glucose and other metabolite levels from insulin levels. Zwilling had shown in the late 1940s that insulin injections into embryonated chick eggs were teratogenic. They produced malformations that he termed "rumplessness" which closely resembled caudal dysgenesis. The possibility that exogenous insulin itself could be teratogenic could not initially be dismissed. Hypoglycemia is demonstrably teratogenic in a variety of animal models. Since many persons in generally poor glycemic control tend to have both very high and very low blood sugar levels, the possibility that transient episodes of hypoglycemia could be etiologic has been entertained.

During early postimplantation embryogenesis, before the development of the chorioallantoic placenta, the embryo is critically dependent upon glycolysis for its energy supply. Interruption of this energy supply can result in congenital malformations. Freinkel et al[35] have used mannose to interfere with glycolysis and produce malformations in rat embryos in vitro. More recent work in mouse embryo culture also documents that a prolonged period (28 hours) of hypoglycemia during neurulation, when the embryo is dependent upon glycolysis, can be teratogenic.[36] Shorter exposures can cause developmental delay, which appears to be largely reversible when the glucose concentration is returned to normal. Equivalent stages of morphogenesis (e.g., neurulation) take considerably longer in the human than they do in the rodent. It seems unlikely that hypoglycemic episodes of sufficient length and severity to disturb normal development occur frequently enough to contribute significantly to the clinical problem of malformations in humans. The possibility that an inhibition of glycolysis could result from some other metabolic disturbance in diabetes, such as elevated butyrate levels, has been raised. Specific investigation of this possibility, however, has shown that butyrate reduces ribose availability from the pentose phosphate pathway and thus DNA synthesis, but does not alter glycolysis.[37]

Work in intact animals showed that the incidence of anomalies among the fetuses of mothers made experimentally diabetic could be reduced by insulin therapy. Thus it seemed that something about the state of poor metabolic control was teratogenic. In vitro whole embryo cultures showed that hyperglycemia alone was not a very effective teratogen. Malformations were not consistently seen until glucose concentrations of 900–1,200 mg/dl were reached. These are levels that are clearly not seen in routine clinical practice.

The landmark studies of Sadler[38,39] showed that the serum of poorly metabolically controlled diabetic rats could be teratogenic in vitro with glucose concentrations of only 600 mg/dl. Subsequently it has been demonstrated that moderately high glucose concentrations in combination with elevated but still physiologic levels of beta-hydroxybutyrate are teratogenic in vitro. Precisely how these metabolites synergize to produce malformation is not yet understood. Possibly they interfere with the early embryonic energy supply by damaging the yolk sac, as suggested by Reece et al.[40] Possibly the effect is mediated through some mechanism involving prostaglandin, as suggested by the fact that the effect can be modified by the administration of supplemental arachidonic acid.[41] Some of the work of Sadler et al suggests that a low molecular weight compound with somatomedin inhibitory action may be instrumental in teratogenesis.[42]

FOLIC ACID SUPPLEMENTATION

Folic acid supplementation beginning preconception has been shown to reduce the incidence of neural tube defects (NTD). Recently, the Medical Research Council of Great Britain published the results of a randomized, well-controlled multicenter trial in patients with a prior pregnancy affected with a NTD.[43] Recruited patients were randomized into 4 groups: folate alone, folate with other vitamins, no folate or vitamins, or vitamins alone without folate. Large doses of folate (4 mg) were used to ensure that if there was an effect from folate, it would be found. Supplementation started at least 14 days before the last menstrual period and continued through the 12th week of pregnancy. Among 514 patients treated with folic acid, there were five recurrences (1%) compared with 18 recurrences among 517 patients (3.5%) without folic acid supplementation. This reduction in the incidence of NTD was highly statistically significant.

The Hungarian Family Planning Program conducted a randomized controlled trial evaluating the effect of folic acid supplementation in preventing the first occurrences of NTD.[44] Treated patients received a multivitamin and mineral tablet containing folic acid 0.8 mg and control patients received a tablet with vitamin C and trace minerals only. There were no NTD among 2104 treated patients compared to six among 2052 controls. Because of these results, the Centers for Disease Control recommend that all women of child bearing age consume 0.4 mg of folic acid daily.[45] Although similar studies have not been performed in women with diabetes, we assume that reductions in the incidence of NTD would occur in their pregnancies as well. Therefore, we treat all women who present for preconception care with folic acid 0.4 mg daily (see Chapter 5).

MANAGEMENT

Glycosylated Hemoglobin

Each patient presenting for prenatal care has a Hb A_1 determination performed at the first visit. If that first visit is before 12 weeks of gestation, then we use the data cited above to counsel each patient regarding her a priori risk for a major malformation. This must be done carefully, stressing the statistical nature of the information. Further specific investigation of the individual pregnancy must wait until later in pregnancy.

We have been concerned over the years that our counseling might lead women to terminate pregnancies that were likely to be normal. A pregnancy with a high Hb A_{1c}, according to the data of Miller et al, still had a 78% likelihood of having no major malformation. We studied 89 consecutive women who presented in the first trimester with an initial Hb A_1 value placing them at approximately a 20% risk of major malformation. The reasons why women elect to terminate pregnancies are, of course, terribly complex and often difficult to discern. Eight of the 89 patients elected to terminate their pregnancies after obtaining knowledge of their initial Hb A_1 values. It was our best judgment, however, that only one of the eight was significantly influenced by her Hb A_1 value. In our experience then, it seems to be a rather rare event for a woman to elect to terminate her pregnancy solely on the basis of a 20% a priori risk of malformation.

Maternal Serum Alpha-Fetoprotein

Maternal serum alpha-fetoprotein (MSAFP) screening in conjunction with human chorionic gonadotropin and unconjugated estriol should be assessed in women with diabetes for the purpose of defining the risk of aneuploidy. In a population which is already being screened by a highly skilled sonographer, the MSAFP may be less useful in identifying congential anomalies. Screening should be performed at 16–18 weeks of gestation, and, to be properly interpreted, the gestational age must be accurately known. There are two special considerations that must be kept in mind for diabetic women.

The normal values for diabetic women as a group tend to be lower than the values for nondiabetic women.[18,46] The median value for a group of diabetic women is approximately 0.8 multiples of the median (MOM) for a nondiabetic group. Thus, the values for diabetic women must be adjusted up slightly before interpretation. This is done simply by dividing the actual value obtained by 0.8 to obtain the adjusted value.

The positive and negative predictive values of any screening test are dependent upon the incidence of the disease under study. Major congenital malformations are several-fold more common among diabetic women. Thus, to assure a diabetic woman that a negative test gives her the same very low probability of an affected child, the cutoff value for a normal test must be lowered. At the Joslin Clinic we use 1.5 MOM as the upper limit of normal rather than the 2.0 MOM, which we use for our nondiabetics.

The lower values of MSAFP seen in diabetic pregnancies do not appear to be related to either White class or to Hb A_1 as shown in Tables IX and X.

After adjustments have been made as noted above, abnormal values should be evaluated, just as they are for nondiabetic patients.

Ultrasound Examination

The value of a carefully performed ultrasound examination by a skilled operator using state of the art equipment cannot be overstated. To optimally visualize the heart and great vessels this exam should be performed in all diabetic women at 18 weeks. Most neural tube defects are readily identified on routine examination with up to 100% sensitivity in some studies.[47–49] Other studies have been less successful.[50] Certain intracranial abnormalities may be more difficult to diagnose.[51] Congenital cardiac abnormalities, particularly milder or progressive ones, may be difficult to diagnose on ultrasound.[52] Evaluation of the sensitivity and specificity of ultrasound in diagnosing congenital abnormalities was performed at the Joslin Clinic and Brigham and Women's Hospital.[11] Thirty-eight major congenital abnormalities occurred among 32 infants. Eighteen major malformations were diagnosed by ultrasound performed between 12 and 23 weeks gestation. All six central nervous system malformations and all five life-threatening cardiac lesions were identified. Lesions not identified by

TABLE IX. Maternal Serum Alpha–Fetoprotein Weight-Adjusted Levels by White Class*

Class	Number	Median MOM
B	32	.76
C	56	.81
D	38	.86
F, FR, R, T	38	.84

*MOM, multiples of the median.

TABLE X. Maternal Serum Alpha-Fetoprotein Levels According to Hb A_1 Concentration*

Hb A_1	Number	Median MOM
≤7.6	45	.85
7.7–8.3	40	.86
8.4–9.3	42	.84
≥9.4	37	.69

*MOM, multiples of the median.

ultrasound included interventricular septal defects, unilateral renal ageneses, abnormalities of hands or feet, and cleft palate without cleft lip. None of these missed abnormalities was life-threatening. Two false positive readings involved diagnoses of mild hydronephrosis which resolved on later examinations during the pregnancies. Overall, the sensitivity was 56% and the specificity was 99.5%. There was a 7.3% incidence of congenital abnormalities in this population, and a positive and negative predictive value of 90% and 97% respectively.

CONCLUSIONS

The key to reducing perinatal morbidity and mortality owing to major malformations remains prevention. Glycemic control in the first trimester is not only relevant, it is critical. Since many women do not recognize their pregnancies until they are well into the first trimester, and since it usually takes several weeks of effort to attain good glycemic control, preconception control must be our goal. Women with diabetes in their reproductive years must be educated and impressed with the fact that they must plan their pregnancies and make a concerted effort to maximize control before conception. Euglycemia is not necessary to keep the risk of malformation to a minimum, but it is imperative that a good level of glycemic control be reached. Unfortunately, it appears that even excellent first trimester glycemic control cannot provide a promise of outcome equal to that for nondiabetic women. Until we can offer this to our patients, there is work to be done.

REFERENCES

1. Joslin EP: Pregnancy and diabetes mellitus. Boston Med Surg J 173:841–849, 1915.
2. Lawrence RD, Oakley W: Pregnancy and diabetes. Quart J Med 11:45–75, 1942.

3. White P: Pregnancy complicating diabetes. Am J Med 7:609–616, 1949.
4. Hanson U, Persson B, Thunell S: Relationship between haemoglobin A_{1c} in early type 1 (insulin-dependent) diabetic pregnancy and the occurrence of spontaneous abortion and fetal malformation in Sweden. Diabetologia 33:100–104, 1990.
5. Gregory R, Scott AR, Mohajer M, et al: Diabetic pregnancy 1977–1990: Have we reached a plateau? J R Coll Physicians Lond 26:162–166, 1992.
6. Gestation and Diabetes in France Study Group: Multicenter survey of diabetic pregnancy in France. Diabetes Care 14:994–1000, 1991.
7. Tchobroutsky C, Vray MM, Altman JJ: Risk/benefit ratio of changing late obstetrical strategies in the management of insulin-dependent diabetic pregnancies. A comparison between 1971–1977 and 1978–1985 periods in 389 pregnancies. Diabetes Metab 17:287–294, 1991.
8. Pedersen LM, Tygstrup I, Pedersen J: Congenital malformations in newborn infants of diabetic women. Correlation with maternal diabetic vascular complications. Lancet i:1124–1126, 1964.
9. Drury MI, Greene AT, Stronge JM: Pregnancy complicated by clinical diabetes mellitus: A study of 600 pregnancies. Obstet Gynecol 49:519–522, 1977.
10. Gabbe SG, Mestman JH, Freeman RK, Goebelsmann UT, Lowensohn RI, Nochimson D, Cetrulo C, Quilligan EJ: Management and outcome of pregnancy in diabetes mellitus, classes B to R. Am J Obstet Gynecol 129:723–732, 1977.
11. Greene MF, Benacerraf BR: Prenatal diagnosis in diabetic gravidas: Utility of ultrasound and maternal serum alpha-fetoprotein screening. Obstet Gynecol 77:520–524, 1991.
12. Soler NG, Walsh CH, Malins JM: Congenital malformations in infants of diabetic mothers. Quart J Med 178:203–213, 1976.
13. Ylinen K, Aula P, Stenman U-H, Kesaniemi-Kuokkanen T, Teramo K: Risk of minor and major fetal malformations in diabetics with high haemoglobin A1c values in early pregnancy. Br Med J 289:345–346, 1984.
14. Simpson JL, Elias S, Martin AO, Palmer MS, Ogata ES, Radvany RA: Diabetes in pregnancy, Northwestern University series (1977–1981). 1. Prospective study of anomalies in offspring of mothers with diabetes mellitus. Am J Obstet Gynecol 146:263–270, 1983.
15. Kitzmiller JL, Cloherty JP, Younger MD, Tabatabaii A, Rothchild SB, Sosenko I, Epstein MF, Singh S, Neff RK: Diabetic pregnancy and perinatal morbidity. Am J Obstet Gynecol 131:560–580, 1978.
16. Ballard JL, Holroyde J, Tsang RC, Chan G, Sutherland JM, Knowles HC: High malformation rates and decreased mortality in infants of diabetic mothers managed after the first trimester of pregnancy (1956–1978). Am J Obstet Gynecol 148:1111–1118, 1984.
17. Kucera J: Rate and type of congenital anomalies among offspring of diabetic women. J Reprod Med 7:61–70, 1971.
18. Milunsky A, Alpert E, Kitzmiller JL, Younger MD, Neff RK: Prenatal diagnosis of neural tube defects. VIII. The importance of serum alpha-fetoprotein screening in diabetic pregnant women. Am J Obstet Gynecol 142:1030–1032, 1982.
19. Mills JL, Baker L, Goldman AS: Malformations in infants of diabetic mothers occur before the seventh gestational week. Implications for treatment. Diabetes 28:292–293, 1979.
20. McCarter RJ, Kessler II, Comstock GW: Is diabetes mellitus a teratogen or a coteratogen? Am J Epidemiol 125:195–205, 1987.
21. Chung CS, Myrianthopoulos WC: Factors affecting risks of congenital malformations. Birth Defects: Original Article Series 11:10; 23–37, 1975.
22. Comess LJ, Bennett PH, Man MB, Burch TA, Miller M:. Congenital anomalies and diabetes in the Pima Indians of Arizona. Diabetes 18:471–477, 1969.
23. Leslie RDG, John PN, Pyke DA, White JM: Haemoglobin A_1 in diabetic pregnancy. Lancet ii:958–959, 1978.

24. Miller E, Hare JW, Cloherty JP, Dunn PJ, Gleason RE, Soeldner S, Kitzmiller JL: Elevated maternal hemoglobin A1c in early pregnancy and major congenital anomalies in infants of diabetic mothers. N Engl J Med 304:1331–1334, 1981.
25. Mills JL, Fishl AR, Knopp RH, Ober CL, Jovanovic LG, Polk BF: Malformations in infants of diabetic mothers: Problems in study design. Prev Med 12:274–286, 1983.
26. Mills JL, Knopp RH, Simpson JL, Jovanovic-Peterson L, Metzger BE, Holmes LB, Aarons JH, Brown Z, Reed GF, Bieber FR, Van Allen M, Holzman I, Ober C, Peterson CM, Withiam MJ, Duckles A, Mueller-Heubach E, Polk BF: Lack of relation of increased malformation rates in infants of diabetic mothers to glycemic control during organogenesis. N Engl J Med 318:671–676, 1988.
27. Greene MF: Prevention and diagnosis of congenital anomalies in diabetic pregnancies. Clinics in Perinatology 20:533–547, 1993.
28. Fuhrmann K, Reiher H, Semmler K, et al: Prevention of congenital malformations in infants of insulin-dependent diabetic mothers. Diabetes Care 6:219–223, 1983.
29. Damm P, Molsted-Pedersen L: Significant decrease in congenital malformations in newborn infants of an unselected population of diabetic women. Am J Obstet Gynecol 161:1163–1167, 1989.
30. Steel JM, Johnstone FD, Hepburn DA, et al: Can prepregnancy care of diabetic women reduce the risk of abnormal babies? Br Med J 301:1070–1074, 1990.
31. Kitzmiller JL, Gavin LA, Gin GD, et al: Preconception care of diabetes: Glycemic control prevents congenital anomalies. JAMA 265:731–736, 1991.
32. Willhoite MB, Bennert HW, Palomaki GE, et al: The impact of preconception counseling on pregnancy outcomes. The experience of the Maine Diabetes in Pregnancy Program. Diabetes Care 16:450–455, 1993.
33. Gregory R, Tattersall RB: Are diabetic pre-pregnancy clinics worthwhile? Lancet 340:656–658, 1992.
34. Grimes DA: After office hours: Unplanned pregnancies in the United States. Obstet Gynecol 67:438–442, 1986.
35. Freinkel N, Lewis NJ, Akazawa S, Roth SI, Gorman L: The honeybee syndrome—Implications of the teratogenicity of mannose in rat-embryo culture. N Engl J Med 310:223–230, 1984.
36. Sadler TW, Hunter ES: Hypoglycemia: How little is too much for the embryo? Am J Obstet Gynecol 157:190–193, 1987.
37. Hunter ES, Sadler TW, Wynn RE: A potential mechanism of DL-hydroxybutyrate-induced malformations in mouse embryos. Am J Physiol 253:72–80, 1987.
38. Sadler TW: Effects of maternal diabetes on early embryogenesis: I. The teratogenic potential of diabetic serum. Teratology 21:339–347, 1980.
39. Sadler TW: Effects of maternal diabetes on early embryogenesis: II. Hyperglycemia-induced exencephaly. Teratology 21:349–356, 1980.
40. Pinter E, Reece EA, Leranth CZ, Sanyal MK, Hobbins JC, Mahoney MJ, Naftolin F: Yolk sac failure in embryopathy due to hyperglycemia: Ultrastructural analysis of yolk sac differentiation associated with embryopathy in rat conceptuses under hyperglycemic conditions. Teratology 33:73–84, 1986.
41. Goldman AS, Baker L, Piddington R, Marx B, Herold R, Egler J: Hyperglycemia-induced teratogenesis is mediated by a functional deficiency of arachidonic acid. Proc Natl Acad Sci USA 82:8227–8231, 1985.
42. Sadler TW, Phillips LS, Balkan W, Goldstein S: Somatomedin inhibitors from diabetic rat serum alter growth and development of mouse embryos in culture. Diabetes 35:861–865, 1986.
43. MRC Vitamin Study Research Group: Prevention of neural tube defects: Results of the Medical Research Council Vitamin Study. Lancet 338:131–137, 1991.

44. Czeizel AE, Dudas I: Prevention of the first occurrence of neural tube defects by periconceptional vitamin supplementation. N Engl J Med 317:1832–1835, 1992.
45. MMWR: Recommendations for the use of folic acid to reduce the number of cases of spina bifida and other neural tube defects. Recommendations and Reports 14. MMWR 41:1–7, 1992.
46. Wald NJ, Cuckle H, Boreham J, Stirrat GM, Turnbull HC: Maternal serum alpha-fetoprotein and diabetes mellitus. Br J Obstet Gynecol 86:101–105, 1979.
47. Campbell J, Gilbert WM, Nicolaides KH, et al: Ultrasound screening for spina bifida: Cranial and cerebellar signs in a high risk population. Obstet Gynecol 70:247–250, 1987.
48. Goldstein RB, Podrasky AE, Filly RA, et al: Effacement of the fetal cisterna magna in association with myelomeningocele. Radiology 172:409–413, 1989.
49. Hashimoto BE, Mahony BS, Filly RA, et al: Sonography, a complementary examination to alpha-fetoprotein testing for fetal neural tube defects. J Ultrasound Med 4:307–310, 1985.
50. Lindfors KK, McGahan JP, Tennant FP, et al: Midtrimester screening for open neural tube defects: Correlation of sonography with amniocentesis results. Am J Radiol 149:141–145, 1987.
51. Pober BR, Greene MF, Holmes LB: Complexities of intraventricular abnormalities. J Pediatr 108:545–551, 1986.
52. Benacerraf BR, Pober BR, Saunders SP: Accuracy of fetal echocardiography. Radiology 165:847–849, 1987.

SECTION V

PERSONAL CONSIDERATIONS

CHAPTER 13

Psychosocial Responses to Pregnant Women with Diabetes

Elisabeth Kay, MSW

INTRODUCTION

Having a chronic illness or a pregnancy evokes a variety of emotional responses. It is crucial to recognize throughout the treatment of the woman who is both pregnant and has diabetes that she will have ongoing and changing attitudes towards both conditions. Each influences the other and both affect her daily life. In this chapter, most attention will be paid to those women whose pregnancy takes place within the context of long-term diabetes. A woman will usually have been managing her illness in her own style for years. She will have developed her own particular psychological adjustment toward having a chronic illness. That is, she will have dealt with some of the emotional stages inherent in grappling with it and its implications for her[1] and she will, as do all women, have her own perceptions of pregnancy, childbirth, and mothering. There is for a period of many months a confluence of both these psychologically laden states—pregnancy and diabetes. The diagnosis of the pregnancy necessarily provokes a crisis since, the woman needs to rework her attitudes toward management of her diabetes and to incorporate the reality of being pregnant. This chapter examines some of the interwoven struggles confronting the woman whose pregnancy is complicated by diabetes. It also probes special issues of the prenatal and postnatal periods. Both the diabetes and the pregnancy are individually important. Sometimes they will be dealt with as separate entities; at other times they become merged. Moreover, as with any crisis, when one member of a family is affected, so are others. Each family member's emotional wherewithal affects his or her response to the pregnancy. Again, the interlocking complexity and structure of the

Diabetes Complicating Pregnancy: The Joslin Clinic Method, Edited by Florence M. Brown, MD and John W. Hare, MD.
ISBN 0-471-11031-0 © 1995 John Wiley & Sons, Inc.

unit affects the capacity of the woman whose pregnancy is complicated by diabetes.

REWORKING ATTITUDES ABOUT DIABETES IN THE CONTEXT OF PREGNANCY

One of the early observations of pregnant women dealing with their diabetes is their immediate awareness that their medical/obstetrical care is distinct from that of their peers. The requirements for more intense care give way to stressors not experienced in the non-diabetic population. At the Joslin Pregnancy Clinic, patients often receive preconception counseling in order to achieve the best glycemic control possible prior to conception. As they work even harder than usual at achieving safe ranges of hemoglobin A_1 to have a healthy baby, the pressure to conceive takes on an added stress. If conception happens quickly, they are likely to feel more like their non-diabetic peers. But if it does not, they find themselves not only monitoring their diabetic control tightly, but also dealing with the awareness that the pregnancy is not happening. One woman reported, "You know, it was as if I was pregnant for fifteen months. Once I knew I wanted a baby, all of my attention needed to be focused on both the diabetes and getting pregnant. I couldn't just be anxious or have fun trying to become a pregnant woman. I felt I had to behave as though I already was pregnant. Each month that I got my period, I was both angry and disappointed."

In addition to preconception watchfulness, appointments with the diabetologist begin early in the pregnancy, whereas their peers may wait until two and a half months gestation before visiting their obstetricians. The interval between visits is weekly, not monthly. Their infants have a greater risk of congenital abnormalities than do infants of women without diabetes. A woman who is working needs to make arrangements to attend the Clinic. She may need to work extra hours or use sick or maternity time benefits. The perception that the patient is taking excessive time off may threaten job security. The choice between economic survival and maternal fetal health and welfare become societal demons with which to wrestle. Spouses or significant others who wish to be present at antenatal appointments encounter the same difficult choices. Wanting to be involved, without the risk of being viewed as an unenthusiastic employee, is not often easily accomplished.

Hospitalizations for pregnancy related complications carry with them the same threats of job insecurity. But equally important is that they can pack an emotional wallop. The separation is upsetting to the family. Older children worry about what is happening to their mother. The under current sibling rivalry, already present at the idea of a new baby, is not helped if they view the hospitalization as an abandonment at a time when they need their mother the most. When a pregnancy related complication occurs, the need for hospitalization carries an inherent threat that something could be happening to the mother or the unborn fetus.

Medical management of a baby in the Neonatal Intensive Care Unit (NICU) for the first 12 to 24 hours of life and the obligatory separation between mother and child can be another stress for the woman with diabetes. A 35 year old woman who had Type I diabetes since age 14 described her experience.

> I had a miserable time getting pregnant in the first place. Not only did I have diabetes, I had also contended with infertility. Throughout my 27 week pregnancy, I was bleeding despite doing everything I was told. When my son was born, he was whisked off to the NICU with tubes everywhere. Miraculously, he is now fine. But I am not. I feel so cheated. I have spent the last year and a half wishing, being anxious, being compliant, and terrified. While I love my son, I wanted just one piece of feeling normal. Perhaps had I been able to hold him immediately after his delivery, I might have felt the joy I missed throughout the pregnancy. Because of his prematurity, the doctors, not I, became his life-savers.

Most women find it helpful when credence is given to the additional burden they must bear. Not only does this validation mesh with their own perception, but it also provides the emotional support necessary to work at the rigors imposed on them throughout the process. Conversely, when there is no recognition of the stressful nature of the pregnancy, women can become resentful and isolated. It is not uncommon for care givers to hear patients long for understanding from friends and family regarding what it is they go through. One of the most commonly agitating comments women speak of is some variation of, "But you should be happy that you have such wonderful providers. You know, it used to be that diabetic women were told they should not get pregnant!"

Reworking their perceptions of their diabetes includes a concern that with each visit they face the potential of learning that it has worsened. Appointments, therefore, often have an anxiety factor built in, whether or not they actually need to contend with any complications. While it is reassuring for most that their diabetes will revert to its pregravid baseline, it is nevertheless a time of threat and worry with specific attention to their disease. They must increase blood sugar and urine monitoring; titrate food, insulin, and exercise, trying to avoid insulin reactions on the one hand and high blood sugars on the other. They make appointments with ophthamologists for care or treatment of eye changes. They bring their sheets which they have filled out giving daily blood sugar levels for the previous week. While intellectually this kind of homework is understood as a mechanism used by their diabetologists to help determine insulin requirements, emotionally many report it feels like an area in which they personally can pass or fail.

As an example, a woman who is having difficulty tolerating the anxiety might present weekly sheets that are filled out with the same pen, have almost normal blood sugars without variation in levels, and, most telling, have no coffee or blood stains. It could be that the physician is looking at a particularly compulsive person who rewrites her log prior to coming to her appointment. But when her clinic blood sugar level and hemoglobin A_1 are high, reflecting poor diabetic control, perhaps then it is a matter that needs further investigation. By misrepresenting the diabetes control, the woman may be expressing a sense of failure she has dealt with all her life. Homework, always difficult, was graded with an "F." Helping the woman to understand that perfection is not the goal without shaming her that she has been "found out" is not easy. The practitioner needs to be aware that the patient is already humiliated at both her high blood sugars and her inability to do her "homework." If the patient reacts defensively to the sensitivity of the physician, there should be no surprise. No one likes to be caught with a hand in the proverbial cookie jar. If, however, in the ensuing weeks, there are no changes, the problem may be rooted in her past and best dealt with by the mental health provider on the team. This woman, as are all attendees, is well aware that the chances for having a healthy baby depend on her vigilance. Working toward resolving her hidden fears permits her to stay with the program in more positive ways.

Most women and providers recognize some psychological advantages of close monitoring of their diabetes. Receiving news of a lowered hemoglobin A_1 level often positively influences women's determination to maintain continued watchfulness. That accomplishment, in and of itself, has a way of improving self-esteem. It empowers them, letting them know that they can actually control and have an impact over their own bodies. It can strengthen the relationship with the team members, for it has been with their cooperative effort that the improvement occurred. Another positive by-product may be a decrease in anxiety about fears of defectiveness in their baby and, hence, a sense of reality that motherhood may actually come to fruition. The relationship between mothers and fathers develops into a richer mutuality, especially if the women have felt their partners have been a source of support for their efforts. In turn, the fathers' role as nurturer can augment their sense of participation in the pregnancy.

For some women and their partners, the need for close attention to their diabetes simply does not coincide with their personality styles or present situation. It requires high-powered organizational skills combined paradoxically with an ability to give up previously attained autonomy of self-regulation. Some women have reported that so much attention is focused on the diabetes that it becomes difficult to remember they are having a baby. Losing sight of the main purpose of intensified control is easily understood. Not infrequently, the partners, feeling left out and helpless, become controlling. If the pregnant women report less than perfect blood sugar results, the over-vigilant potential fathers notice every morsel the women ingest, how many times they forget to exercise, and stand by waiting to pounce when the home-monitoring numbers are too high. Rather than feeling supported by the partners' concern, the women report feeling resentful and infantalized. The goal for the couple is to develop a sense of mutual empowerment within the context of her diabetes and their pregnancy.

There is tremendous frustration for women who have unstable or brittle diabetes. Many arrive at the clinic already with a sense of failure, for despite their efforts, their control is labile. They are relieved when their physicians understand it is the diabetes and not themselves that subverts the regimen. This understanding is crucial, but it does not relieve the anxiety of delivery, since this group, probably more than any other, understands the relationship between near-normal glycemic control and a healthy baby.

A crisis can occur with early detection of abnormalities. The choice to terminate a pregnancy inevitably evokes ethical questions with which parents grapple. While the technology is available, societal support for electing a termination for a defective fetus is still in its infancy. The choice to terminate is often a terribly private one. It might be met by intense disapproval if others knew. Respecting this right to privacy is necessary regardless of the health team's individual and collective wish even if it is different from the couples'. Some termination services provide special counseling intervention in such situations. If the anomaly appears to be related to the diabetes, then helping the woman with her guilt becomes a part of the focus of the mental health intervention.

There is also a group of women whose diabetes complications make termination of the pregnancy inevitable. These women may be suffering from severe renal compromise, gastroparesis, or, rarely, coronary artery disease. The decision to intervene is made with regard to the health of both mother and fetus. At this point, the women are usually hospitalized. Most feel sick and lethargic. The psychological ramifications can be profound. Some of these patients have not known of the existence of renal disease before the pregnancy. This may be because it was not diagnosed or because of a psychological need to deny the reality. In either case, they need to come to grips that their management will now hinge on how their kidneys are functioning. These patients face the threat that their body cannot support a pregnancy. In addition, they must cope with the feelings that the pregnancy caused their kidneys to malfunction. Self-blame and rage are common emotions, subdued sometimes only because of lack of energy. Ambivalence about the pregnancy and the baby abound since they feel threatened with their own mortality. Some days they want to have the pregnancy terminated; other days they are willing "to do anything" to maintain it. It needs to be anticipated that these women will regress in their behavior, since so much is now out of their control. Moreover their family members are also upset. Some partners are able to put aside their own inner turmoil to stay empathic toward their women's angst. Others go through similar emotional swings, blaming the health team or their partner for the deteriorating conditions.

If the critical medical situation necessitates termination of a pregnancy, a new reality needs to be addressed. The couple will need a great deal of support for themselves as they begin grieving for a lost pregnancy. Encouragement of this process is crucial. While stressing the fact that it was the disease, not the woman, that caused the loss, this does not mitigate the profound sense of sadness, fear, and narcissistic injury. The process of healing the hurt from their lost dreams will come in its own time and place; it will often be uneven and develop its own idiosyncratic nature. Medical and obstetrical providers, who are aware that each couple will react differently, can help by validating what they hear as normal, given the special circumstances for the termination. At the appropriate time, the couple will need to be advised about future pregnancies.

In summary, then, this population, in facing pregnancy, needs to give new attention and sometimes new meaning to their diabetes. It is a complex process, sometimes dependent on their psychosocial situation, their own physiology, or the interweaving of the two.

PSYCHOSOCIAL PROCESSES OF PREGNANCY WHEN DIABETES IS PRESENT

It is well established that pregnancy is "a period of psychologic unrest."[2] Psychoanalytic researchers have identified a variety of developmental tasks for women in order to achieve optimal maturation during pregnancy. Bibring pointed out the need for women to accept the concept that they are temporarily at one with another human being. Once the physical and psychological symbiosis is accepted, the next step is preparing for the separation that occurs at the time of delivery. While integrating these complex feelings toward the fetus, they are altering their relationship with the father of the infant. Women must now add to their self-concepts the role of motherhood. Finally, pregnancy offers an opportunity to begin to change the relationship that women have with their own mothers, as they become colleagues in the role of raising a family.[3] A patient who is working on this latter task said, "Now that I know I am having a daughter, I have suddenly become less willing to criticize my mother."

Caplan outlined similar tasks for women. He described the importance of accepting the pregnancy, developing an attachment to the fetus, and adopting a realistic relationship with the newborn.[4] All investigators point out that the women's ability to reach their optimal developmental maturity within the pregnancy period influences their initial successful parenting of the newborn.

For some women with diabetes the initial acceptance of their pregnancy is the most difficult task. They come to the Clinic with certain beliefs about themselves and their disease that need major alterations. Some women have been told that their diabetes precludes conception. In accepting the notion of infertility, they have not availed themselves of proper birth control methods in order to have a planned pregnancy. The may feel resentful and out of control of their reproductive lives or may disbelieve that they are pregnant. The psychological task is to integrate the reality that they are indeed pregnant, despite their previous view of themselves as incapable of becoming so.

Other misinformed women believe that a pregnancy would be life-threatening to themselves or to the fetus. Learning from a health team that it is almost as likely that they and their fetus can do as well as the non-diabetic population is welcome news. It takes time, however, to trust this reality.

One woman who was encouraged to maintain her pregnancy by our team reported her difficulty in making the adjustment.

> My diabetes has been taken care of by my internist for years. He strongly recommended that I never become pregnant. He's seen me through four hospitalizations and one episode of ketoacidosis. Is he not competent? Why would he tell me not to have children? If I follow your advice does this mean I need to give him up?

Thus, for particular groups of women, the tasks of initial acceptance can be confusing and complicated.

Family members may also contribute to their sense of fragility and vulnerability. Clinicians have been particularly aware of the fears of mothers for their daughters, who are now pregnant and have diabetes. The women, looking to bridge the collegial gap that Bibring wrote about, are unable to do so since their mothers are remembering frightening episodes of uncontrolled diabetes during their daughters' childhood and adolescence. Rather than being able to support their daughters' wish for children, they themselves become the ones who need support. The medical team can be enormously helpful by speaking to the mother, explaining what is likely to happen in a particular pregnancy. Even if complications can be expected, the decision to continue the pregnancy is one made now by the daughter as an autonomous adult. If diabetes has existed in the family and caused serious complications, it is not surprising that the pregnant daughter with diabetes becomes the victim of over-protectiveness in a way that is unsupportive. The kind of relationship between mother and pregnant daughter may indicate that a joint session with a mental health provider would be a useful intervention. Alternatively, the most help might be to aid the daughter to work through the sadness of having an unsupportive mother.

As noted in an earlier section, partners, too, may be unable to give the emotional support needed to help their women in ideal ways. Their overinvolvement or underinvolvement may leave the women isolated. Conversely, it may be very difficult for some pregnant women to accept the support of their partners. If they have minimized their diabetes as their way of normalizing their lives or as a way to avoid fear of rejection, becoming pregnant defies inattentiveness to their chronic diabetes. All women need support during this critical time; a woman with diabetes needs more of it.

In addition to grasping the idea of being pregnant with new demands upon relationships, there is also the process of attachment to the fetus. It can be related to the experience that women have had with previous pregnancies. If they have had successful outcomes, they may manage quite well with the present one. If, however, they have had any kind of pregnancy or perinatal loss, the ability to attach themselves emotionally to the fetus is usually altered. Women will often feel a sense of relief when a pregnancy has surpassed the time in gestation that they lost an earlier one. It is useful to acknowledge those difficult periods, both as a way of validating fears and helping to differentiate between now and then. As long as they are comfortable with their feelings toward the fetus, there is usually no reason to intervene. Mental health referrals are indicated if women are becoming overwhelmed with guilt at their nonattachment.

One woman sought help when she continued to feel nothing about the pregnancy or the fetus, despite her ability to go through the rigors of the regimen. Her reaction was particularly disturbing to her since she had become very involved with her first pregnancy two years earlier. That child, however, had been anencephalic and died soon after birth. Not feeling anything for her present unborn infant was her adaptive protection against the hurt of another loss. Realizing that she would first need to see for herself that this baby would survive, she allowed herself to remain detached until delivery. Her guilt subsided as she was assured her reactions were normal. She focused on her blood sugar results since she knew the anencephaly had been related to her diabetes. At six weeks postpartum, she reported that it had taken her some weeks to feel comfortable with her daughter. She was pleased that she could monitor her own growth in her capacity to feel, rather than only the cognitive monitoring of her glucose.[5]

As time for labor and delivery approaches, women become physically and psychologically prepared for the separation between themselves and the fetus. When an induction or Cesarean section is based on fetal lung maturity, amniocentesis takes on special meaning. Women, who feel ready to meet their newborn, are invariably disappointed if the amniocentesis results require a delay in delivery. It is our experience that women, whose pregnancies have been marked by additional complications such as bleeding, polyhydramnios, or hypertension, are more anxious to be delivered; they have a greater need to know that the infant is safe.

Delivery is, of course, the culmination of all the work to ensure both their and the infants' optimal health. Pain is one aspect of labor and delivery. Women, especially those without medical complications, sometimes measure their self-worth by their behavior during this time. They report feeling ashamed if they do not perform according to their own or others' expectations. Using anesthesia or being deprived of a natural birth, similarly, can produce feelings of inadequacy.[6] Women with diabetes often have fewer available choices and higher rates of Cesarean sections. They tend to focus less on their behavior and route of delivery than they do on knowing the health of the baby. Prevalent issues such as birthing rooms and natural childbirth, are less significant than in the general population. More important is the need for ongoing reassurance from those present in the labor and delivery suite. They realize that their bodies are truly out of control and express feelings of being frightened. They also elaborate on the overwhelming joy and excitement of the birth itself.

The final phase of pregnancy, the immediate postpartum period, is also part of a complicated process of change. The parents begin to integrate the newborn into their evolving sense of family, with all its joys as well as worries. Initially, the new mother needs to tend to her own recovery, whether this be from a vaginal or surgical birth. Decisions about breast or bottle feeding need attention. This choice is carefully made by the woman, her family, and her providers. If breast feeding is not suitable, shame can easily be provoked. The risk of this occurring can stress the already fearful new mother. At the time of discharge from the hospital, the new unit leaves the intensity of professional care and begins to operate on its own.

An interesting phenomenon has been reported by a number of patients at their six-week postpartum visit. They speak of missing the comfort of their weekly appointments. At the beginning of the pregnancy, most had difficulty accepting the need for close monitoring. But during the process of the careful supervision they felt quite safe. Moreover, strong ties to particular team members have been broken with the end of the pregnancy. The team had become an integral part of the patient's support system. A loss is incurred.

The postpartum period also brings a variety of changes. Often a mother will experience lability of moods stemming from normal hormonal shifts, blood sugar level swings, and sleep deprivation. Dr. Anderson's term, "general maternal fatigue" succinctly defines the way mothers describe not having a clue how their day went by so quickly, without being able to describe anything they accomplished. For previously working women, adjustments are complex. For some, being on maternity leave brings with it a sense of serenity as they learn about themselves and their baby. For others, the adjustment is different. They miss the self-esteem work provided. Since it is hard to explain how the time passed with this newborn, they wonder how they managed to accomplish what they used to when they worked all day. One woman ruefully said, "You know, my plan had been that once I was on my maternity leave I would make a gourmet dinner every night. My son is six weeks old and I haven't done a thing." Concern about how to integrate motherhood, a return to work, and management of a chronic disease play important roles in the psychological dynamics of postpartum women with diabetes.

Allowing a period to review the entire pregnancy usually alleviates any residue of uncomfortable feelings and helps promote a healthy integration of the baby into the family. If, instead, women present with postpartum depression, immediate psychiatric attention is indicated.

When a baby is delivered prematurely, or with one or a series of congenital anomalies, the parents are faced with the possibility of prolonged anxiety and stress. Initially, most women are ill-equipped to take on the neonatal illness, since they are also recovering from the birthing experience. The sensitivity of the Neonatal Intensive Care Unit is critical in helping parents cope with the roller coaster experience that often occurs with these infants. Here, too, the women lose the connection to their former health team members; new ones, the neonatal staff, become vital.

Despite the advances in obstetric, diabetic, and pediatric management, which reduce the chances of neonatal and intrauterine fetal demise, there are occasions when sudden or even anticipated losses still happen at delivery or after arduous hopeful weeks when the infant is in the NICU. Careful attention to the bereavement experience must be given to these women and their families, both because of the current tragedy, as well as for the impact it can have on future pregnancies and the capacity to parent. Ample literature supports the necessity of formalizing the grieving process of infant loss.[7–9] Since diabetes is often implicated in these deaths, guilt and rage are often seen intermingled with profound sadness. According to May, the group treatment model has been particularly useful since it 1) gives permission to discuss the infant and cause of death, 2) decreases the sense of being the only couple who has experienced such an event, 3) provides a forum for sharing emotions and 4) is a place where couples can address their discomfort over the reactions of friends and family members.[9] If parents cannot avail themselves of a bereavement group, members of the health care team can be helpful by encouraging an open environment for discussion while appreciating the vulnerability these losses engender. It is important to allow for differences between the couple to "get over" the feeling of loss. While a variety of books and articles have been written about grief, each individual experience is unique. The grief will be over when it is over. Pressuring one or the other partner to "get on with things" merely increases a sense of isolation. It is more worrisome if there is no sign of mourning resulting from the trauma. Respecting the defensive nature of parental shock can be difficult for the health team which has less and less time in today's early discharges from the hospital to establish trusting relationships with their patients. It is nevertheless useful to let patients know that even if they feel little grief now, they may become overwhelmed with feelings when they get home. The name of the social worker or mental health provider should be made available as part of the discharge process. If they find they continue to have a kind of numbness about them for weeks at a time, they should also contact a mental health provider.

PERSONALITY STYLES

Given all the physical and emotional changes that occur throughout the months of pregnancy, it is well to keep in mind that each woman's personality style colors how she perceives her experience. In addition, it defines her ability to deal with health team recommendations.[10] A particularly obsessive woman used an insulin pump as a way to keep control of her blood sugars. She insisted on maintaining low blood sugar levels despite frequent unconscious reactions, one of which resulted in an automobile accident. She realized that she was annoying her doctors by her obstinate behavior, but she felt powerless to do otherwise. Her older sister who also had diabetes, was seen in the family as a baby killer, since years ago as a teenager she had delivered a stillborn. It was the family's understanding that the sister had caused the death because of her inattention to her blood sugars. This patient would not endure the guilt that her sister had. Moreover, her husband who was equally fearful, watched her every move. Though he felt he was being supportive, his rigidity was motivated by his own helplessness in the face of her pregnancy.

On the other side of the psychological spectrum was a woman who insisted that she could not keep to the diabetic program because she maintained that she had a "sugar addiction." She regularly bought several candy bars at a time, saved them until she could no longer tolerate the deprivation, and then ate them all in one sitting. She did not wish to hurt her infant, but the strength of her "addiction" got in the way. Intensive psychotherapy helped her to associate prior parental abuse with her need to soothe herself with sweets. She learned that her anxiety about an unsuccessful pregnancy outcome echoed childhood fears. She became more able to forgo her outmoded coping mechanism and use the health care team to deal directly with her fears.

MAJOR PSYCHIATRIC DISORDERS

With severe psychiatric disorders such as schizophrenia or manic depressive illness, pregnancy represents even more of a challenge for the woman and her health care providers. The team needs to become larger, incorporating a psychiatric provider as well as diabetologists and obstetricians. Issues of psychopharmacological medications and their potential teratogenic effects on the fetus versus the benefits to the mother need assessment. Discharge planning, if the woman cannot manage her infant safely, needs to begin early. With fewer and fewer state and local resources to help psychiatrically disturbed families, ethical dilemmas are increased for everyone. It can be especially difficult for health care providers with time constraints to maintain a nonpunitive stance toward these unfortunate women. Yet it is exactly what they need if they are to be successful in producing as healthy a baby as possible. Continuity of care providers is optimum.

TEENAGE PREGNANCIES

Just as pregnancy in women with rigid personality styles and major psychiatric illness elicits the need for special care, teenage pregnancy complicated by diabetes compels health care providers to understand a myriad of psychological mechanisms. Bibring writes that pregnancy in the adult woman represents a crisis. What happens when adolescents or young adults already having their own identity crises become pregnant? The late Erik Erikson defined adolescence as a period of identity versus role confusion. He believed that the reason young people fall in love was "less a sexual matter than an attempt to arrive at a definition of one's identity by projecting one diffused ego image on another and by seeing it thus reflected and gradually clarified."[11] Thus, sexual activity is not a wish to become pregnant, but a wish to help define oneself. These young people are struggling for autonomy and independence. Peer identification is heightened, with most of them dressing alike, eating the same foods, enjoying their own music, and often testing out alcohol and illicit drugs. If one adds parental alienation or family dysfunction to this already chaotic state, there is another element of crisis.

Adolescence is often a period of moderate to poor diabetic control. The need to be seen as normal, within the context of one's peer group, is powerful. This can be altered by the timing of the diagnosis of diabetes, how well it is integrated into one's self-concept, and how well the internal and external supports for its management are handled. When a teenager becomes pregnant, the emotional maelstrom of adolescence is added to the crisis of pregnancy.

The complex issues for the health care team in providing medical, obstetrical, psychological, and societal help take place in the context of a confused young woman. Often too overwhelmed, she cannot hear physician advice. A major issue, which appears hardest to address, is whether she wants to maintain or to terminate the pregnancy. Too often, the assumption that she will want to have a child—either to keep or to give up for adoption—does not permit an informed choice. Her right to choose involves proper counseling, which includes a reality check on what she will gain and give up as she becomes a parent. There is no one right decision; she can only make the best decision given accurate information. Some teens are hopeful that having a baby will increase their autonomy. In general, despite programs such as WIC (Women's, Infants, and Children), subsidized housing, and welfare, they are set back to a position of relying on the very parental structure from which they were fleeing. If they choose to continue with the pregnancy, they need to be instructed as to the expectations of the Clinic, appreciating that their freedom to experiment with their peer group may be curtailed. They will need to explore and develop their supports outside the health care team, so that a fallback system is in place after delivery.

Education about contraception for the teenager with diabetes should be an on-going part of her medical care. A young woman already on birth control pills, had diabetes, cerebral palsy, and asthma. Because of side effects, she was taken off her birth control pills without any substitution. She quickly became pregnant, adding another trauma to her already vulnerable body.

While some authors describe teenagers as "immature,"[12] they fail to recognize that they are doing what teenagers are supposed to do—working out their own identity issues and establishing real relationships. The natural course of this process is bumpy and irregular. Coping with all the stresses of a diabetic pregnancy, on top of the normal age appropriate fluctuations, justifies a referral to the mental health provider of the team. However, getting the teen to show up for appointments with a therapist is much easier said than done. One social worker explained how a normal adolescent might look like a borderline personality if the behavior occurred in an adult. All attempts at breaking through a particular young woman's arrogant defenses were impossible. Despite her hostility, noncompliance, spiteful personality, and high blood sugars, she delivered a healthy baby. Five years later, she returned to the Clinic, again pregnant. The "borderline" had had a metamorphosis; she changed into a lovely butterfly, had a five year old in tow, and was fully attached to both the program and the pregnancy. Only then she was able to talk about her terror the first time around and why it was so very difficult to engage with anyone who tried to get close to her. She also acknowledged that despite her reluctance to participate actively, knowing there was someone who was there was reassuring.

CONCLUSION

The above illustrations are only a few representations of the variety of combinations of people and situations that present themselves for care. It must be remembered that each individual has her own story that will need understanding above and beyond the medical/obstetrical concerns to insure optimum psychological and physical outcomes. The patients have not only their own psychology, but their family constructs, their pregnancy histories, their perception of their health, and their private longings and yearnings.

ACKNOWLEDGMENTS

The author wishes to thank Barbara Anderson, Ph.D., Clinical Psychologist at the Joslin Diabetes Center and Anne M. Korpi, MSW, Clinical Social Worker at the Brigham and Women's Hospital, Boston, MA and formerly a consultant at the Joslin Pregnancy Clinic for their guidance and encouragement.

REFERENCES

1. Holmes DL: Diabetes in its psychosocial context. In Marble A, Krall LP, Bradley RF, Chrislieb AR, Soeldner JD (eds): "Joslins's Diabetes Mellitus," 12th edition. Philadelphia: Lea & Febiger, pp 882–906, 1985.
2. Merkatz RB, Budd K, Merkatz IR: Psychologic and social implications of scientific care for pregnant diabetic women. Semin Perinatol, 2(4):373–381, 1978.
3. Bibring GL: Some considerations of the psychological process in pregnancy. Psychoanal Study Child 14:113–121, 1957.
4. Caplan G: Emotional implications of pregnancy, and influences on family relationships. In Stuart HC, Prugh DG (eds): "The Healthy Child." Cambridge: Harvard University Press, pp 72–81, 1960.
5. Hare JW, Kay E: Giving birth. Diabetes Forecast. p 26, Jan–Feb. 1981.
6. Coleman AD, Coleman LL: Labor and delivery. In "Pregnancy: The Psychological Experience. " New York: Herder and Herder, pp 79–84, 1971.
7. Borg S, Lasker J: "When Pregnancy Fails." Boston: Beacon Press. pp 3–10, 1981.
8. Lewis E: The management of stillbirth. Coping with an unreality, Lancet 2:619–620, 1976.
9. May R: Paper presented to the Ninth Annual Symposium for the Advancement of Social Work with Groups. Boston Park Plaza, October, 1987.
10. Kay, E: The emotional experience of pregnant diabetic women: Its impact on health care professionals. Diabetes Educator 9(2): 35s, 1983.
11. Erikson, EH: "Childhood and Society." New York: Norton, p 262, 1993.
12. Papatheodorou, NH: Diabetes and pregnancy: A psychological perspective. In Nuwayhid BS, Brickman CR III, Lieb SM (eds): "Management of the Diabetic Pregnancy." New York: Elsevier, 1987.

Index

KU-208-332

Element. cycling 181
Carbon cycle. 68, 69
Nitrogen cycle. 68, 71

Environmental Soil Science

BOOKS IN SOILS, PLANTS, AND THE ENVIRONMENT

Soil Biochemistry, Volume 1, edited by A. D. McLaren and G. H. Peterson
Soil Biochemistry, Volume 2, edited by A. D. McLaren and J. Skujiņš
Soil Biochemistry, Volume 3, edited by E. A. Paul and A. D. McLaren
Soil Biochemistry, Volume 4, edited by E. A. Paul and A. D. McLaren
Soil Biochemistry, Volume 5, edited by E. A. Paul and J. N. Ladd
Soil Biochemistry, Volume 6, edited by Jean-Marc Bollag and G. Stotzky
Soil Biochemistry, Volume 7, edited by G. Stotzky and Jean-Marc Bollag
Soil Biochemistry, Volume 8, edited by Jean-Marc Bollag and G. Stotzky

Organic Chemicals in the Soil Environment, Volumes 1 and 2, edited by C. A. I. Goring and J. W. Hamaker
Humic Substances in the Environment, M. Schnitzer and S. U. Khan
Microbial Life in the Soil: An Introduction, T. Hattori
Principles of Soil Chemistry, Kim H. Tan
Soil Analysis: Instrumental Techniques and Related Procedures, edited by Keith A. Smith
Soil Reclamation Processes: Microbiological Analyses and Applications, edited by Robert L. Tate III and Donald A. Klein
Symbiotic Nitrogen Fixation Technology, edited by Gerald H. Elkan
Soil-Water Interactions: Mechanisms and Applications, edited by Shingo Iwata, Toshio Tabuchi, and Benno P. Warkentin
Soil Analysis: Modern Instrumental Techniques, Second Edition, edited by Keith A. Smith
Soil Analysis: Physical Methods, edited by Keith A. Smith and Chris E. Mullins
Growth and Mineral Nutrition of Field Crops, N. K. Fageria, V. C. Baligar, and Charles Allan Jones
Semiarid Lands and Deserts: Soil Resource and Reclamation, edited by J. Skujiņš
Plant Roots: The Hidden Half, edited by Yoav Waisel, Amram Eshel, and Uzi Kafkafi
Plant Biochemical Regulators, edited by Harold W. Gausman
Maximizing Crop Yields, N. K. Fageria
Transgenic Plants: Fundamentals and Applications, edited by Andrew Hiatt
Soil Microbial Ecology: Applications in Agricultural and Environmental Management, edited by F. Blaine Metting, Jr.
Principles of Soil Chemistry: Second Edition, Kim H. Tan
Water Flow in Soils, edited by Tsuyoshi Miyazaki
Handbook of Plant and Crop Stress, edited by Mohammad Pessarakli
Genetic Improvement of Field Crops, edited by Gustavo A. Slafer
Agricultural Field Experiments: Design and Analysis, Roger G. Petersen
Environmental Soil Science, Kim H. Tan

Additional Volumes in Preparation

Mechanisms of Plant Growth and Improved Productivity: Modern Approaches, edited by Amarjit S. Basra
Selenium in the Environment, edited by W. T. Frankenberger and Sally Benson
Plant–Environment Interactions, edited by Robert E. Wilkinson
Handbook of Plant and Crop Physiology, edited by Mohammad Pessarakli
Handbook of Phytoalexin Metabolism and Action, edited by M. Daniel and R. P. Purkayastha
Seed Development and Germination, edited by Jaime Kigel and Gad Galili

Environmental Soil Science

Kim H. Tan
The University of Georgia
Athens, Georgia

Marcel Dekker, Inc. New York • Basel • Hong Kong

Library of Congress Cataloging-in-Publication Data

Tan, Kim H. (Kim Howard)
Environmental soil science / Kim H. Tan
p. cm. — (Books in soils, plants, and the environment)
Includes bibliographical references (p. 255) and index.
ISBN 0-8247-9198-3 (acid-free paper)
1. Soil science. 2. Soils. 3. Soil ecology. 4. Soil pollution.
I. Title. II. Series.
S591.T35 1994
631.4—dc20 94-2466
CIP

The publisher offers discounts on this book when ordered in bulk quantities. For more information, write to Special Sales/Professional Marketing at the address below.

This book is printed on acid-free paper.

Copyright © 1994 by MARCEL DEKKER, INC. All Rights Reserved.

Neither this book nor any part may be reproduced or transmitted in any form or by any means, electronic or mechanical, including photocopying, microfilming, and recording, or by any information storage and retrieval system, without permission in writing from the publisher.

MARCEL DEKKER, INC.
270 Madison Avenue, New York, New York 10016

Current printing (last digit):
10 9 8 7 6 5 4 3 2

PRINTED IN THE UNITED STATES OF AMERICA

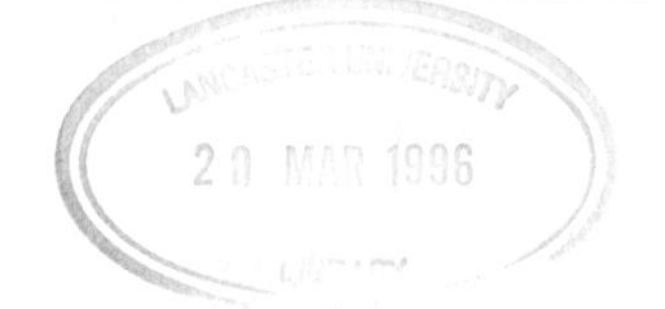

95 07146

PREFACE

The tremendous pressure on our soils and the environment by the industrial and agricultural expansion of the last few decades has created a new burst of questions on environmental quality. The intensive use and misuse of our soil, water, and air resources due to population expansion and the increasing level of pollution that accompanies an increasing standard of living have augmented the hazard of declining soil productivity. The use of fertilizers, insecticides, and herbicides in agriculture has expanded tremendously; and the pollution of streams and lakes and the contamination of soils and groundwater with toxic chemicals have become more widespread. These trends have resulted in an increased sense of awareness of environmental issues.

A large amount of information is, in fact, available on environmental problems and the use of soil for disposal of organic wastes. However, most such books on soil science are based on the traditional concepts of soil conservation and erosion. Until now there has not been a book relating the principles of recent environmental issues to soil science because information on global warming, ozone depletion, and acid rain has been scant.

Environmental soil science, which can be defined as the science of soils in relation to the environment, examines how soils are the product of the environment and how their properties are closely associated with environmental factors. Those who acquaint themselves with environmental principles in soil science are better able to prevent or to recognize an environmental problem when it arises and to find ways to solve it intelligently. This book is written with the purpose of relating environmental principles and soil science in plain language, easy to comprehend by a wide range of agricultural and environmental scientists, soil remediation specialists, microbial ecologists, horticulturists, engineers, geologists, foresters, and professionals and students in related disciplines.

The organization of the book does not follow the traditional division into the physical, chemical, and biological characteristics of soil, since this book is not intended to provide another version of the many textbooks existing on *basic soils*. Instead, the chapters are arranged according to the different soil constituents, e.g., solid, liquid, and gas. This format helps elucidate the natural coexistence of basic soil properties with environmental science. The soil constituents control soil characteristics and reactions, and many of these soil reactions affect the environment. Therefore, the text starts with an attempt to show the effect of environmental factors in the formation of different kinds of soils, and the dominant impact of climate and vegetation in determining the distribution of these soils in the world. This is followed by chapters 2 through 5, in which the soil constituents in the solid, liquid, and gas phases are discussed in terms of their interactions with the environment. The effects of environmental factors on weathering of primary minerals and formation of clay minerals are stressed in chapter 2. The organic components, biochemical reactions, and interrelationships with the environment are highlighted in chapter 3. Gaseous components, biochemical reactions in aerobic and anaerobic conditions, and their implications in pollution of soil and atmospheric air are featured in chapter 4. Soil water, dissolved macro- and micronutrients, and their relationship to environmental processes, e.g., eutrophication, are discussed in chapter 5. The reactions of dissolved inorganic and organic solids, and dissolved CO_2 and O_2 gas, are included as they are important in affecting environmental quality. Chapter 6 discusses the electrochemical properties of clay and humic acids and their significance in pollution. Chapter 7 examines efforts in crop production and the consequent changes they bring to soils and the environment, whereas chapters 8 and 9 summarize alternative methods in crop production, e.g., soilless agriculture and biotechnology. The final chapter concerns soil and pollution, assessing the implications of agricultural and industrial wastes for environmental quality. Acid rain, the greenhouse effect, and the depletion of ozone are among covered topics.

I want to thank Dr. Harry A. Mills, Professor of Horticulture, University of Georgia, and Dr. J. B. Jones, Jr., Director, Macro-Micro International, Inc., Athens, GA, for their review and constructive criticism. Appreciation is extended to Ms. Nickie Whitehead for reading and editing the manuscript and to Dr. Juan Carlos Lobartini and Mr. John A. Rema for their assistance with the laser printer in the development of this book. Thanks are extended to Dr. D. H. Marx, Director, Institute of Tree Root Biology, USDA—Forestry Science Laboratory, Athens, GA; Dr. M. F. Brown, University of Missouri, Columbia, MO; Tousimis Research Corp., Rockville, MD; Potash and Phosphate Institute, Atlanta, GA, and to the various publishers, scientific societies, and fellow scientists who gave permission to reproduce photographs. Special recognition also goes to the many unnamed persons who have assisted in the development of the book. Finally, I want to acknowledge the support and understanding of my wife, Yelli, who stood by with great enthusiasm and a lot of encouragement.

Kim H. Tan

CONTENTS

CHAPTER 1

SOILS AND THE ENVIRONMENT

1.1 DEFINITION AND CONCEPT OF SOILS

Soil is a term understood by almost everyone, yet the meaning of this term may vary among different people and soil can be defined in many ways (Brady, 1990; Foth, 1990). The farmer, engineer, chemist, geologist, and layman bring different viewpoints or perspectives to their concepts of soil. Environmentalists may even define soil differently than soil scientists. With the introduction of the pedological concept in soil science during the beginning of the 20th century, these differences have diminished considerably. Yet, even now, a commonly accepted definition of soil is still missing, notwithstanding the fact that most people agree that soils are products of the environment. Of the several definitions of soils that can be found in the literature, the definitions of Kellogg (1941) and the USDA Soil Survey Staff (1951; 1990) perhaps most closely reflect the relationship of soils to the environment. According to these definitions: "Soils are considered natural bodies, covering parts of the earth surface that support plant growth, and that have properties due to the integrated effect of climate and organisms acting upon the parent material, as conditioned by relief, over a period of time". Several soil scientists, notably Buol et al. (1973), may object to this definition, but the definition does show the dependency of soils on several environmental factors. It may be noted that this definition does not recognize moon or lunar material as soil. Lunar material, which is not affected by organisms, is excluded from the definition, but it may qualify as a parent material or regolith (Ming and Henninger, 1989).

The above definition of soils agrees closely with an earlier formulation of soils. In his famous book, *Factors of Soil Formation*, Hans Jenny (1940) reported that soils could be characterized by the formula:

$$S = f\,(cl, o, p, r, t)$$

In this equation, S = soils, f = function, cl = climate, o = organisms, p = parent material, r = relief, and t = time.

Climate, organisms, parent material, relief, and time are considered the five major factors in soil formation. According to such a formulation, these environmental factors are the main variables that determine *the state of the soil.* In other words, soils are formed by the combined effect of these factors. The nature of soils can be changed only when the variables cl, o, p, r, and t change individually or in combination. In such a formula the factor S (soil) cannot be changed to modify such variables as climate, organisms, or parent material, which is in practice true to a certain extent. For example, a change in the nature of soils will not result in a change of the parent material. However, it may apply to the variable o, organisms. Under certain cases, a deterioration of soil conditions brings about drastic changes in vegetation and/or other organisms. It is more difficult, however, to show a clear-cut relationship with the variable cl, climate, but a change in the nature of soils may sometimes result in a change in climate. A good illustration of this type of change is the formation of desert and savannah types of climate due to deforestation and the consequent degradation of soils in tropical regions of Africa.

1.2 PEDOLOGIC CONCEPT OF SOILS

Soil science is sometimes divided into *edaphology*, the science of soils as media for plant production, and *pedology*, the science of soils as biochemically synthesized bodies in nature (Brady, 1990). The concepts of these two branches in soil science are embraced by the above definitions of soils. The difference between them is only in their application or use. Edaphology applies to soil science mainly in crop production, as indicated earlier, whereas pedology studies the characterization, genesis, morphology, and taxonomy of soils. Nevertheless, the basic concept of soils in pedology still constitutes the key for perception of soils in edaphology.

According to the pedologic concept, the soil is a three-dimensional body in nature, showing length, width, and depth. An individual soil body, briefly called soil, occurs in the landscape side by side with other soils like the pieces of a jigsaw puzzle. Each soil is considered an independent body with a unique morphology as reflected by a soil profile. The soil profile is defined by specific series of layers of soils, called soil horizons, from the surface down to the unaltered parent material. It is formed by the integrated effect of the soil formation factors.

Measured by area, the soil can be small in size or a few hectares in extent, and it is common and more convenient in research and analysis to deal with a small representative part of the soil. The smallest representative unit of a soil body is called a *pedon* (Figure 1.1). A pedon has three dimensions and is comparable in some ways to the unit *cell* of a crystal. One soil body consists of contiguous similar pedons. This group of contiguous similar pedons in one soil body is called a *polypedon*. The polypedon or soil body is bordered on all sides by other pedons with different characteristics. The size of a pedon is measured

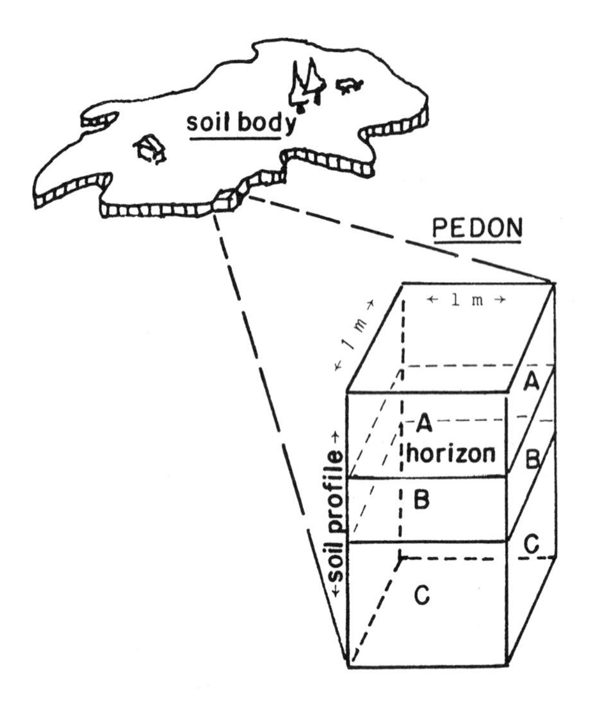

Figure 1.1 The relationship of a pedon to a soil body.

by its surface area, with the smallest measuring 1 m^2. A pedon is bordered on its sides by vertical sections of soils, the *soil profiles* (Figure 1.2). Each soil profile, extending from the surface down to the parent material, is composed of several soil horizons. The soil profile characterizes the pedon, hence it identifies the soil. The horizons tell much about the soil properties. They provide information on color, texture, structure, permeability, drainage, biological activity, and other attributes of importance in soil characterization, formation, fertility, crop

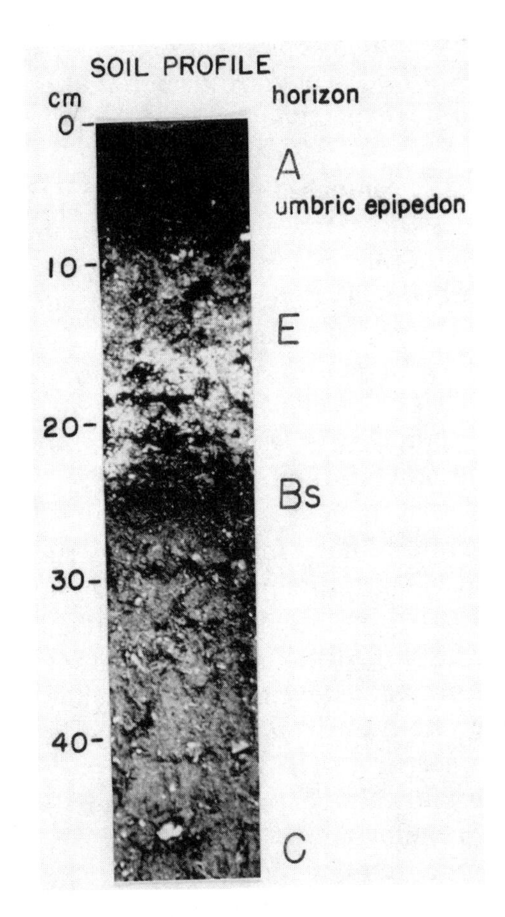

Figure 1.2 A soil profile of a sandy, mixed, frigid Entic Haplorthod (spodosol), showing the effect of the environment in its formation. The soil profile is characterized by an A horizon, rich in humus, underlain by an E horizon, which is bleached in color because of eluviation of humus and iron. The Bs horizon is dark in color because of illuviated humus and iron. The C horizon is the parent material.

production, and engineering. Six main groups of horizons, called *master horizons*, have been identified. They are designated by the symbols O, A, E, B, C, and R, respectively.

1. O horizons are organic deposits composed of dead, partially decomposed and decomposed vegetative material. This horizon, lying on the surface above the mineral horizon, is in many cases very thin, and only in undisturbed soils covered by vegetation can it assume considerable thickness. The name for this horizon, assigned by the U.S. Soil Taxonomy, is *histic epipedon* (Soil Survey Staff, 1990, 1992). The O horizon can be subdivided into O_i (non- to slightly decomposed), O_e (intermediately decomposed), and O_a (highly decomposed) horizons.

2. A horizons are the topmost mineral horizons lying below the O horizon. They are composed of large amounts of inorganic material intimately associated with humified organic matter, e.g., sand, silt, and clay. Because of its organic matter content, the A horizon is usually darker in color than the horizons below. In the absence of an O horizon, the A horizon is frequently the surface horizon. When the properties of the A horizon result from cultivation or related human activities, the horizon is designated by the symbol Ap (p = plow).

In the U.S. Soil Taxonomy, a number of A horizons are considered diagnostic for classifying soils. They are called *diagnostic epipedons*, from the Greek words epi (over), and pedon (soil). Four major diagnostic epipedons are of importance in soils of the USA. The first one is the *mollic epipedon*, a thick, dark-colored A horizon, which is rich in organic matter, and has a base saturation > 50% and a strong structure. *Umbric epipedon* is the second epipedon and is similar to a mollic, except for the presence of a base saturation that is lower than 50%. The third is the *ochric epipedon*, a light colored A horizon, which is low in organic matter and may be hard and massive when dry. The fourth epipedon, *histic epipedon*, has been defined earlier as a surface horizon (above the A horizon) rich in organic matter. This epipedon may be wet during some part of the year. A fifth diagnostic epipedon, of importance in Western Europe, should be added: *plaggen epipedon*. This is a human-made surface layer, more than 50 cm thick, that has been formed by long, continued manuring.

3. *E* horizons are mineral horizons located under the A horizon. They are the zones of maximum leaching or *eluviation*, zones of removal of soil constituents, e.g., clay, humus, Fe, and Al compounds. E horizons are white, pale, light, or bleached in color. White E horizons are called *albic* horizons in Soil Taxonomy. A horizons grading into E horizons are transitional horizons and carry the symbol AE. Similarly, E horizons grading into underlying B horizons are designated by the symbol EB.

4. *B* horizons are located underneath E horizons. In the absence of an E horizon, the A horizon lies directly above the B horizon. B horizons, frequently referred to as subsoils, are the zones of *illuviation* (accumulation) of soil materials removed from A and E horizons. Illuvial concentration of silicate clays, Fe, Al, or humus alone, or in combination may be present. B horizons grading into underlying C horizons are transitional horizons and carry the symbol BC.

Many of the B horizons are also diagnostic for characterizing soils. They are called *diagnostic subsurface horizons*. Some of the most important diagnostic subsurface horizons are the (1) *argillic* horizon (Bt), a B horizon enriched with silicate clays; (2) *spodic* horizon (Bh or Bhs), a horizon enriched with humus and Fe and Al oxides; (3) *cambic* horizon (Bw), a young B horizon, recently changed by physical and chemical reactions; and (4) *oxic* horizon, a highly weathered B horizon, containing Fe, Al oxides and 1:1 lattice type (kaolinitic) clays. For a complete list of these diagnostic horizons and their characteristics, refer to

Keys to Soil Taxonomy (Soil Survey Staff, 1992).

5. *C* horizons are located under the B horizons, and are considered parent materials of soils. They are mixtures of weathered rocks and minerals, and are largely unaffected by soil formation processes. These materials may rest upon the rocks from which they have been formed, or they may lie upon an unrelated geologic formation.

6. *R* horizons are the underlying solid rock formation with little evidence of weathering.

Soils may differ from one another in the nature and arrangement of horizons. The kind and sequence of horizons determine the *soil orders* and *soil series* in Soil Taxonomy. A farm may have several soil series, each of which responds differently to soil cultivation. By studying soil profile characteristics, these differences can be identified and inferences made as to the proper management practices. In general, road banks or preserved soil sections, called *soil monoliths*, can be used to examine soil profiles. One can also dig a pit, exposing a vertical section of the pedon, for this purpose.

1.3 SOIL ORDERS

As discussed in the preceding pages, soil profiles are also important in identifying soil orders. The order is the highest (broadest) category in the U.S. Soil Taxonomy system (Soil Survey Staff, 1990). This classification system divides orders into *suborders*, suborders into *great groups*, great groups into *subgroups*, subgroups into *families*, families into *series*, and the latter into *soil types*.

Eleven groups of soil orders (Table 1.1) are recognized. Placement in a particular soil order is based on differences in soil formation processes, as reflected in the nature and sequence of soil horizons. Each soil order contains soil profiles, whose properties are almost similar. The names of these orders are derived from Latin or Greek terms, and have a common suffix: *sol*, for soil.

1.3.1 Entisols

Entisols are young and shallow soils, and hence are characterized by A/C or A/R profiles. They are still immature soils and have profiles in which B horizons have not yet developed. The soils do not have many horizons for various

Table 1.1 Soil Orders

Order name	Derivation (meaning)	Formative elements carried to suborders[1]
Entisols	Recent, young	ent
Inceptisols	L. *inceptum*, beginning	ept
Mollisols	L. *mollis*, soft, friable	oll
Spodosols	Gk. *spodos*, woodash	od
Alfisols	Al = aluminum, fi for Fe = iron	alf
Ultisols	L. *ultimus*, ultimate weathering	ult
Oxisols	oxidation, highly oxidized	ox
Aridisols	L. *aridus*	*id*
Vertisols	L. *verto*, turn, invert	ert
Andisols	from andosols, Japanese an=black, do = soil	and
Histosols	Gk. *histos*, tissue	ist

[1] Formative elements are abbreviations from order name, and are used as suffixes in suborders names, e.g., psamment, aquept, ustoll, humod, etc. L. = Latin, and Gk.= Greek.

reasons, e.g., short formation time, occurrence on steep or actively eroding slopes, receiving frequent deposits from flooding, etc. Entisols with A/C profiles profiles are the entisols over sand deposits (Psamments). They occur extensively in the coastal plains of South Georgia, Florida, and Alabama. In contrast, entisols with A/R profiles are entisols over hard rocks (Orthents). These entisols are more common in the Rocky Mountains and other regions where rock formations can be found, such as the Blue Ridge Mountains, and the Piedmont Plateau.

The fertility of entisols varies considerably, depending on the conditions, from very low to very high. For instance, the alluvial floodplains of the Mississippi river are composed of fertile entisols, whereas the coastal plains of the USA have entisols with low fertility.

1.3.2 Inceptisols

Inceptisols mark the beginning of a mature soil and are characterized by A/Bw/C profiles. The B horizons are in the stage of formation and are called *cambic* horizons (B_w). As such, these soils are in a more advanced stage of development than are entisols. These soils are widely distributed in the world. Large areas of inceptisols are found in the United States in the Blue Ridge Mountains and the Piedmont Plateau. The natural fertility of inceptisols also varies widely. Inceptisols in New York and Pennsylvania are low in fertility, whereas those in the U.S. Pacific Northwest are quite fertile (Brady, 1990).

1.3.3 Mollisols

Mollisols are mature soils characterized by A/Bk/C profiles. The A horizon is typically a *mollic epipedon*, whereas the B horizon is usually a *calcic B* horizon, which carries the symbols Bk (k for the accumulation of calcium carbonates). Mollisols develop by a soil formation process called *calcification* under semihumid climates and tall grass vegetation. They are important *grassland soils*, and occur extensively in the Great Plains, west of the Mississippi River. Large areas of mollisols are also found in the great plains of Canada, and in Ukraine, where they are called *chernozems*.

Mollisols are very fertile and are considered to be among the world's most important agricultural soils. They contribute toward the development of the cornbelt in the USA and the wheatbelts in Canada and Russia.

1.3.4 Spodosols

Spodosols are mature soils with profiles characterized by a sequence of A/E/Bh or Bhs/C horizons. They are formed by a soil formation process called podzolization, typically in cool humid regions under a coniferous or mixed conifer-hardwood vegetation. Exceptions to the above may be present, such as the occurrence of spodosols in Florida and in the plains of the Amazon River in Brazil. Under the influence of acid leaching, Al and Fe compounds and/or humus are translocated to the B horizon, creating a *spodic B* horizon. When this B horizon is enriched, mainly with humus, a Bh horizon is formed. This type of spodosol is called a *humod* (hum = humus and od = formative elements from spodosol) in the U.S. Soil Taxonomy. On the other hand, when a mixture of Al and Fe compounds and humus is accumulated in the B horizon, a Bhs horizon is formed. Under certain conditions, Fe is the dominant illuvial constituent, and in this case a Bs horizon is formed. A spodosol with a Bs horizon is called a *ferrod* in the U.S. Soil Taxonomy.

Large areas of spodosols are found in the northeastern part of the United States and Canada, and in northern Europe, Russia, and Siberia. In Europe, these soils are called *podzols*. These soils are very acidic in reaction, and in the United States they are used for pastures in dairy farming. Limited spodosol areas in northern Maine are used successfully for potato production (Brady, 1990).

1.3.5 Alfisols

Alfisols are mature soils with profiles characterized by a sequence of A/E/Bt/C horizons. They are formed by a combination of podzolization and laterization processes in cool to warm temperate humid regions, usually under hardwood forest. These soils are affected by a more drastic leaching process than mollisols and are, therefore, in a more advanced stage of profile development. The surface soil varies in color from gray-brown to reddish brown. Alfisols with gray-brown surfaces were once called *gray-brown podzolic soils*. This name is still used in Canada, Australia, and parts of Europe. Because of the eluviation process, the B horizon is enriched with illuvial clay and is called an *argillic* horizon (Bt). Alfisols are highly productive soils with a percentage base saturation in the subsoil of > 35%, which ranks them medium in fertility.

1.3.6 Ultisols

Ultisols are mature soils with A/E/Bt/C profiles. They are formed by a combination of laterization and podzolization, with the emphasis on laterization, in warm humid regions to the humid tropics, where leaching processes are very pronounced. Under these conditions, the soils are highly weathered and the A horizons may accumulate varying amounts of Fe oxides, which impart their yellow to red colors. Enrichment of the B horizon with illuvial clay has also caused the formation of argillic horizons (Bt). Because of the drastic leaching process, the soils exhibit a very low base status, with a percentage base saturation in the subsoil < 35%.

Ultisols occur extensively in the southern region of the continental United States, Hawaii, and Puerto Rico. In other parts of the world, e.g., northern Australia, these soils are called *yellow podzolic, red-yellow podzolic*, or *red podzolic soils* according to the color of the surface soil. Because of their acidic condition and low base status, these soils have a very low fertility. They also exhibit a low degree of stable aggregation and are therefore sensitive to erosion. Nevertheless, with adequate liming, the addition of organic matter, fertilizer applications, and proper management, these soils can become quite productive in the southern region of the United States.

1.3.7 Oxisols

Oxisols are mature soils with A/B/C profiles. Formed by a laterization process in warm humid and tropical regions, they are typically highly weathered, even more than the ultisols. The B horizons of oxisols are *oxic horizons*, defined earlier as subsurface horizons containing large amounts of hydrous-oxide clays or sesquioxides and 1:1 layer type (kaolinitic) of clays. Because the electrical charges of these clays are highly variable, the soils are sometimes referred to as *soils with variable charges* (Theng, 1980). Many alfisols and ultisols are frequently included in this group of soils.

Large areas of oxisols occur in Central and South America and in Africa, Southeast Asia, and Australia. They are highly leached; therefore, they are acidic in reaction and low in bases. Nevertheless, the potential of many of these soils for agricultural production is far in excess of that currently realized, as has been demonstrated in Brazil and central Africa (Brady, 1990). Although they have very high clay contents, these soils have stable granular structures and are frequently nonsticky, loose and friable. Often they can be cultivated even under heavy tropical downpours. However, depending on the iron content, some oxisols can be converted into *laterites*, in which the formation of iron pans may inhibit the growth of plants.

1.3.8 Aridisols

Aridisols are mature soils with profiles characterized by a sequence of A/Bk/C, A/Bn/C, or A/Btn/C horizons. They are formed in arid and semiarid regions, where the dry conditions favor the accumulation of salts and other compounds in the surface and subsoil. When the B horizon is enriched with illuvial carbonates, it is called a Bk horizon. If sodium is the illuvial soil constituent, it is called a Bn (n for natrium, European for sodium) horizon. When both clay and sodium have accumulated in the subsoil, the horizon is designated by the symbol Btn.

In the western part of the USA, these soils are distinguished sometimes into *white alkali soils* and *black alkali soils*. The white alkali soils are blanketed with a white crust of salt crystals on their surface, whereas the black alkali soils are not covered by white crystals of salts and are black or darker in color. Extensive areas of aridisols are also found in the Sahara Desert of Africa, in the Gobi and Taklamakan Deserts of China, and in the deserts of Turkestan, the Middle East, and Australia. In Russia, the soils are called *solonchaks*, which are the equivalent of white alkali soils, and *solonetz*, the equivalent of black alkali soils.

Frequently the limiting factor for cultivation of aridisols is water. In areas where irrigation can be provided, such as with center-pivot irrigation in the arid regions of the USA, the soils can be made productive.

1.3.9 Vertisols

Vertisols are mature soils that are characterized by A/B/C profiles. Their name denotes their high swell-shrink capacity, which induces a natural plowing effect on the soil. This effect is caused by the presence of smectite or montmorillonite in the clay fraction, known for its high degree of swelling and shrinking. Wide and deep cracks are formed when the soil shrinks during dry condition, and surface soil materials may then crumble down or slough off into the bottom of the cracks. Upon wetting, these soils swell and subsoil materials are worked up again. The overall effect is like the "turning" effect of a plow.

The formation of vertisols are not limited to a particular type of climate. They are found all over in the world, especially where conditions favor the formation of smectites. Large areas of vertisols are present in India, Ethiopia, South Africa, and northern Australia. In addition, these soils are also located in Indonesia, Mexico, Venezuela, Paraguay and Bolivia. In the USA, these soils are found in east central (Houston) and southern Texas, and to a lesser extent in eastern Mississippi and western Alabama.

Physically these soils are very poor, making them less suitable for crops and engineering. In addition to their high swell-shrink capacity, the soils are sticky when wet and very hard when dry. Nevertheless, extensive areas of vertisols are cultivated with success in India and Africa for sorghum, millet, cotton, and corn production. In Indonesia, sugar cane is grown satisfactorily on vertisols.

1.3.10 Andisols

Andisols are young soils with A/B/C or A/C profiles (Soil Survey Staff, 1992), which were formerly called *andepts*, or *andosols* (Soil Survey Staff, 1975; Tan, 1984). Today they are defined by the U.S. Soil Taxonomy as soils with *andic* properties, which specify among others the presence of < 25% organic carbon content, 2% or more acid oxalate extractable Al and Fe, and a P retention of > 25% (Soil Survey Staff, 1990, 1992).

The original andosols are volcanic ash soils rich in organic matter, which imparts to the A horizon the distinctive dark to black color from which the name is derived. The original name andosol was derived from Japanese (an = black and do = soil). The B horizon often has the characteristics of a cambic horizon (Bw). The soils, first identified in Japan, were originally called *ando soils*. This name was later changed to andosol (Tan, 1984). In many other parts of the world and in the FAO soil classification system, the soils are still known as andosols. Using the new USDA criteria for andic properties, many red colored soils that do not resemble andosols are now "misplaced" in the new andisol order. Since the new name "andisol" was coined from the old term "andosol", the distinctive properties that give the original soil its name should be recognized and maintained, hence the criteria for andic properties adjusted accordingly. If not, it is suggested that the name andisol be deleted completely, and a new order name be created that does not have any association with the original name andosol.

Andosols occupy about one hundred million hectares, or 0.76% of the world land area (Dudal, 1976). However, on a global scale, they often do not occupy large areas in any one place. Instead they are associated with the presence of volcanoes, and hence are frequently scattered all around in small areas.

The presence of large amounts of organic matter — together with amorphous and paracrystalline clays, allophane, and imogolite — is the reason for the many unique properties of andosols. These constituents are responsible for their variable charges, extremely high waterholding capacity, and low bulk density. In Indonesia, andosols are fertile soils, and are a key factor in successful horticultural and many agricultural operations. Tobacco and the best tea plantations are found on andosols, whereas the more rugged part of the country covered by andosols is planted with pine trees. In Japan, andosols also constitute fertile agricultural soils. In a few cases, it has been reported that the soils are either low in phosphates or exhibit high P fixation capacity (Tan, 1965, 1984; Amano, 1981).

1.3.11 Histosols

Histosols are characterized by O/C or O/Ab (b for buried) profiles. The soil's O horizon is relatively thick and contains at least 12% organic carbon (Soil Survey Staff, 1975). It may lie on a mineral C or a buried A horizon. Histosols, therefore, are organic soils, and are typically formed in a water-saturated environment, where conditions are favorable for development of thick peat and muck deposits.

The presence of these soils is not limited to any climatic region. They may occur in environments ranging from the cold tundra to the tropical regions in the Amazon River delta. Large areas of histosols are found in the USA near the Great Lakes and in the coastal areas of the South, especially in Florida. With proper drainage, the histosols in Florida are successfully used in growing vegetables. In the Great Lakes region of the US, potatoes and flowers are grown on histosols. In the Netherlands, histosols are the sites for growing tulips and other cut flowers. Of particular concern with cultivated histosols is the problem of *subsidence*, the sinking or falling of the soil's surface below its original level. This phenomenon is caused by the continuous decomposition of the organic matter brought about by the better aeration.

1.4 RELATION OF SOIL ORDERS WITH THE ENVIRONMENT

As discussed above, several of the soil orders are formed under the dominant influence of climatic and vegetational factors. After formation, they are in equilibrium with the prevailing environment. Such soils were once called *zonal* soils (Thorp and Smith, 1949), and their geographic distribution follows climatic and vegetational zones in the world. Moving south on the northern hemisphere from the tundra circle to the Equator, a sequence of soils from spodosols to oxisols can be noticed. Their occurrence reflects the intimate relationship of the soils to the environment.

South of the tundra circle, the climate changes first into a cold-cool humid climate. Such a climate, together with a coniferous vegetation, favors podzolization and the consequent formation of podzols or spodosols. The type of forest, composed of coniferous trees called the *taiga forest* in Russia, stretches from northern Europe, Russia, and Siberia, to Alaska and Northern Canada. Here then is the zone of podzols or spodosols.

Next to this zone at a lower latitude is a zone with a temperate climate and a mixed stand of coniferous and hard-wood forests. This is the zone of gray-brown podzolic soils or alfisols. Further south on a latitudinal basis, a zone exists with a warm temperate humid climate and a hardwood forest, which favors the formation of red-yellow podzolic soils or ultisols. The next zone to the south, before the Equator, is a desert zone characterized by desert soils or aridisols. On both sides of the Equator lie the tropical zones with warm humid climates and tropical rain forests. These are the zones for laterization, hence the zones of lateritic soils or oxisols. This sequence of soils according to latitudinal zones with changing climates and vegetation will be repeated again in the southern hemisphere. Such a geographic distribution of soils corresponds with the distribution of soils in the USDA general soil map of the world (Brady, 1984).

A similar sequence of soils according to changing environment can also be noticed from east to west in the continental United States. The eastern seaboard of the USA, characterized by a humid climate, has a mixed stand of conifers and hardwoods in the Northeast and hardwood forests in the South-east. The Northeast is the major zone of spodosols and alfisols, whereas the Southeast is the main zone of ultisols. Moving from the eastern seaboard to the Great Plains in the west, a zone will be encountered with a semihumid climate and tall grass vegetation. This is the zone of mollisols, or more specifically the *udolls*. Further westward, the region is characterized by a semiarid climate and short grass vegetation. This is the zone of *ustolls*, or mollisols formed under dryer conditions. Lastly, next to this zone in the far West lies the zone of aridisols in the arid regions. Such a distribution of soils in the United States, in accordance with the changing environments from east to west, is reflected by the USDA general soils map of the United States (Foth, 1990).

CHAPTER 2

INORGANIC SOIL CONSTITUENTS

The soil system is composed of three phases: a solid, liquid, and gas phase. The solid phase, a mixture of inorganic and organic material, makes up the skeletal framework of soils. Enclosed within this framework is a system of pores, shared jointly by the liquid and gaseous phase. In *mineral soils*, the inorganic material is present in large amounts, whereas the organic fraction is found in substantially smaller amounts. Mineral soils are defined in *Soil Taxonomy* (Soil Survey Staff, 1990) as soils that contain by weight 80% or more inorganic and 20% or less organic material. On the other hand, in *organic soils*, the amount of organic matter far exceeds that of inorganic material. Organic soils contain by weight 80% or more of organic matter and 20% or less of inorganic material. These soils are formed only where the conditions are favorable for the accumulation of large amounts of organic residue, e.g., low temperatures and/or the presence of excessive amounts of water due to poor drainage. Since mineral soils are the most abundant in nature, the use of the term *soil* usually refers to mineral soils.

Inorganic material, organic matter, water, and air are considered the four major soil constituents (Brady, 1990). Their concentrations may differ from soil to soil, or from horizon to horizon. A soil with a loam texture and that is in optimum condition for plant growth is reported to have a volume composition of 45% inorganic material, 5% organic matter, 25% water, and 25% air (Brady, 1990). As indicated earlier, water and air are present in the pore spaces; thus a soil excellent for plant growth is composed of 50% solid space and 50% pore space.

The spatial arrangement in soils of the solid particles and associated pores is called the *soil fabric* (Figure 2.1). Kubiena (1938), who introduced the concept of soil fabric, believed it to be comparable with rock fabric, the arrangement of mineral grains in rocks. The coarse inorganic grains, together with coarse organic fragments (>2 μm), form the *soil skeleton* (Stoops

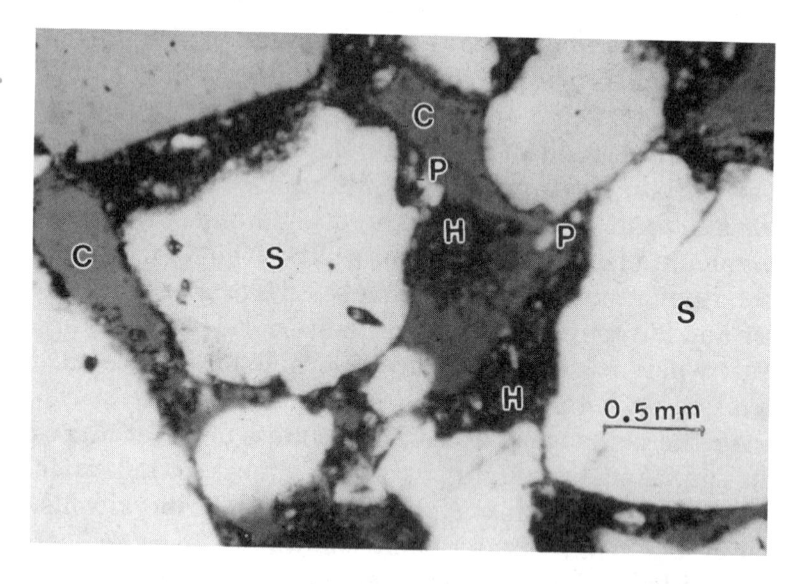

Figure 2.1 A thin section of soil showing a soil fabric, composed of sand grains (S), clay (C), humus (H), and associated pores (P). The sand grains form the skeleton of the soil fabric, whereas the clay and humus are the inorganic and organic plasma, respectively.

and Eswaran, 1986; Brewer and Sleeman, 1988). This can then be distinguished into inorganic and organic skeletons. All other materials smaller than 2 µm constitute the *soil plasma.* Skeleton grains may, of course, weather to produce plasma. The pattern produced by the arrangement of these soil constituents in association with pores creates the soil fabric. Many different kinds of soil fabrics can be formed, depending on the various combinations of size and shape of the soil constituents and on their occurrence as single grains or as aggregates. For more details on the different types of soil fabrics reference is made to Brewer and Sleeman (1988).

2.1 SOIL COMPOSITION

The inorganic fraction in soils is derived from the weathering products of rocks and consists of rock fragments and minerals of varying sizes and composition. Rock fragments are usually not considered soil constituents, but will yield soil constituents upon weathering. Separated according to size, the inorganic soil fraction can be distinguished into three major soil fractions: *sand, silt* and *clay* (Table 2.1), collectively called the soil separates. The particles with a diameter larger than 2 mm are gravel, stones, and boulders, and as indicated above are not considered soil constituents. They are rock fragments which upon weathering may yield sand, silt, and clay. Sand grains are irregular in size and shape, and are not sticky and/or plastic when wet. Their presence in soils promotes a loose and friable condition which allows rapid water and air movement. They are chemically inert and do not carry electrical charges, hence have low water-holding and cation exchange capacities. Silt particles are intermediate in size and possess characteristics between those of sand and clay. Some silt particles may be capped or coated by clay films as a result of the weathering of silt surfaces. Because of this, silt may exhibit some plasticity, stickiness, and adsorptive capacity for water and cations. Clay is the smallest particle in soil and has colloidal properties. It carries a negative charge and is chemically the most active inorganic constituent in soils. The presence of clay gives to the soil a high water-holding and cation exchange capacity. However, clay is sticky and plastic when wet. In the concept of soil fabrics, clay constitutes the inorganic plasma.

Table 2.1 Size Limits (Diameter) of Major Soil Separates According to the USDA and International System

Soil separate	USDA system	International system
	------------- mm	-------------
Very coarse sand	2.00 - 1.00	
Coarse sand	1.00 - 0.50	2.00 - 0.20
Medium sand	0.50 - 0.25	
Fine sand	0.25 - 0.10	0.20 - 0.02
Very fine sand	0.10 - 0.05	
Silt	0.05 - 0.002	0.02 - 0.002
Clay	< 0.002	< 0.002

Source: Soil Survey Staff (1962).

The inorganic soil fraction is composed of soil minerals, hence this component is also referred to as the *mineral fraction* of soils. *Minerals* are by definition inorganic substances in nature, possessing definite physical characteristics and chemical composition. In many other textbooks and in medical science, the term mineral refers to nutrient elements, such as N, P, K, Ca, Mg, etc. However, in soil science a clear distinction is made between minerals and nutrient elements. The term *mineral* may be defined as a compound composed of two or more elements, whereas a nutrient element is an element that can be used as food by plants.

The soil minerals can be distinguished into primary and secondary minerals. *Primary minerals* are minerals that have been released by weathering from rocks in a condition that is chemically unchanged. These minerals constitute the sand fraction of soils. *Secondary minerals* are minerals that have been derived from the weathering of primary minerals. They are present in the clay fraction of soils. The use of the terms primary and secondary minerals may frequently create some concern among soil scientists, since secondary mineral deposits are sometimes regarded as primary on a pedological basis.

2.2 MINERAL COMPOSITION

The composition of soil minerals is very variable, and depends on the composition of the rocks. The rocks from which the minerals originate are composed mostly of the elements O_2, Si, Al, Fe, Ca, Mg, Na, and K (Table 2.2). The soil minerals are, therefore, made up of these elements. Most of the minerals are either *silicates* or *oxides*. The Si in soil silicates is present in the form of *silica tetrahedrons*, which constitute the basic units of the crystals. On the basis of the arrangement of the SiO_4 tetrahedra in the crystal structure, six types of soil silicates can be distinguished. Listed in alphabetical order, they are (Figure 2.2): cyclosilicates, inosilicates, nesosilicates, phyllosilicates, sorosilicates, and tectosilicates (Tan, 1982, 1993). Most of the minerals in the sand and a major part of the silt fraction are cyclosilicates, inosilicates, nesosilicates, sorosilicates, or tectosilicates. Since they are coarse in size, they have low specific surface areas and do not exhibit colloidal properties. They participate in a number of chemical reactions and exhibit some adsorption, but are not really active in chemical reactions. Most of the minerals in the soil clay fraction are phyllosilicates. Other minerals may also be present, such as quartz and other primary minerals in particle sizes of < 2 μm, sesquioxides, talc, sulfides, sulfates, and phosphates.

Table 2.2 Chemical Composition of Basaltic and Granitic Rocks*

	Basalt	Granite	Average
		%	
SiO_2	50.4	69.5	60.0
Al_2O_3	16.9	15.7	16.3
Fe_2O_3	2.8	2.6	2.7
FeO	6.9	0.7	3.8
MgO	7.5	0.9	4.2
CaO	8.2	1.0	4.6
MnO	0.1	–	0.05
K_2O	1.6	2.8	2.2
Na_2O	3.3	2.6	3.0
TiO_2	1.4	0.9	1.2
H_2O+	0.8	1.0	0.9

*Source: Clarke (1924); Mason (1958); Mohr and Van Baren (1960); and Mohr et al. (1972).

2.3 PRIMARY MINERALS

Although numerous primary minerals are found in nature, only a few contribute to soil formation. Major primary minerals found in soils are listed in Table 2.3.

Quartz. This mineral, classified as a tectosilicate can occur as a primary or secondary mineral in soils. As a primary mineral, it is believed to be the last mineral to crystallize from the magma. The fact that quartz crystallizes at lower temperatures makes it fairly stable at earth temperatures. A quartz crystal does not exhibit cleavage, but will fracture upon impact. Although it is very resistant to weathering, eventually quartz grains can become rounded in nature.

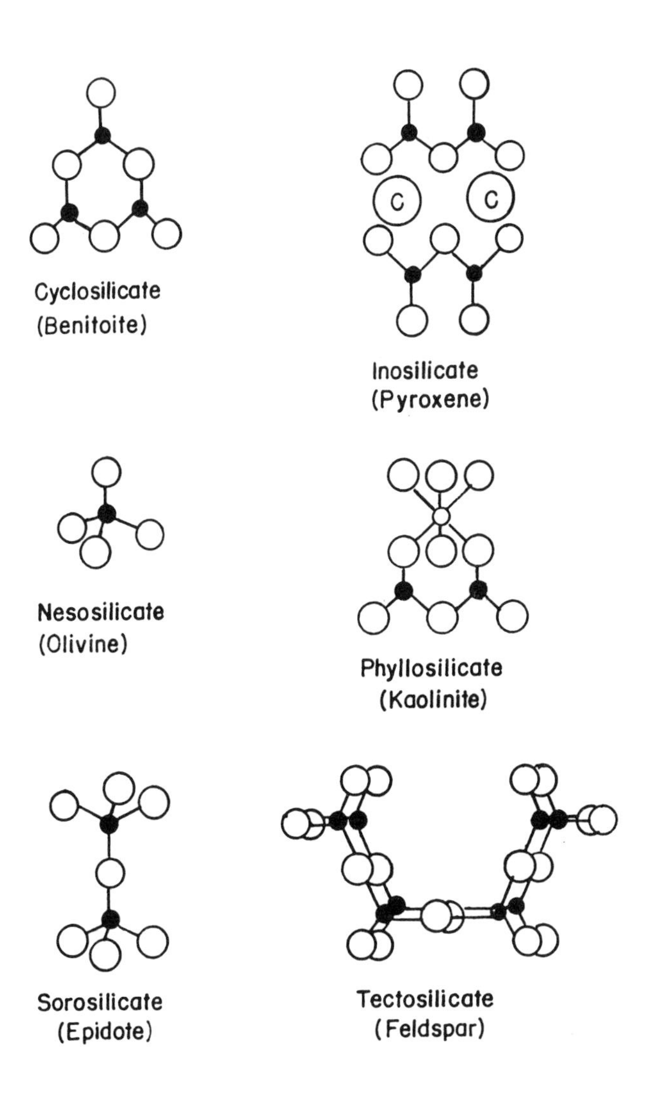

Figure 2.2 The molecular structure of soil silicates distinguished by the different arrangement of SiO_4 tetrahedra.

Feldspars. Feldspars are also members of the tectosilicates. They can be distinguished into two groups: (1) potash feldspars, e.g., orthoclase and microcline with a general composition of $KAlSi_3O_8$ as indicated in Table 2.3, and (2) plagioclase, e.g., albite and anorthite ($CaAl_2Si_2O_6$). Feldspar minerals are considered solid solution minerals with a framework of silica tetrahedra, in which the cavities are occupied by K, Na, and Ca. The minerals are almost as hard as quartz, but due to the presence of non-framework ions, they weather very easily.

Mica. The mica group belongs to the phyllosilicates, and exhibits a sheet structure similar to that of clay minerals. As indicated in Table 2.3, two types of mica minerals, muscovite and biotite, are recognized. Because of their sheet structure, these minerals exhibit cleavage and are easily attacked by water. Because of the presence of Fe and Mg in biotite, this mineral is less resistant to weathering than muscovite.

Ferromagnesians. Ferromagnesians, the dark colored minerals, are classified as inosilicates or nesosilicates. Two important groups of minerals in the inosilicates are pyroxenes, with single chain Si tetrahedra, and amphiboles, with double chain Si tetrahedra. The most common mineral species in the pyroxene group is augite, $Ca(Mg,FA,Al)(Al,Si)_2O_6$, whereas that in the amphibole group is hornblende. Olivine belongs to the nesosilicates, and is a common mineral in dark colored igneous rocks, such as gabbro and basalt. The presence of nonframework Ca-O, Mg-O, and Fe-O bonds forms weak spots in the structure.

Magnesium Silicates. These minerals are correctly called *serpentine* minerals. They belong to the phyllosilicates (Hurlbut and Klein, 1977). Major minerals in the group are antigorite and chrysotile, both characterized by the composition for serpentine, $H_4Mg_3Si_2O_9$, as listed in Table 2.3. The name *serpentine* refers to the green, serpent-like clouding of the minerals,

Table 2.3 Common Primary Minerals in Soils

Primary mineral	Chemical composition
1. Quartz	SiO_2
2. Feldspar	
Orthoclase, microcline	$KAlSi_3O_8$
Albite (plagioclase)	$NaAlSi_3O_8$
3. Mica	
Muscovite	$H_2KAl_3Si_3O_{12}$
Biotite	$(H,K)_2(Mg,Fe)_2(Al,Fe)_2Si_3O_{12}$
4. Ferromagnesians	
Hornblende	$Ca(Fe,Mg)_2Si_4O_{12}$
Olivine	$(Mg,Fe)_2SiO_4$
5. Magnesium silicate	
Serpentine	$H_4Mg_3Si_2O_9$
6. Phosphate	
Apatite	$(Ca_3(PO_4)_2)_3.Ca(F,Cl)_2$
7. Carbonates	
Calcite	$CaCO_3$
Dolomite	$CaMg(CO_3)_2$

whereas the name *antigorite* is derived from antigorio in Italian, and chrysotile from the Greek terms for golden and fiber.

Phosphate Minerals. This very large group of minerals does not belong to the silicates. Most of their members are so rare that they are seldom mentioned. Of the many types of phosphate minerals, perhaps only the apatite group is common in soils. Three types of apatite minerals can be distinguished: *fluorapatite, chlorapatite*, and *hydroxylapatite*, containing F, Cl, and OH, respectively. Of the three, fluorapatite is the most common. The apatite mineral is used in the manufacture of phosphate fertilizers. To render the P more soluble, the mineral is treated with sulfuric acid, H_2SO_4, and converted into the fertilizer superphosphate. The residue from the production of superphosphate contains large amounts of gypsum, $CaSO_4$, which is a valuable source of liming material.

Carbonates. Carbonates can be distinguished into three groups: *calcite, aragonite*, and *dolomite*. They are not silicates and are, rather, compounds composed of triangular groups of metal-carbonate, $-(CO_3)^{2-}$, complexes. Calcite is one of the most common minerals in soil formation. The name *calcite* comes from *calx*, the latin term for burnt lime. Aragonite is less common because it is less stable than calcite under atmospheric conditions. It is usually formed at higher temperatures than calcite. In experimental conditions, aragonite is precipitated from warm carbonated water, whereas calcite will precipitate in cold carbonated water (Hurlbut and Klein, 1977). For this reason, aragonite occurs near hot springs, and is also a major component of coral reefs and the pearly layers of oyster shells. Aragonite was first discovered in Aragon, Spain, hence its name. Dolomite is reported to have been formed from limestone, $CaCO_3$, by the substitution of some of the Ca for Mg. The mineral is named in honor of Dolomieu (1750-1801), a French chemist.

2.4 WEATHERING OF PRIMARY MINERALS

Primary minerals are affected by weathering processes. *Weathering* is defined as the disintegration and alteration of rocks and minerals by physical, chemical and biological processes. *Physical weathering* involves the disintegration of rocks and minerals into smaller particles. *Chemical weathering* is the decomposition and alteration of rocks and minerals into new materials with a completely different chemical composition, such as the secondary minerals. The chemical reactions responsible for chemical weathering are hydrolysis, hydration-dehydration, oxidation-reduction, carbonation and dissolution. For more details on the reaction processes reference is made to Brady (1990), Donahue et al. (1983), and Birkeland (1974). In *biological weathering*, physical and chemical decomposition processes are assisted by living organisms. For example, in a warm humid climate, plant growth is abundant and large amounts of humus are formed, containing humic acids and a variety of other organic and inorganic acids. The chelating capacity of these acids is important in the decomposition of soil minerals (Tan, 1986). In many cases, the effect of chelation or complex reactions on mineral weathering may exceed that brought about by hydrolysis (Birkeland, 1974).

The weathering of primary minerals not only causes new minerals to be formed, as indicated above, but also releases soluble materials. Many of the materials released are elements that can serve as plant nutrients, e.g., K, Ca, Mg, Fe, and P, and their release can, therefore, improve soil fertility. Potash feldspar, and muscovite, for example, are potential sources of soil K, whereas biotite can enrich the soil with K and Fe. Ferromagnesians are potential sources of soil Fe, Mg, and Ca, and apatite minerals are the main inorganic sources of soil P. Several of the elements released also have an important bearing in soil formation:

1. Si, Al, and Fe contribute to clay formation,
2. Fe and Mn are essential in reduction and oxidation processes,
3. K, and Na are dispersing agents in soils, and
4. Ca and Mg have strong flocculating powers, hence they contribute to the formation and stabilization of soil structure.

2.4.1 Environmental Factors in Weathering

The weathering of these primary minerals to form secondary minerals is quite complex and depends upon the climate, biotic factors, and a number of other parameters. Climate is perhaps the most important factor in mineral weathering. In arid climates, physical weathering predominates. Chemical alteration is at a minimum due to lack of water, and not much clay is formed. On the other hand, in a warm humid climate, both moisture content and temperature are favorable for chemical weathering, and large amounts of clay are produced. The biotic factors of importance in the weathering of primary minerals include aerobic decomposition of organic matter, respiration of plant roots and micro-organisms, biological nitrification process, and the presence of humic acids and other organic acids. Both aerobic decomposition of organic matter and respiration of plant roots produce CO_2, which increases the dissolution capacity of soil water. Under warm humid conditions favoring abundant plant growth, respiration is perhaps more important than aerobic decomposition, although the latter does contribute to the production of CO_2 in soil air. The process of respiration is represented by the reaction below:

$$C_6H_{12}O_6 + 6O_2 \rightarrow 6CO_2 + 6H_2O + \text{energy} \tag{2.1}$$

In this reaction, carbohydrate is oxidized by micro-organisms to obtain the energy needed for performing metabolism and growth. The CO_2 is a byproduct of the oxidation reaction and must be discarded from the plant body into soil air. This reaction increases the CO_2 content in soil air to ten to several hundred times more than is found in atmospheric air. The CO_2 content in the earth atmosphere is approximately 0.03%, or 300 ppm. The CO_2 released in the soil dissolves in soil water to form carbonic acid, H_2CO_3. The latter, a weak acid, is capable of dissociating its proton, which increases the dissolution power of soil water. The reactions of formation and dissociation of H_2CO_3 are represented as follows:

$$CO_2 + H_2O \rightarrow H_2CO_3 \tag{2.2}$$

$$H_2CO_3 \rightarrow H^+ + HCO_3^- \tag{2.3}$$

Nitrification also increases the dissolution capacity of soil water by yielding protons during the reaction. Nitrification, the conversion of ammonium, NH_4^+, into nitrate, NO_3^-, takes place in two steps. In the first step, ammonium is converted into nitrite by *Nitrosomonas* bacteria. In the second step, nitrite is transformed into nitrate by *Nitrobacter* bacteria. As indicated by the reactions below, protons are produced during the first step of the process:

$$2NH_4^+ + 3O_2 \rightarrow 2NO_2^- + 2H_2O + 4H^+ + \text{energy} \tag{2.4}$$

$$2NO_2^- + O_2 \rightarrow 2NO_3^- + \text{energy} \tag{2.5}$$

Humic acids and a variety of organic acids, formed during the decomposition of soil organic matter, also serve as sources of protons that enhance the dissolution power of soil water. When abundant plant growth results in the formation of large amounts of plant residue, large amounts of humic acids and other organic and inorganic acids are produced. These acids not only release protons, they also enhance chelation and complex reactions, important forces in the physical and chemical weathering of soil minerals as indicated above.

In addition to the aforementioned climatic and biotic factors, mineral weathering also depends on three general factors: (1) the physical properties of the minerals, (2) their chemical characteristics and crystal chemistry, and (3) the saturation of the environment.

2.4.2 Physical Properties of the Minerals

Crystal size, shape, hardness, and crystal imperfection are some of the physical characteristics affecting mineral weathering (Ollier, 1975). Large minerals are more resistant than small minerals due to the greater surface areas of smaller particles. Larger surface areas provide more sites for contact with water and other weathering agents. Therefore, the smaller the particles, the faster the rate of weathering.

Hardness depends upon the bond strength between the elements in the structure of the mineral. Bond strength will be discussed in the next section on the effect of chemical properties on weathering. The degree of hardness of minerals is frequently rated on the *Mohs scale* from 1 to 10, with 1 indicating the softest mineral, such as talc, and 10 the hardest mineral, such as diamond (Hunt, 1972; Tan, 1986). Minerals with a hardness > 7, such as topaz, corundum and diamond, are uncommon in soils. Therefore, the degree of hardness of most soil minerals ranges from 1 to 7. Quartz, with a hardness of 7, is generally the hardest mineral in soils and is very resistant to weathering.

Crystal shape is another important physical property that affects mineral weathering. Platy crystals with perfect geometrical shapes are more resistant than imperfect crystals. Loose bonds are perhaps the cause of crystal imperfections. Porosity and cleavage in crystals are additional physical factors in weathering. Rocks and minerals with high porosity tend to weather more rapidly than do those that are more dense and solid. Both porosity and cleavage allow solutions to penetrate deeply into the crystal structure.

2.4.3 Chemical Characteristics and Crystal Chemistry

As discussed earlier, the fundamental units of silicate minerals are silica tetrahedrons, which can be joined together in several ways. As cited earlier, the silica tetrahedrons in quartz are joined together by a mutual sharing of tetrahedral oxygen atoms. This sharing produces a Si-O-Si linkage, called the *siloxane bond*, which is considered the strongest chemical bond in nature (Sticher and Bach, 1966; Tan, 1992). This is the reason why quartz is the hardest mineral in soils. In other minerals, single or several units of silica tetrahedra can be linked together by cations. These cations are nonframework ions, and form weak spots in the mineral structure. For example, in ferromagnesians, double chains of silica tetrahedra are linked together by Ca and Mg atoms (Figure 2.2). These cations can be made soluble by water, resulting in a collapse of the mineral structure. For a more detailed treatise on stability of minerals and bond strength, reference is made to Tan (1982, 1992), Sticher and Bach (1966), and Keller (1954).

2.4.4 Saturation of the Environment

The removal of weathering products by leaching, precipitation, and absorption by plant roots are critical to the process of mineral decomposition. Mineral weathering may stop when the soil solution bathing the minerals becomes saturated as decomposition progresses. For example, dissolution of calcite releases Ca in the soil solution. When the released Ca is not removed from the soil solution, the latter is soon saturated with Ca. The resulting state of equilibrium prevents further weathering of calcite. Stability regions, based on supersaturation, saturation, and undersaturation of soil solutions, have been developed for major soil minerals (Tan, 1993). Some of the stability and phase relation diagrams are very complex (Garrels and Christ, 1965).

Because of the aforementioned factors, some minerals

weather rapidly, whereas others weather slowly. Quartz, a hard mineral, is very resistant to weathering, and may accumulate in the soil's sand fraction. Other minerals, such as the ferromagnesians and plagioclase, weather more rapidly. A large number of weathering sequences have been formulated, and one is given below as an example:

most resistant → least resistant

quartz > muscovite > feldspars, biotite > plagioclase, ferromagnesians

2.5 SECONDARY MINERALS

2.5.1 Environmental Factors Affecting Formation of Secondary Minerals

As indicated in preceding sections, secondary minerals are formed by the weathering of primary minerals. They are microscopically small (< 2 μm) and make up the clay fractions of soils, or the soil inorganic plasma. The primary minerals are broken down and altered into secondary minerals under the influence of climate and biological activity (Ollier, 1975; Birkeland, 1974). The original (primary) minerals can be completely or partially dissolved, and transformed into new materials, the clay minerals. The resulting products are generally in equilibrium with the newly imposed physico-chemical environment. One of the chemical reactions important in the breakdown of feldspars is hydrolysis. By definition, it is the reaction of the mineral with water (hydro is the Greek word for water). The process in a generalized or simplified form can be written as follows:

$$\underset{}{KAlSi_3O_8} + H_2O \rightarrow \underset{\text{precursor of clay}}{HAlSi_3O_8} + \underset{\text{soluble material}}{KOH} \tag{2.6}$$

As shown above, orthoclase is altered by hydrolysis into clay, while at the same time a soluble compound is produced. The formation of clay minerals is, however, very complex and will be affected by many factors, e.g., climatic, and lithologic factors. In temperate regions, hydrolysis of feldspars tends to form more illitic than kaolinitic type of clays. This reaction can be stated as:

$$3KAlSi_3O_8 + 2H^+ + 12H_2O \rightarrow \underset{\text{illite}}{KAl_3Si_3O_{10}(OH)_2} + 6H_4SiO_4 + 2K^+ \quad (2.7)$$

However, in warm humid regions, such as the subtropics and tropical regions, hydrolysis of orthoclase, producing kaolinitic types of clays, is more prevalent:

$$2KAlSi_3O_8 + 2H^+ + 9H_2O \rightarrow \underset{\text{kaolinite}}{H_4Al_2Si_2O_9} + 4H_4SiO_4 + 2K^+ \quad (2.8)$$

Lithologic differences may also produce different types of clays. Duchaufour (1976) postulated that the types of clays produced by weathering of basic rocks differed from those produced by weathering of acid rocks. According to his hypothesis

basic rocks → ferromagnesians, feldspars → smectite → kaolinite

acid rocks → quartz, feldpars → kaolinite

The minerals that make up the basic rocks are composed of large amounts of ferromagnesians which are rich in bases. These minerals release sufficiently high amounts of bases upon weathering to create the basic environment required for the formation of smectite. In contrast, acid rocks contains minerals that produce relatively low amounts of bases upon weathering. Quartz, a major component of acid rocks, is composed mainly of SiO_2, and is resistant to weathering. On the other hand, the small amounts of K released by feldspar are hardly sufficient to create the basic environment needed to form smectite. Consequently, kaolinite is formed in this relatively more acidic environment.

2.5.2 Major Types of Secondary Minerals

The major secondary minerals present in soils are listed in Table 2.4 (Tan, 1993; Mackenzie, 1975).

Allophane. Allophane is noncrystalline in nature, and several definitions for this mineral are present today (Tan, 1992). It is classified as amorphous clay because it is amorphous to x-ray diffraction analysis, meaning x-ray diffraction of the mineral yields featureless curves. Its chemical composition is postulated to be:

$$SiO_2.Al_2O_3.2H_2O \quad \text{or} \quad Al_2O_3.2SiO_2.H_2O$$

The presence of allophane gives unique properties to the soil. Allophane has a large variable negative charge and behaves amphoterically. It also exhibits a high P fixation capacity. The mineral interacts with humic matter, and soils containing allophane usually have black A horizons, rich in organic matter.

Table 2.4. Major Clay Minerals in Soils

Major minerals	Layer type	CEC (cmol(+)/kg)	Major occurrence
Amorphous/paracrystalline clays			
Allophane		35	Volcanic ash soils, spodosols
Imogolite		35	Volcanic ash soils, spodosols
Crystalline silicate clays			
Kaolinite	1:1	8	Ultisols, oxisols, alfisols
Halloysite	1:1	10	
Smectite	2:1	70	Vertisols, mollisols, alfisols
Illites	2:1	30	Mollisols, alfisols, spodosols, aridisols
Vermiculite	2:1	100	Accessory mineral in many soils
Chlorite	2:2	0	Accessory mineral in many soils
Sesquioxide clays			
Goethite, α-FeOOH		3	Oxisols, ultisols
Hematite, α-Fe_2O_3		3	Oxisols, ultisols
Gibbsite, $Al(OH)_3$		3	Oxisols, ultisols
Silica minerals			
Quartz, $n(SiO_2)$		–	Accessory mineral in many soils
Crystobalite, $n(SiO_2)$		–	Accessory mineral in volcanic ash soils

These soils, in the past, were called *andosols* or *ando soils*, from the Japanese word *ando* for black.

Imogolite. Imogolite was found for the first time in 1962 in weathered volcanic ash or pumice beds called *imogo* (Yoshinaga and Aomine, 1962). Since then it has been detected in many other volcanic ash soils, and in the Bh horizons of spodosols, derived from nonvolcanic materials. It has also been synthesized under laboratory conditions (Inoue and Huang, 1984). Imogolite is frequently closely associated with the presence of allophane in soils. The intermediate phase between allophane and imogolite, or imogolite-like allophane, is called *proto-imogolite* (Figure 2.3). In many respects, the chemical characteristics of imogolite are similar to those of allophane. Its chemical composition is assumed to be

$$SiO_2.Al_2O_3.2.5H_2O$$

However, in contrast to allophane, the crystal structure of imogolite is better defined. Electron microscopy shows imogolite to have hairlike or spaghetti-like structures (Figure 2.3), hence this mineral is classified as paracrystalline clay.

Kaolinite. Kaolinite, a phyllosilicate mineral, is called ***kandite*** in the British literature. It is characterized by the following general chemical composition per unit cell:

$$2SiO_2.Al_2O_3.2H_2O$$

Structurally they are 1:1 lattice type minerals. As illustrated in Figure 2.4, each crystal unit of kaolinite is composed of one

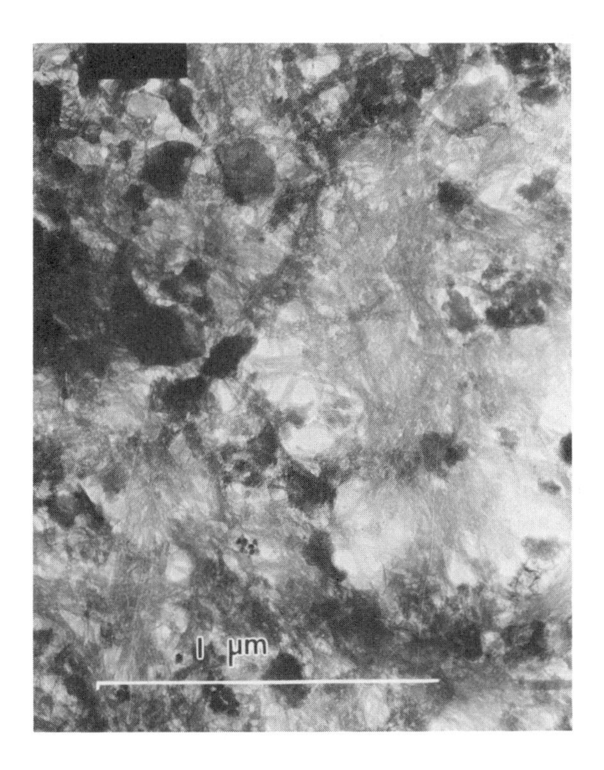

Figure 2.3 Transmission electron micrograph of imogolite in the clay fraction of an andosol derived from volcanic ash in Indonesia.

octahedral sheet stacked above one tetrahedron sheet. The two crystal units, making up one kaolinite particle, are held together by hydrogen bonds, and the intermicellar space has, therefore, a fixed dimension. Since the crystal units are rigidly held, and since very little expansion and contraction are exhibited by the intermicellar space, kaolinite displays low plasticity. Little isomorphous substitution occurs in the crystal

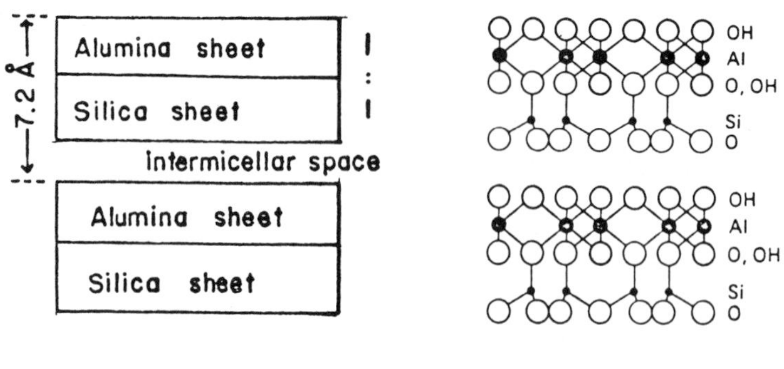

Figure 2.4 The structure of kaolinite, composed of alumina octahedron and silica tetrahedron sheets, stacked into a two-layer crystal unit. This is the reason kaolinite is grouped as a 1:1 layer type of clay.

and, consesequently, its permanent charge is very small. However, kaolinite has a variable or pH-dependent negative charge attributed to the dissociation of protons from exposed OH groups. As a result, its cation exchange capacity may vary with pH. Usually it is in the range of 1 to 10 cmol(+)/kg (= me/100g). Members of the kaolinite group are kaolinite, dickite, and nackrite. Kaolinite is an important mineral in the clay fractions of ultisols and oxisols.

Halloysite. Halloysite is also a 1:1 layer type of clay. It has a general composition of $Al_2O_3.2SiO_2.4H_2O$, and is similar in structure as kaolinite. However, in contrast to kaolinite, halloysite exhibits some expansion and contraction, and contains interlayer water. Upon heating, halloysite is irreversibly dehydrated and the mineral is converted into metahalloysite. The mineral is considered a precursor of kaolinite, as can be noticed from the following weathering sequence:

igneous rocks $\rightarrow$ smectite $\rightarrow$ halloysite $\rightarrow$ metahalloysite $\rightarrow$ kaolinite.

Smectite. Smectite is an expanding 2:1 layer type of clay, and is one of the most common minerals in the smectite group. Formerly, this mineral was called *montmorillonite*. Two other minerals of importance in this group are *beidellite*, with a high Al content, and *nontronite*, an Fe rich smectite. Frequently, the term *bentonite* is used for smectite minerals. However, bentonite is a clay deposit from which commercial grade smectite is produced. The chemical composition of smectite is variable, but it is usually expressed as $Al_2O_3.4SiO_2.H_2O + xH_2O$. The crystal unit is composed of two silica tetrahedron sheets with one alumina octahedron sheet sandwiched in between (Figure 2.5). The crystal units making up a smectite clay particle are loosely bonded together by water in the intermicellar space. Hence, this space may expand or contract depending on soil moisture conditions. Accordingly, the crystal units can move in either direction, causing the high plasticity of the mineral. When wet, smectite is very sticky and the mineral may exhibit internal swelling. Smectite clay is especially prevalent in vertisols, mollisols, and some alfisols. The high plasticity and swell-shrink potential of the mineral make these soils plastic when wet and hard when dry. The dry soil is difficult to till and displays wide cracks.

Illite. Illites are micaceous types of clays and are variously identified as *hydrous micas* and *hydrobiotite*. However, because illite is of secondary origin, and because of its different chemical

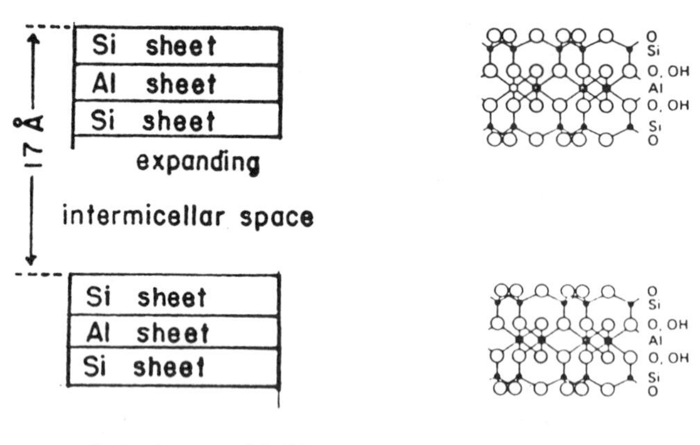

Figure 2.5 The structure of smectite (montmorillonite) composed of an alumina octahedron sheet sandwiched between two silica tetrahedron sheets, forming a three-layer crystal unit. This is the reason why smectite is grouped as a 2:1 layer type of clay.

composition, illite differs from true micas. Illite contains more SiO_2 and less K than muscovite. Structurally, it is similar to smectite, and varies from smectite only because of the presence of interlayer K (Figure 2.6). The crystal units are held strongly together by the K ions, and the mineral, therefore, has a lower swell-shrink potential than smectite. Illite is usually considered the nonexpanding type of clay in the 2:1 group. Its close relationship with smectite can be illustrated by the reaction

$$\text{Illite} \leftrightarrow \text{Smectite} + K^+$$

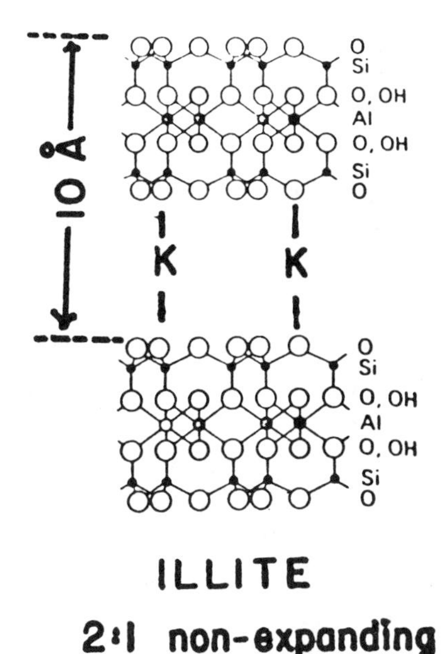

Figure 2.6 The structure of illite with K in the intermicellar space between the crystal units. Illite is also a 2:1 layer type of clay.

Consequently, in soils affected by high precipitation, the mineral tends to be altered into smectite because of leaching of the interlayer K. Illite is an important mineral in the clay fraction of mollisols, alfisols, spodosols, aridisols, inceptisols, and entisols.

Vermiculite. Vermiculite can be distinguished into *true vermiculite* and *clay vermiculite*. True vermiculite is a rock-forming mineral, that becomes twisted and curled upon heating. After heating, the mineral usually expands to 20 to 30 times its original size. It is used as packing or potting material. On the other hand, clay vermiculite is of pedogenic origin, and is sometimes called *soil vermiculite, pedogenic vermiculite*, or *14 Å mineral*. It is a 2:1 layer type of clay with Mg in octahedral positions between the two silica tetrahedron sheets. When $Al(OH)_3$ or gibbsite is present in the intermicellar spaces, the mineral is called *hydroxy aluminum interlayer vermiculite* or *HIV*.

As noticed in Table 2.4, vermiculite is one of the clay minerals with the largest CEC among the inorganic soil colloids. The mineral is known to exhibit *wedge-zones*, attributed to marginal curling of layers on the mineral surface (Tan and McCreery, 1975; Raman and Jackson, 1964). These wedge-shaped zones provide partially enlarged interlayer spacings for entrapment of organic matter (Figure 2.7), or for fixation of K, NH_4^+, and other cations. The high K and NH_4^+ fixation capacity in many soils is attributed more to the presence of vermiculite than to that of smectite or illite. Vermiculite usually occurs as accessory minerals in the clay fractions of ultisols, mollisols and aridisols. It is formed more in well-drained soils, in contrast to smectite which requires a gley condition for formation.

<u>Chlorites</u>. Chlorites are hydrated Mg and Al silicates that are similar to mica minerals in appearance. Structurally, they are related to vermiculite, but a recent trend is to use the term 2:2 layer for chlorite. This term reflects the fact that both the octahedral sheet sandwiched between the silica tetrahedral sheets, and the intermicellar space are filled with $Mg(OH)_2$, called brucite layers. The replacement of Mg by Al in the brucite layers creates positive charges, which practically neutralize all negative charges. Consequently, chlorite has no charge or only a very small charge, hence, a small CEC. The abundance and occurrence of the mineral are very low. Chlorites are usually detected as accessory minerals in the soil's clay fractions.

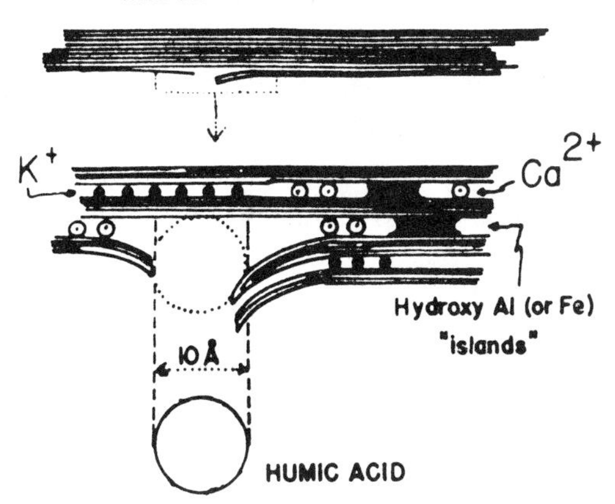

Figure 2.7 Wedge-zones in clay mineral structures, attributed to curling of layers on mineral surfaces. These wedge-shaped zones provide enlarged interlayer spacings for entrapment of cations and humic acids (Tan and McCreery, 1975).

Interstratified Clays. Soil clays exist in nature as a mixture of different types of clays stacked together in a packet. The process of stacking is called *interstratification*, and the clays are called *mixed layer* or *interstratified clays*. The different types of clays cannot be separated from the stacks or packet by physical means as is the case with an ordinary physical mixture of clays. Interstratification can occur *randomly* or *regularly (systematically)*. Interstratified clays are present in a large variety of soils in cold, temperate, and tropical regions. In the soils of the humid regions, interstratification often takes place in the sequence smectite-chlorite-mica, or mica-illite. In soils of the subtropical regions of the United States, interstratified clay, composed of smectite-kaolinite or vermiculite-kaolinite, has also been detected.

Sesquioxides. The sesquioxide clays do not belong to the phyllosilicates, but are oxides of iron and aluminum and/or their hydrates (Table 2.4). Sesquioxide minerals are amphoteric in character and exhibit variable charges. Therefore, these clays, together with amorphous clays, are also known as *clays with variable charges*, whereas the soils are called *soils with variable charges*. The minerals are also known for their high phosphate and metal fixing capacity.

The sesquioxide minerals usually occur in highly weathered soils, e.g., in oxisols and ultisols. *Goethite* and *hematite* are responsible for the yellow and red colors of the oxisols and ultisols, whereas the *gibbsite* content is used to indicate the degree of weathering, as formulated in the oxidic ratio (Soil Survey Staff, 1975):

$$\text{oxidic ratio} = (\%\text{extractable } Fe_2O_3 + \%\text{gibbsite})/\%\text{clay}$$

Soils are considered to be highly weathered if the value of the oxidic ratio is ≥ 0.2.

The iron oxide minerals have also been reported to influence the physical properties of soils. Iron oxides can be adsorbed on soil mineral surfaces, inducing a cementation effect that leads to the development of strong aggregation and to the formation of concretion and crust (Baver, 1963). This enhanced stable aggregation causes oxisols in the tropics to be friable, rather than sticky and plastic as would have been expected from their high clay content.

Silica Minerals. Silica minerals are also not phyllosilicates. They are composed entirely of silica, and structurally they belong to the tectosilicates. The coarse silica minerals are constituents of the silt and sand fractions, whereas the particles ≤ 2 µm belong to the clays. Two groups of silica minerals are usually recognized, *noncrystalline* and *crystalline*. *Opaline silica* belongs to the noncrystalline group. It is of biological origin, formed from the silicification of grasses and parts of deciduous trees. The crystalline group is composed of quartz, tridymite,

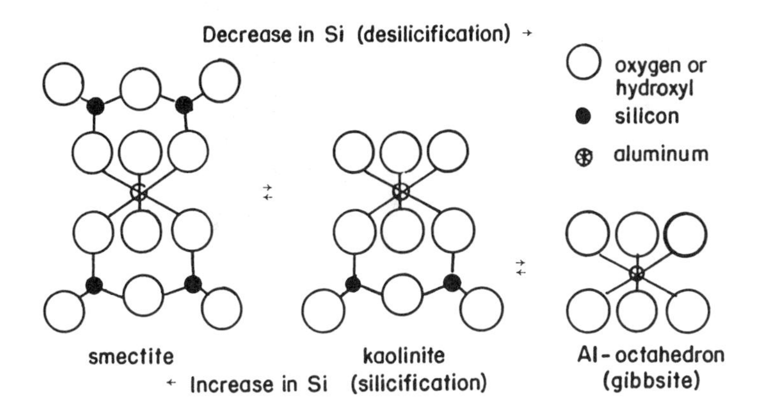

Figure 2.8 Transformation of smectite into kaolinite and gibbsite by a desilicification process. The reverse process, silicification, is the addition of silica to gibbsite and kaolinite to form smectite.

and crystobalite. These minerals occur in a wide variety of soils. Their presence and content are related to parent materials and to the degree of weathering. Inceptisols and entisols can be rich in quartz, but this may be a lithologic effect, or the effect of the parent material. Crystobalite is often volcanic in origin, and its presence is of importance in many volcanic ash soils.

2.5.3 Weathering of Secondary Minerals

Because the clay minerals are the results of weathering processes, one may infer that they are stable or in equilibrium

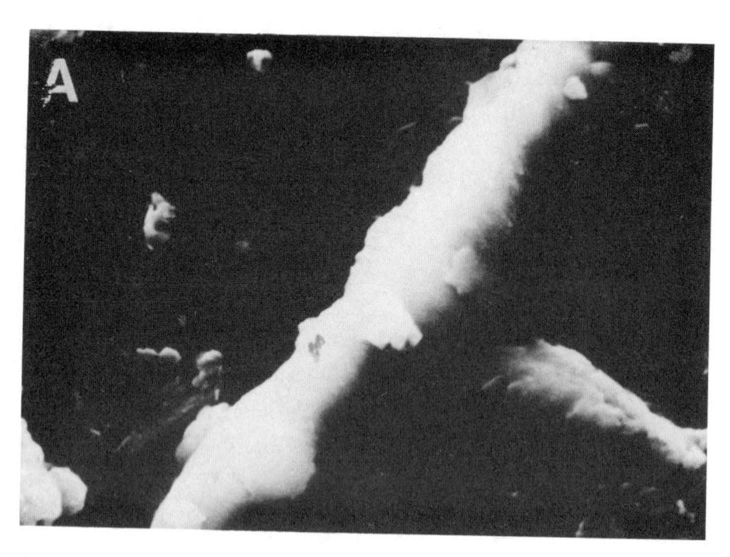

Figure 2.9 Scanning electron micrographs showing the conversion by neoformation of imogolite (A) into kaolinite pseudomorphs (B) stacked into an accordion-like pattern. The clay minerals have been detected in the C horizon of an ultisol derived from volcanic ash in Indonesia (Goenadi and Tan, 1991).

with the prevailing environmental conditions. Nevertheless, these minerals are subject to further weathering. Under changing physico-chemical conditions, clay minerals can be converted from one type to another, a process referred to as *alteration.* Two main processes of alterations can be distinguished: *transformation*, and *neoformation*. Transformation is defined by Singer (1979) as an alteration process of clay minerals that occurs without changing the basic layer structure. This process can further be differentiated into *degradation* and *aggradation*. A degradation process involves loss of substances by destruction, whereas in aggradation, substances are added to the mineral

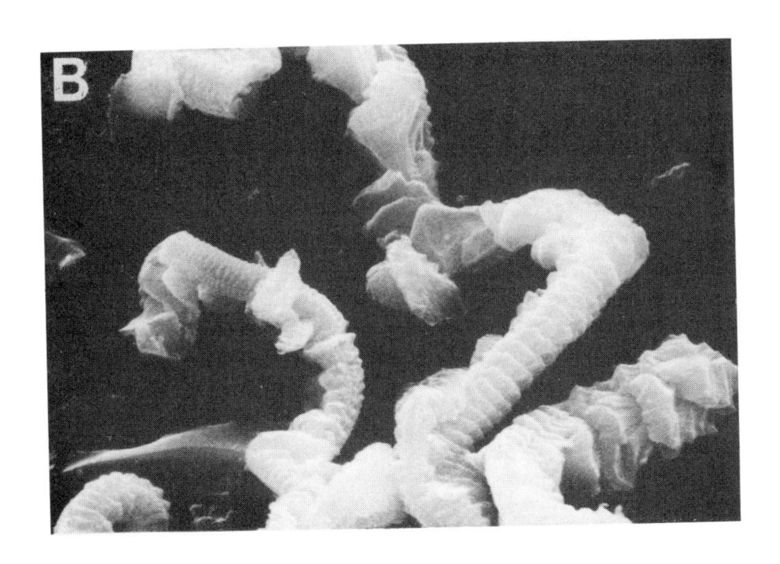

structure to form the new clay minerals (Millot, 1964). Under warm and humid conditions, desilicification and silicification are the two main trends of transformation processes (Figure 2.8).

Desilicification commonly takes place during a laterization process in soils where drainage is not restricted, and Si can be leached. Laterization gives rise to formation of ultisols and oxisols rich in kaolinite and sesquioxides. Over geologic time periods, a continued desilicification process will ultimately transform these minerals into bauxite. Under conditions with a more restricted drainage, silica will not be leached, but will rather be added. This process, called *silicification*, favors formation of smectitic minerals. On the other hand, *neoformation* is the synthesis of clay minerals from other secondary minerals with different structure, and/or from primary minerals by pseudomorphic replacement, or by direct crystallization from solutions or colloidal gels. Figure 2.9 provides examples of neoformation, showing the conversion of imogolite into kaolinite pseudomorphs, and eventually into discrete kaolinite units (Goenadi and Tan, 1991).

CHAPTER 3

ORGANIC CONSTITUENTS

The organic fraction of soils, also called *soil organic matter*, is derived from the soil biomass, and strictly speaking it consists of both living and dead organic matter. The dead organic matter is formed by chemical and biological decomposition of organic residue. It can be distinguished into (1) organic matter in various degrees of decomposition, but in which the morphology of the plant material is still visible, and (2) completely decomposed material. The latter consists of numerous organic compounds, but only a few are present in detectable amounts in soils. Some of them are *nonhumified*, whereas others are *humified* compounds (Stevenson, 1967,1982; Flaig, 1971; Tan, 1993). The nonhumified compounds have been released by decay of plant, animal and microbial tissue in their original or in a slightly modified form. They include carbohydrates, amino acids, proteins, lipids, nucleic acids, lignins, pigments, hormones, and a variety of organic acids. The humified compounds are products that have been synthesized from these nonhumified substances by a process called *humification*. They consist of a group of complex substances such as humic and fulvic acids. The nonhumic and humic material are collectively called *soil humus*.

The soil organic fraction as described above affects the

physical, chemical, and biological conditions in soils. Physically, it increases organic matter content, and imparts darker colors to soils with an increase in organic carbon content. It improves aggregation of soil particles, resulting in the development of stable soil structures. Chemically, it increases the cation exchange capacity, and the waterholding capacity of soils. It affects soil fertility by increasing the soil's nutrient content, especially N and S content. Organic matter is the main source of N in soils. Biologically, soil organic matter is the main source of food and energy for soil organisms. The population of soil organisms will decline with a decrease in organic matter content. In the absence of soil organisms many, if not all, biochemical reactions will come to a standstill.

3.1 SOIL BIOMASS

There are several definitions for biomass, and one definition states that the biomass is composed of microbial tissues only. It can be estimated by microbial counts and a knowledge of cell weights using the following relationship (Stevenson, 1989):

$$\text{Biomass} = \text{number of cells} \times \text{volume} \times \text{density}$$

Another definition indicates that the biomass is the total mass (dry weight) of living organisms (Paul and Clark, 1989; Brady, 1990). The latter is composed of the live *soil fauna* and *flora*, each of which consists of a macro and micro group. This definition appears to be used by a great number of people, because the definition shows that all organisms, not only micro-organism cells, contribute toward formation and accumulation of organic matter in soils.

The biomass is constantly being generated by growing organisms. When the organisms die, their bodies are decomposed, compounds are released, oxidized and degraded, and the final products contribute to the group of compounds that polymerize to form humic matter. Under these conditions, humic matter in soils are slowly but constantly being formed and decomposed at the same time.

3.1.1 Macrofauna

The macrofauna are the higher animals, and their importance in soils is primarily through (1) the breakdown of organic matter, and (2) the cultivation effect. They are, therefore, essential participants in the natural cycle of organic matter. Dead leaves and twigs are chewed by these animals, and moved from one to another place in the soil. Holes and burrows are made into the soil by some animals, such as earthworms, moles, chipmunks, and prairie dogs. In doing so, surface material is brought down, whereas subsoil material is worked up. This has a similar effect as soil cultivation with the plow, hence the term *cultivation effect*. The earthworm is perhaps of special importance in the cultivation effect. Under the tropical rain forest in Nigeria, the earthworm population can amount from 30 to 210 worms per m^2, which translates to 9×10^5 earthworms per hectare (Ghuman and Lal, 1987). By digging their way through the soil, earthworms consume organic matter and soil alike, which are thoroughly mixed and ground in their body. At the same time, this inorganic-organic mixture is subjected to the digestive action of the stomach enzymes. The soil turnover from earthworm activity under a tropical rainforest in Africa is estimated to be 21.5 Mg (tons)/ha per year (Ghuman and Lal, 1987). Earthworm casts are reported to be very high in organic matter, N, P, K, and Ca content, hence can improve soil fertility. The amount of casts produced is substantial, and is estimated to be 250 Mg/ha per year (Brady, 1990). In addition, earthworms may have an important effect on the physical condition of soils. The holes left serve as channels for air and water passage. The two common earthworm species of importance in the USA are *Lumbricus terrestris*, a red colored deep-boring species which was imported from Europe, and *Allolobophora caliginosa*, a pinkish shallow-boring earthworm.

3.1.2 Microfauna

The microfauna are the microscopically small animals, and two of the major species in soils are nematodes and protozoa.

Nematodes are very small thread worms, normally of a size of 1 - 2 mm in length, although exceptions may occur. They can be distinguished into (a) saprophytic, (b) predatory, and (c) parasitic nematodes (Brady, 1984). They are all essential in the natural recycling process of soil organic matter. The *saprophytic nematodes* consume dead organic matter, whereas the *predatory nematodes* feed on other nematodes, and also on a number of microorganisms, such as bacteria, algea, and protozoa. *Parasitic nematodes* feed on live plant roots, causing *nematode disease* in cultivated crops. The parasitic nematodes are attracted to plant roots by a chemical compound secreted by the roots. Therefore, only plants that can produce chemicals attractive to parasitic nematodes can be affected, e.g. soybean, and tomato. If the larvae of parasitic nematodes fail to migrate to the root surface, it will die naturally in soils. As can be noticed in Figure 3.1, the parasitic nematodes have needle-like organs in their mouth to inflict damage and penetrate the root tissue in which they multiply. Although the parasitic nematodes can become harmful for cultivated crops, they are an essential part in the natural recycling process of soil organic matter. They are the major food source of predatory nematodes, whose population will grow or decrease with abundance and decline in parasitic nematodes. Therefore, in nature a certain balance exists between the number of beneficial and harmful organisms. In other words, the population of parasitic nematodes is kept under control by the predatory nematodes. If by human interference, however, conditions are created favorable for the growth of parasitic nematodes, an outbreak of a nematode disease occurs. Rootknot disease caused by infection with the rootknot nematode *Meloidogyne* sp., can cause heavy damage in soybean plants. Today, studies have been conducted to cultivate the predatory nematodes in vitro for use in the biological control of nematode diseases in cultivated crops.

<u>*Protozoa*</u> are considered the most elementary form of animal life in soils. They are microscopically small, and include *amoeba, ciliates*, and *flagellates*. Some of them are pathogenic to animals and humans, whereas others will feed on organic residue and other microorganisms, e.g., rhizobium bacteria (Jones, 1983). The opinion exists that the population of protozoa in soils is often not sufficiently large to influence the recycling of organic matter (Brady, 1990).

3.1.3 Macroflora

The macroflora are the higher plants, including the cultivated crops. All of them will affect the physical, chemical and biological properties of soils. Physically, they are capable of increasing organic matter content in soils when left alone in nature to grow and complete their life cycle.

Roots can enhance development of soil structure. They also grow through cracks, and when they die will leave channels for air and water passage. Chemically, plant residue will affect the nutrient content of soils, and as such the macroflora plays an important role in nutrient cycling, a process that preserves and maintains soil fertility. In this process, the organic residue decomposes, releasing nutrients into the surface soil where they are taken up again by growing plants. Roots can also absorb from subsoils the nutrients that have been leached from surface soils. These nutrients are accumulated in the plant tissue, and will be released in the surface soil with leaf-fall or when the plants die and decompose. Plants grown deliberately for

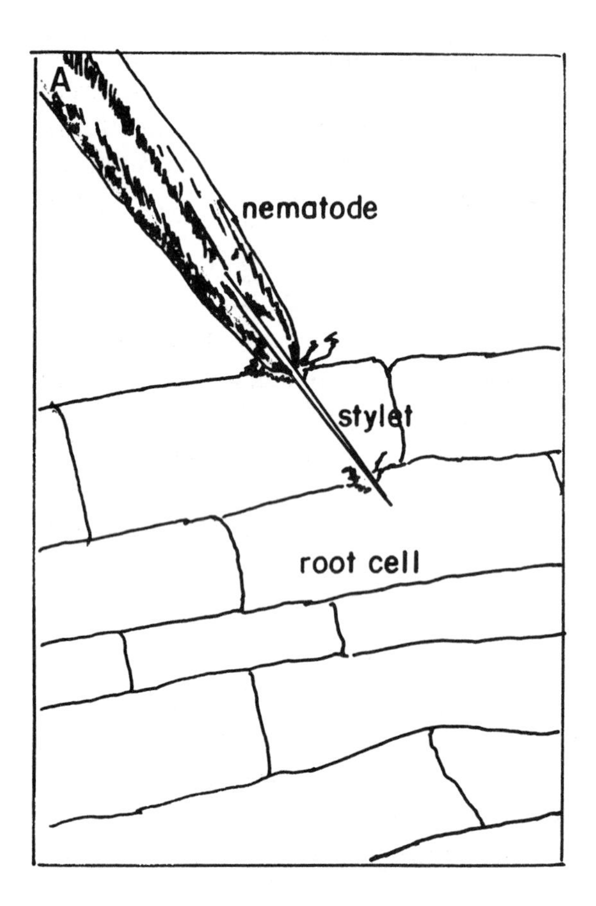

Figure 3.1 (A) Schematic drawing of a parasitic nematode inflicting damage to root cells. (B) Reproductive organs of a rootknot nematode, *Meloidogyne* sp. (J. Plaskowitz, USDA, courtesy Tousimis Research Corp., Rockville, MD).

improving soil fertility, e.g. improving nutrient content and physical conditions of soils, are called *green manures*. The macroflora finds also application in protecting the surface soil against erosion and other destructive forces in the environment.

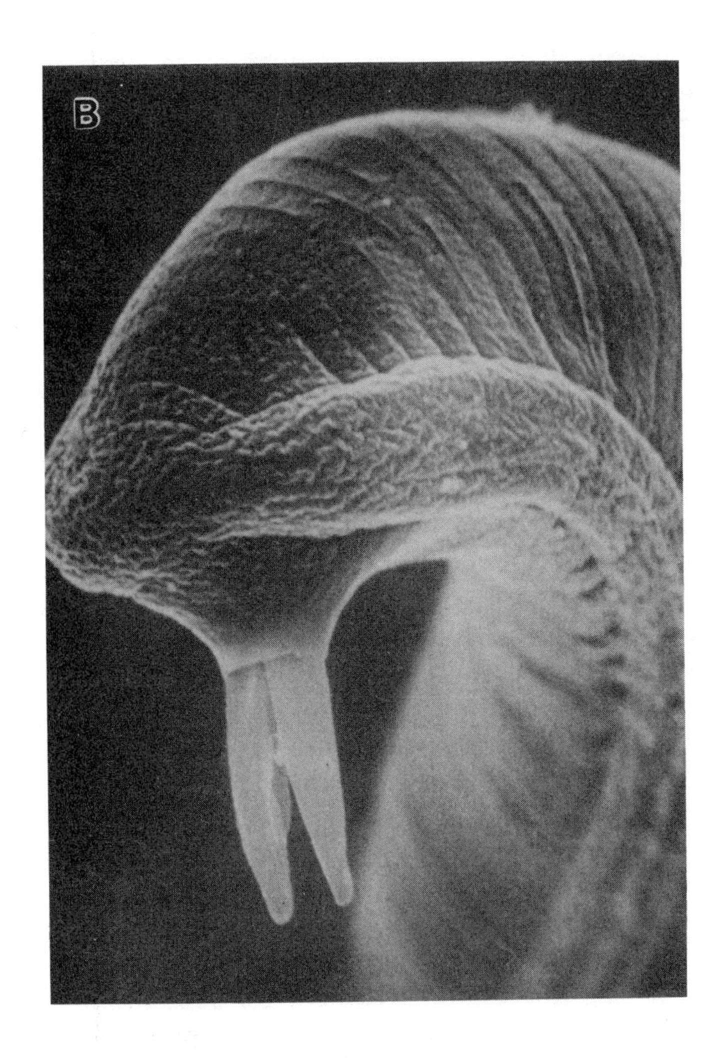
B

Plants grown to protect soil surfaces against these harmful forces are called *cover crops*.

Biologically, higher plants affect the life of almost all organisms, macro and micro alike. From the standpoint of soil microorganisms, a large number of these organisms are congregating around the surfaces of roots. They are attracted to the root surface because of chemical compounds secreted by live roots, which are vital sources of food and energy for the microorganisms. They are called *root exudates* and can be distinguished into three groups (1) *mucigel* or *mucilage*, a mixture of polysaccharides and uronic acids, enveloping especially the root tips, (2) a variety of organic acids, amino acids, and simple sugars excreted by root hairs, and (3) cellular organic substances produced by senescence of root epidermis. Because of these substances, the number of microorganisms is noted to be more abundant near the root surface than in the bulk soil. Nematodes and rhizobia alike are attracted to the root surface because of the chemicals produced by growing roots. However, the population of pathogenic organisms may also increase and may cause the development of root diseases, e.g., nematode disease. This zone of soil in the immediate vicinity of the root surface is called the *soil rhizosphere* (Rovira and Davey, 1974). Many of the soil chemical and biochemical reactions, vital for the growth of plants, occur in the soil rhizosphere. Soil pH is generally lower in the rhizosphere, whereas denitrification is believed to be more rapid close to the root surface. This is due to a greater respiration in this zone by the larger population of microrganisms. In turn, an increased respiration produces a greater reducing condition necessary for the denitrification process. The root exudates are also capable of dissolving and chelating metal compounds. Such a reaction is believed to be the process by which roots obtained their iron.

3.1.4 Microflora

The microflora are the lower plants, or the microscopic small plants. Numerically, they are the most abundant of all the living organisms in soils. They are usually present in large numbers near feeder roots of plants and play a vital role in many dynamic microbial reactions. On the basis of their feeding habit, they can be saprophytic, parasitic, pathogenic or symbiotic in nature. Most of them are present mainly in the surface soil or the root zone (Table 3.1). The population of microorganisms decreases rapidly with depth in the soil. In the subsoil and/or C horizon only minimal amounts of these microorganisms can be detected. Although a large variety of microorganisms exist in soils, only a few major species will be discussed in this book (Table 3.2).

Table 3.1 The Number of Microorganisms in a Well-Drained Soil

Soil horizon	**Aerobic bacteria**	**Anaerobic bacteria**	**Fungi**	**Actino-mycetes**	**Algae**
		----------------	x 10^3 g/g soil	----------------	
A	7500	2000	150	2000	30
B	2	1	2	tr	–

Source: unpublished data of the author.

Table 3.2 Some Common Soil Microflora

I. Bacteria	1. heterotrophic 2. autotrophic
II. Fungi	1. mold 2. yeast 3. mycorrhizae
III. Actinomycetes	
VI. Algae	
VII. Lichen	

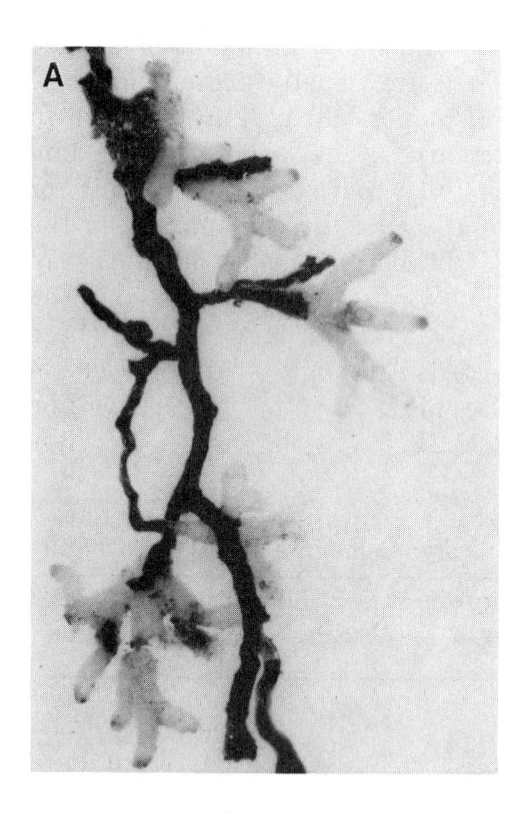

Figure 3.2 (A) Ectomycorrhizae in pine root (courtesy D.H. Marx, USDA-Forestry Science Laboratory, University of Georgia, Athens, GA). (B) Endomycorrhizae (courtesy M.F. Brown, University of Missouri, Columbia, MO).

Bacteria are the simplest form of plant life in soils, and are composed of single cells, usually 5 μm in size. They lack nuclear membranes and their nucleoplasm is, therefore, not separated from the cytoplasm. Hence, they are called *prokaryotic* (Paul and Clark, 1989). The majority of bacteria species are *hetero-trophic* or *organotrophic*. These are bacteria that need organic

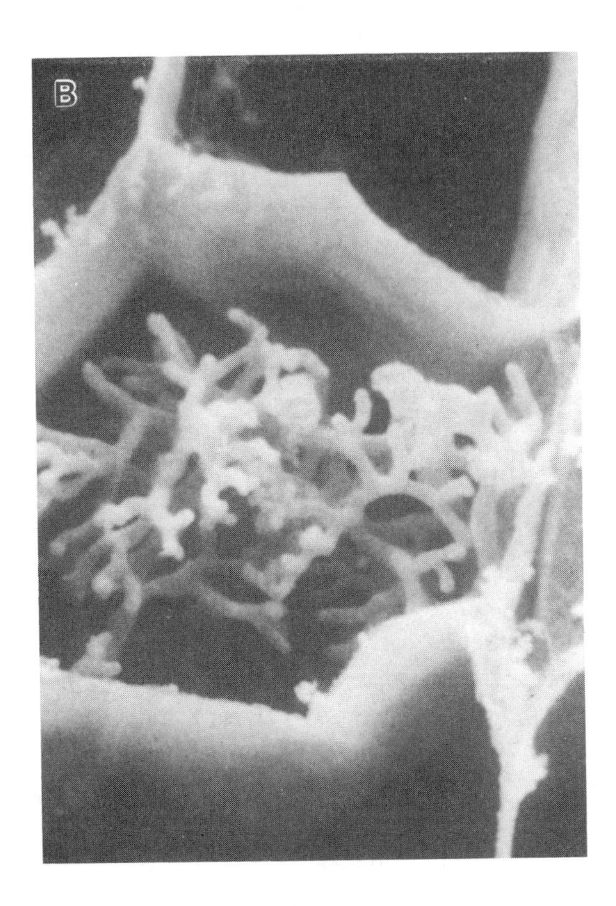

matter for food and energy, or in scientific terms: the cell carbon is obtained by the bacteria from an organic substrate. On the other hand, *autotrophic* or *lithotrophic* bacteria are bacteria that use inorganic matter, such as NH_4^+, Fe^{2+}, SO_4^{2-} and/or CO_2 for food and energy.

Bacterial cells are often distinguished into *gram positive* (G^+)

and *gram negative* (G^-) cells. The term G^+ is given to cells that become crystal violet after treatment with a *gram staining solution*, containing KI, whereas the term G^- refers to cells which destain readily (Paul and Clark, 1989).

Bacteria takes part in many, if not all, organic transaction of importance to soil fertility and the growth of higher plants. They are responsible for a number of enzymatic reactions, e.g., nitrogen fixation and nitrification. These reactions will be discussed in a later section of this chapter.

Fungi are also elementary forms of plant life in soils. The individual cells have a nucleus and, in contrast to bacteria, they are *eukaryotic* organisms. The cells may be linked together into filaments called *hyphae*, which are collectively called *mycelium* (Paul and Clark, 1989). Fungi must depend for their food and energy on organic matter in soils. As with bacteria, fungi also lack *chlorophyll*, the green substance essential for photosynthesis. Because of the absence of chlorophyll, fungi have developed into saprophytes, pathogens, parasites or symbionts in nature. Saprophytic fungi contribute to nutrient cycling in soils. Together with bacteria, they share the responsibility of decomposing organic residue in soils, breaking it down into simpler forms, which then become available again to plants. Rotting of food, paper, wood, and household goods is a type of organic and/or nutrient cycling, although this rotting process is considered harmful from a human standpoint. As parasites or pathogens, fungi may cause diseases in plants and animals. Fungal diseases in plants have been known for a long time, but it was the disastrous impact of potato blight in Ireland in the middle of the 19th century that started the science of *plant pathology* (Webster, 1975). Many types of fungi are used today in the food and pharmaceutical industries. Some types of fungi are edible, whereas others are used in the fermentation of wine, bread, and cheese. Production of antibiotics and other chemicals are additional examples of the usefulness of fungi. Penicillin, an antibiotic medicine had been isolated originally from the fungus *Penicillium notatum* or *P. chrysogenum*. Currently, fungi also find application in improving plant growth and soil fertility. The roots of many plants are infected with a type of root fungus called *mycorrhizae*. Three groups of mycorrhizae are recognized today: (a) ecto-, (b) ectendo-, and (c) endomycorrhizae (Harley, 1969; Marx and Krupa, 1978). *Ectomycorrhizae* is a root fungus (Figure 3.2A) that forms an intercellular fungal network in the root cortex called the *Hartig net*. Often, the fungus forms a sheath around feeder roots, hence the term ecto (outside). It is living in symbiosis with pine, spruce, fir, birch, hemlock, beech, and oak trees, and hence is sometimes referred to as *tree-mycorrhizae*. *Endomycorrhizae*, on the other hand, is living in symbiosis within the root tissue (Figure 3.2B). This group is more numerous and more widespread of the mycorrhizaes, and is found in almost any cultivated crop, to name a few: in roots of wheat, corn, cotton, rice, apple, cacao, coffee, rubber, citrus, maple, and poplar. The walls of root cells in these plants are penetrated by the mycelium, and inside the cells the fungus forms highly branched small structures called *arbuscules*. This is the reason why this type of fungus is also referred to as *vesicular arbuscular* (VA) mycorrhizae. The *ectendo* group has the characteristics of both the ecto- and endomycorrhizae.

The beneficial effect of mycorrhizae to plants is noticed in increased nutrient uptake, and protection against pathogenic attack (Marx, 1969). As can be seen from Figure 3.3 (see also Figure 3.2A), the fungus sends out fine filamentous mycelium into the soil, which translates into increasing substantially the surface area of plant roots. It has been estimated that the active surface area of roots is increased to as much as 10 times by the mycelium, which in turn may result in an increase in water and nutrient uptake. The advantage of mycorrhizae is especially noticed in infertile soils, where the fungus can assist the host plants in nutrient uptake. Some of the fungus is known for its capacity to extract P from soils low in P, or from unavailable P

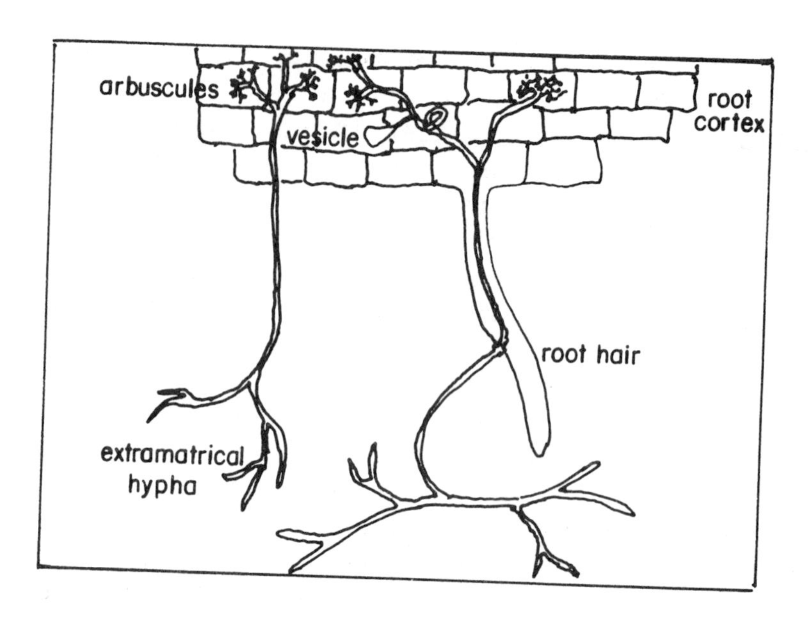

Figure 3.3 Schematic drawing of endomycorrhiza mycelium growing into the soil, increasing in this way the surface area of plant roots.

sources, e.g., *Pisolithus tinctorius*. The latter fungus is well adapted for extracting P from soils low in P, hence allowing the host plant to grow in soils too infertile for other plants.

Actinomycetes. In many books, *actinomycetes* are defined as lower plants with properties in between those of bacteria and fungi. Like the fungi, actinomycetes have cells that also develop into filamentous hyphae, but their mycelial threads break up into spores resembling bacterial cells. For this reason, they are sometimes referred to as *thread bacteria* (Brady, 1990). Paul and Clark (1989) classify them also within the bacterial group *Streptomyces*. Actinomyces are present in moist, well-drained soils. They are very sensitive to changes in soil reactions, and grow well at pH levels of 6.0 to 7.0, but will disappear in soils with lower pHs. Most actinomycetes are important in the decomposition of soil organic matter, which can be noticed from the musty smell in decomposing straw piles or freshly plowed land. Some actinomycetes can cause damage on cultivated crops. These parasitic actinomycetes are especially harmful in potato crops by causing potato scab disease. However, since the pathogen is sensitive to low pH levels, this disease is usually controlled by growing the potatoes at lower soil pH by treatment of the soil with powdered S. Many of the actinomycetes are also used in the pharmaceutical industry because of their capability to produce antibiotics, e.g. antiviral, antibacterial, antifungal, antiprotozoal, and antitumor compounds (Paul and Clark, 1989). For example, streptomycin is an antibiotic that was isolated originally from *Streptomyces* by S.A. Waksman in 1942. He was awarded the Nobel prize for this discovery.

Algae are the lower plants that contain chlorophyll. Of all the green plants, they are perhaps the most widely distributed chlorophyll-containing plants on earth. Though mostly aquatic in nature, terrestrial forms of algae, called moss, exist on rocks, soils, stems, barks and leaves. These types of algae grow best in wet condition. Aquatic algae includes seaweed and plankton, whereas soil algae are composed of *green, blue-green, brown*, and *red algae*, and *diatoms* (Brady, 1990). Diatoms are characterized by stiff cell walls rich in Si, coated by organic matter. A number of microbiologists consider bluegreen algae to belong to the *cyanobacteria* (Paul and Clark, 1989). The blue-green algae frequently grow in ponds and inundated paddy soils. They are capable of fixing nitrogen from the air. In the tropics, the blue green algae often grow in close association (symbiosis) with the *Azolla* plant (Figure 3.4), an aquatic fern commonly found

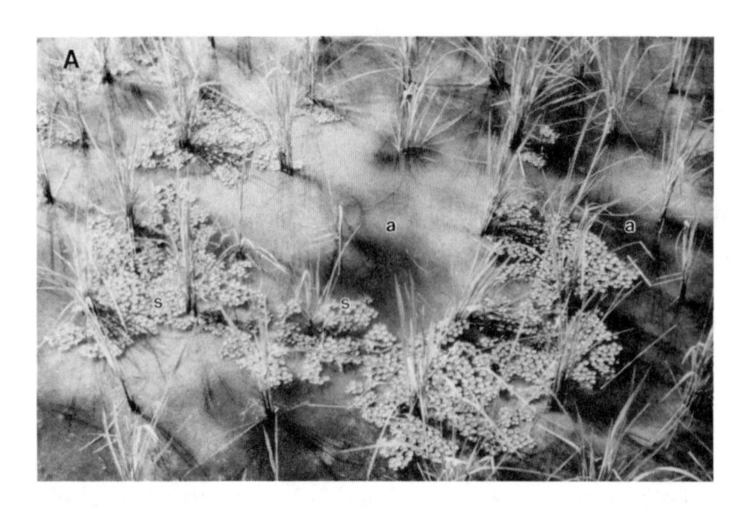

Figure 3.4 (A) Algae growth (a) and *Salvinia* sp. (s) mixed with some *Azolla* sp. in a paddy rice field in Bogor, Indonesia. (B) Closeup of *Azolla* sp. plant.

in paddy soils. Such an association is sometimes called a *phototropic* association (Paul and Clark, 1989). They are the reason for the *Azolla* to enrich paddy soils with N compounds. As will be discussed in another chapter, algae also finds application in the food and health industry.

<u>*Lichens*</u> are symbiotic associations of fungi and algae, and according to Webster (1975) belong to the *Lecanorales* group. The fungus and the algae form a single *thallus* called *lichen thallus* (Paul and Clark, 1989). In most lichen thalli the algae are confined to a special region, called the *algal zone*, which is interspersed by fungal hyphae. It is believed that the fungus provides mineral nutrients to the algae, which in turn supply the fungus with carbohydrates, and if the algae is a blue-green algae also with nitrogen compounds. Lichens can grow on rock surfaces or infertile soils, and as such they are considered pioneer plants, contributing to soil formation. They also inhabit

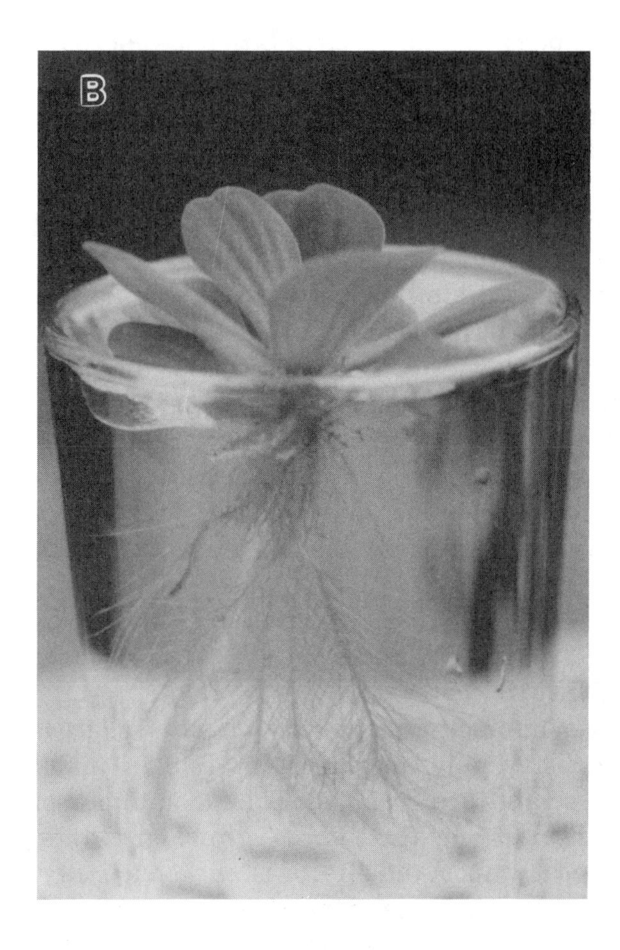

other surfaces, such as roof tops, tree trunks and stems, and fence posts. Their growing range is not limited to any climatic condition, since they are found from the arctic to the humid tropics. In the arctic region, lichens form the staple food for reindeer and arctic hares, whereas in the temperate region they constitute part of the winter forage of caribous, deer and other grazing animals.

Viruses, whose importance is becoming clear, are listed here for completeness. It is not clear yet whether this can be called an organism and/or whether it is an independent group of organisms separate from the microflora. They are either the simplest organisms on earth, or, since they do not have metabolism, are mainly very complex molecules, composed of protein coated RNA or DNA molecules (Paul and Clark, 1989). Whatever they are, viruses exhibit properties of living matter, and will grow and multiply only in the cells of a host organism. They have attracted worldwide attention because of their capability to produce diseases in plants, animals and humans. It appears that this pathogenic attribute can be used to our advantage in the biological control of weeds and insects, and in combatting plant, animal, and human diseases. Not much is yet known how they survive and multiply in soils.

3.2 BENEFICIAL EFFECT OF SOIL MICROORGANISMS

As indicated above, microorganisms are present in great numbers in the soil. They play an important role in many physiological processes, and are responsible for a number of biochemical reactions vital for the life of growing plants. Perhaps one of the most important effects is *carbon cycling*, which includes the biochemical reactions *decomposition* and *mineralization*. Another effect of equal importance is *nitrogen cycling*, including the biochemical reactions, *nitrogen fixation*, *ammonification*, *nitrification*, and *denitrification*. Many, if not all, of these effects and reactions are interrelated. For example, the N-cycle is in essence part of the *nutrient cycling*. In turn, nutrient cycling is closely related to mineralization. It is not in the scope of this book to discuss all the cycles present in soils. Only the carbon and nitrogen cycles will be presented in the following sections. For the various cycles of the many other nutrients reference is made to Stevenson (1986).

3.2.1 Carbon Cycle

The *carbon cycle* is the perpetual movement of organic carbon from the air into the soil and back into the air. It is nature's way to clean the environment by recycling the organic waste, which is mediated by the microorganisms. Many complex diagrams have been developed to depict this cycle, and the overuse of detailed reactions usually tends to cloud the basics of the cycle. In principle, the cycle starts when CO_2 gas in the atmosphere is absorbed by plants and converted into carbohydrates by a process called *photosynthesis*, which can be represented by the reaction

$$CO_2 + H_2O \rightarrow \text{carbohydrates} + O_2 \tag{3.1}$$

This reaction will take place only in the presence of chlorophyll and sunlight. These carbohydrates are the sources for formation of other organic compounds in the plant body, e.g., protein and lignin. With leaf-fall or when plants die, the vegetative remains are subject to decomposition and mineralization processes, which return the carbon from the soil to the air as CO_2 gas.

3.2.2 Decomposition and Mineralization

In the *decomposition* process all organic remains in soils are broken down first into their organic constituents, and finally into CO_2 and H_2O. Some nutrients are also released in inorganic forms. The decomposition process can take place in *aerobic* and *anaerobic* conditions. Aerobic decomposition is characterized by a gradual breakdown of organic waste. The less resistant material is broken down first, whereas the breakdown of the more resistant material, such as lignin and protein, takes place in several stages. Part of the organic compounds released in soils will be converted into *humus* or *humic matter* by the *humi-*

fication process. Eventually humic matter will also be broken down by this process. The end product of aerobic decomposition is CO_2, H_2O, NO_{3-}, and SO_4^{2-} (Stevenson, 1986). On the other hand, *mineralization* is defined as the immediate breakdown of organic waste into CO_2 and H_2O, which is accompanied by the direct release of nutrients in the soil in inorganic (mineral) forms. Although the end product is similar to that of aerobic decomposition, a gradual decay with the subsequent release of "intermediate" organic constituents is absent in mineralization. Therefore, humic matter can not be formed as a result of a mineralization process. In anaerobic decomposition, anaerobic degradation, called *putrification*, of organic waste takes place, and additional organic byproducts are formed, e.g., methane and other foul-smelling compounds. The formation of methane can be illustrated by the reaction

$$C_6H_{12}O_6 \rightarrow \underset{\text{methane}}{3CH_4} + 3CO_2 \quad (3.2)$$

Methane gas is often produced in swampy conditions, and in land fills where it becomes a hazard and an environmental issue. Since the reaction is an anaerobic reaction, efforts in creating a more aerobic environment in land fills can perhaps control the situation. In some cases, the decomposition process can also yield ethyl alcohol or methyl alcohol, as illustrated by the following reaction:

$$C_6H_{12}O_6 \rightarrow \underset{\text{ethanol}}{2C_2H_5OH} + 2CO_2 \quad (3.3)$$

This reaction forms the basis for the production of alternative sources of fuel. In industry, sugars from sugar cane are used for ethanol production, such as in Brazil. Starches from corn and potato, $(C_6H_{10}O_5)_5$, can also be used as inexpensive sources for production of ethanol by fermentation with yeast. From the above, it can be noticed that the soil is a natural producer of the polluting gases CH_4 and CO_2. Both gases are responsible for contributing to the *greenhouse effect* on earth. However, the amount of these gases released by a natural decomposition process is very small compared to that produced by the combustion of fossil fuel in automobiles, industry, and large-scale burning of the tropical rainforest. Most of the CO_2 produced naturally will be "filtered" from the atmosphere by green plants, and used again in photosynthesis for the production of carbohydrates, as conditioned by the carbon cycle.

3.2.3 Nitrogen Cycle

Very simply defined, the *nitrogen cycle* is the movement of nitrogen from the atmosphere through the plants into the soil before it is returned to the atmosphere in its original gaseous state. It is closely associated with the carbon cycle, but can also be considered part of the nutrient cycle. It is believed that a nitrogen cycle as such does not exist in nature, because the soil has a N_2 cycle of its own, called the *inner cycle*, and because the N atom can be transferred from one to another oxidation state in a random fashion (Stevenson, 1986; Paul and Clark, 1989). The cycle is composed of a sequence of biochemical reactions as illustrated in a very generalized diagram in Figure 3.5. The *outer circle* represents the more overall N_2 cycle, whereas the inner circle displays the cycle occurring in soils.

3.2.4 Nitrogen Fixation

Nitrogen fixation is a process by which atmospheric N_2 gas is captured by microorganisms and converted into nitrogen com-

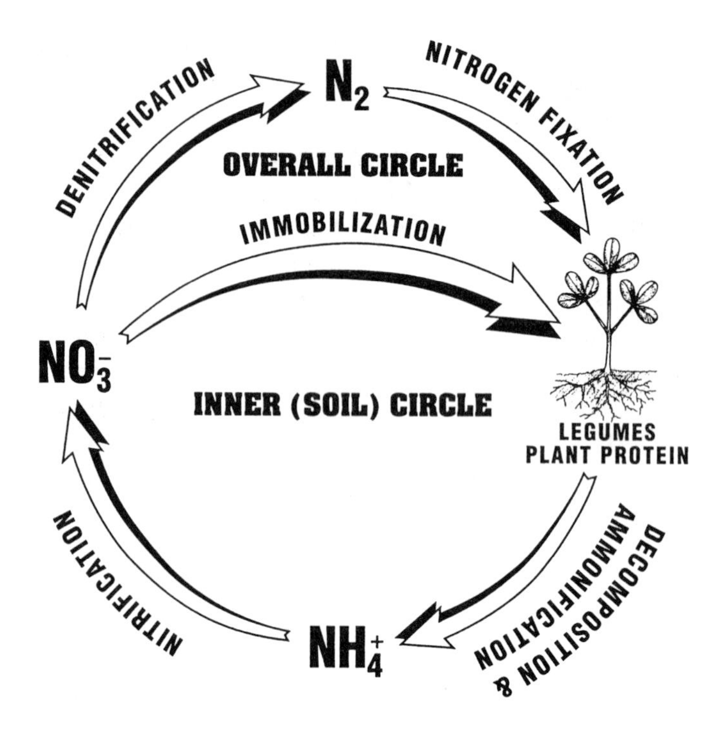

Figure 3.5 Generalized diagram of the nitrogen cycle, showing the overall and inner cycle. Drawing by W. G. Reeves, art coordinator, University of Georgia.

pounds available to plants. The atmosphere contains an abundant supply of nitrogen (70%), but in the form of gas it is unavailable to higher plants. Many people believe that nitrogen fixation is the only process by which soil can be enriched naturally with nitrogen compounds vital for the growth of plants.

Other scientists indicate that the plants containing these organisms in fact deplete soil N (LaRue and Patterson, 1981). The N_2 fixation process can be distinguished into a symbiotic and nonsymbiotic nitrogen fixation process.

Symbiotic Nitrogen Fixation. Symbiotic nitrogen fixation is carried out by the heterotrophic *Rhizobium* bacteria, that live in root nodules of legume plants (Nutman, 1965). When a root hair comes into contact with a rhizobium bacteria, curling of the root hair takes place. The cell walls in the root hair tissue are dissolved enzymatically by the bacteria, and an infection thread is formed that invades the root cortex. Once inside, the rhizobium multiplies into *bacteroids*, which are nourished by the host plant with the necessary nutrients for growth. In turn, the host plant receives N compounds produced by the bacteria from N_2 gas. On its own the host plant is unable to obtain the nitrogen for growth. Such an association to the mutual benefit of each others is called *symbiosis*, hence the term symbiotic N fixation. The O_2 requirement of the bacteria is supplied by a substance similar to hemoglobin in blood called *leghemoglobin*, surrounding the bacteroids in the nodule tissue. The exact reaction for the conversion of N_2 gas into N_2 compounds is not known, and many reaction processes have been proposed involving complicated electron transfer and conversion of ATP into ADP. Nevertheless, it is believed that the first product is ammonium, NH_4^+, the formation of which can be illustrated by the generalized reaction as follows:

$$N_2 + 8H^+ + 6e^- \rightarrow 2NH_4^+ \quad (3.4)$$

Both poor drainage conditions in soils and the application of nitrogen fertilizers, especially nitrates, are noted to inhibit nodulation and N_2 fixation. Most of the *Rhizobium* are very specific and can inoculate only a specific plant. For example, *R. japonicum, R. trifolii, R. meliloti, R. lupini*, and *R. phaseoli* are strains that are found only in soybean, clover, alfalfa, lupine, and beans, respectively. *Cross inoculation* (meaning infecting) for example, soybean with *R. trifolii* is very difficult. However, Clark and Paul (1989) reported that the *Rhizobium* in cowpeas can be used to nodulate a variety of legumes without the specificity encountered in the common legumes of temperate regions.

Recently, symbiotic N_2 fixation has also been reported in a number of non-legume plants, e.g., alnus of the cool temperate regions and casuarina in the subtropics and tropical regions. The non-legume plants can be nodulated or non-nodulated. The organism in the nodules of non-legume plants is identified as an actinomycete called *Frankia* (Havelka et al., 1982; Stevenson, 1986). The plants are usually *pioneer plants* growing in very poor soil conditions. They can establish themselves in infertile soils because of their association with the N_2 fixing organisms.

Nonsymbiotic Nitrogen Fixation. Nitrogen fixation can also be conducted by microorganisms that live independently in soils. This process, called nonsymbiotic nitrogen fixation, is carried out by two groups of organisms, bacteria and blue-green algae (Jensen, 1965). The bacteria of importance are *Azotobacter* and *Clostridium*, both of which are free-living *organotrophic* organisms. They need, therefore, an organic substrate as a source of energy. The blue-green algae, on the other hand, are *phototrophic* organisms, meaning they can utilize CO_2 from the air and also take up nutrients. The *Azotobacter* lives in aerobic soil condition, whereas the *Clostridium* is usually found in anaerobic soils. Recently, an *Azotobacter* species has been detected to grow in close association with *Paspalum notatum*, a tropical grass in Brazil, which is called *Azotobacter paspali* (Dobereiner and Day, 1975). This *A. paspali*-grass association is frequently compared with the symbiotic algae-azolla association, which is perhaps somewhat inaccurate. Whereas the algae appears to be an "integral" part of the *Azolla* tissue, the azotobacter lives in the moist space between the leaf-sheath and the stem of the grass and between the root system. The similarity is only in the fact that it is also supplying N_2 compounds to the plant.

Nitrogen Addition by N_2 Fixation. The amounts of N_2 added to soil by biological N_2 fixation are substantial, although they vary from plant to plant (Table 3.3). The data indicate that the

Table 3.3 Annual Nitrogen Addition by N_2 Fixation

	kg N/ha
Rainfall	1 - 10
Nonsymbiotic	45
Symbiotic:	45 - 260
Alfalfa	260
Red clover	170
White clover	130
Peanut	130
Soybean	120
Field peas	54

Source: Nutman (1965), Jensen (1965), LaRue and Peterson (1981), and Stevenson (1986).

symbiotic N_2 fixing organisms are more efficient than the free living (nonsymbiotic) N_2 fixers in enriching soils with N_2 compounds, especially *R. meliloti* in alfalfa. To be able to obtain the maximum benefit, alfalfa plants have to be plowed under before they reach the flowering stage. At this stage, the plants are not woody and are still succulent, so that they will decompose rapidly in soils, releasing in this way all the N_2 compounds that have been produced.

The data in the Table also list the annual addition of N_2 from rainfall. The amount is relatively small, and it comes from oxidation of atmospheric N_2 by lightning, photochemical oxidation, and fast moving meteorites (Hutchinson, 1944). The electrical discharge by lightning, the most significant of the three, oxidizes N_2 gas in the air into NO_2, which dissolves in raindrops to form nitric and nitrous acids. The reactions can be written as follows:

$$N_2 + O_2 \rightarrow 2NO \quad (3.5)$$

$$2NO + O_2 \rightarrow 2NO_2 \quad (3.6)$$

$$2NO_2 + H_2O \rightarrow \underset{\text{(nitric and nitrous acid)}}{HNO_3 + HNO_2} \quad (3.7)$$

This phenomenon is a form of *acid rain*, which occurs naturally during heavy thunderstorms.

3.2.5 Ammonification

Ammonification is a biological process by which organic nitrogen compounds are converted into ammonia. This is the point where the overall N_2 cycle starts to interface with the inner (soil) N_2 cycle (see Figure 3.4). Organic residue is broken down by decomposition, and the large molecules of protein, amino acids, amino sugars, and ureases unavailable for plant uptake are recycled into simple inorganic N compounds available to plants. Stevenson (1989) considered this process to be a mineralization process. The reaction can be illustrated as follows:

$$R\text{-}NH_2 + H_2O \rightarrow R\text{-}OH + NH_3 + \text{energy} \quad (3.8)$$

where $R\text{-}NH_2$ = ammino acid. The reaction is an enzymatic reaction, and a wide variety of enzymes are involved, each acting on a specific type of nitrogen compound (Stevenson, 1989; Ladd and Jackson, 1982), e.g., proteinases to break the peptide bonds in proteins, and dehydrogenases and oxidases to break the amino group from the amino acid.

3.2.6 Nitrification

Nitrification is the conversion of ammonium into nitrate. The process was first discovered in 1856 by J.T. Way, and twenty years later Warington reported that it was a biological reaction. It was Winogradsky who in 1890 finally isolated the bacteria responsible for the reaction (Alexander, 1965; Brady, 1990). Currently, it is known that nitrification occurs into two steps. In the first step, *Nitrosomonas* bacteria are producing nitrite from ammonium, which is immediately followed by the second step, in which the *Nitrobacter* bacteria transformed the nitrite into nitrate. The reaction processes have been presented earlier as reactions 2.4, and 2.5, respectively. Nitrification is affected by a number of soil conditions, e.g. aeration, temperature, moisture content, pH, soil fertility, and C/N ratios of organic compounds. Most of these factors should be in optimum conditions for bacterial growth.

Agricultural and Environmental Significance of Nitrification. The final product, NO_3^-, is the most soluble form of N_2 in soils, and has an undesirable effect on the environment. Nitrate is an anion, and will not be adsorbed by negatively charged clay minerals, hence will not accumulate in soils. It tends to be leached from soils and may turn up in streams, rivers, lakes, swamps, and in groundwater, which is undesirable from an environmental quality standpoint. If, because of leaching of NO_3^-, denitrification or immobilization of nitrate can not take place, it may disrupt the N_2 cycle, and nitrogen may be lost from soils. To reduce these losses in agricultural operations, nitrate or nitrification inhibitors have been developed. These are artificial chemicals that inhibit the nitrification process so that most of the N_2 fertilizers stay in the NH_4^+ form. Since ammonium is a cation, it can be adsorbed by negatively charged clay surfaces. Slow-release N_2 fertilizers are also applied to control losses of N in soils because of nitrification. In this case, the fertilizer releases only small amounts of inorganic N at a time, giving time to the plants to absorb it.

3.2.7 Denitrification

Denitrification is the conversion of nitrates into N_2O and N_2 gas, and represents the last step in the overall N_2 cycle. By this process the nitrogen is returned to the atmosphere in the form of gas. The process, sometimes called *enzymatic denitrification*, is a reduction process mediated by anaerobic bacteria, e.g., *Pseudobacter, Achromobacter, Bacillus*, and *Alcaligenes* (Broadbent and Clark, 1965; Paul and Clark, 1989; Brady, 1990). The sequence of reduction can perhaps be presented as follows (Stevenson, 1986):

$$\underset{5+}{NO_3^-} \rightarrow \underset{3+}{NO_2^-} \rightarrow \underset{2+}{NO} \rightarrow \underset{1-}{N_2O} \rightarrow \underset{0}{N_2}$$

Environmental Implications of Denitrification. The release of nitrous oxide, N_2O, gas into the air has caused some concern among environmentalists. It is one of the gases that causes the development of acid rain. In addition, nitrous oxide is reported to contribute in the reactions destroying the ozone, O_3, layer that protects the earth from ultraviolet radiation from the sun. However, as in the case with the issue of CO_2 production, it is the accelerated production of N_2O gas by industry that is more significant than the natural process.

Chemodenitrification. Denitrification can also occur without the help of microbial enzymes, and this nonenzymatic process is called *chemical denitrification* or *chemodenitrification*. This reaction takes place in aerobic conditions, and is sometimes also referred to as *aerobic denitrification*. The final products are NO and NO_2, and the NO gas may in turn be oxidized into NO_2. The latter can dissolve in soil water to form nitric and nitrous acid. These processes can be illustrated by the reactions

$$2NO + O_2 \rightarrow 2NO_2 \tag{3.9}$$

$$2NO_2 + H_2O \rightarrow HNO_3 + HNO_2 \tag{3.10}$$

The reactions are similar to those responsible for acid rain (see equations 2.14 and 2.15). It only differs from acid rain in that chemodenitrification causes soil acidity to increase and does not result in the development of acid rain.

Environmental Significance of Chemodenitrification. The opinion exists that this kind of denitrification is not of too much importance in nature. It will not result in a substantial return of soil N_2 to the atmosphere, hence is insignificant in the last step of the N_2 cycle. The nitrogen remains in the soil because the gases formed are rapidly dissolved in soil water to form the acids as shown above. However, it is reported to be a harmful process in agriculture. Because by this process, application of N_2 fertilizers, such as urea, can result in considerable losses of N_2, consequently the fertilizer loses its efficiency in promoting plant growth. The reaction below illustrates the decomposition of the fertilizer by chemodenitrification.

$$2HNO_3 + CO(NH_2)_2 \rightarrow CO_2\uparrow + 3H_2O + 2N_2\uparrow \quad (3.11)$$

The large amounts of CO_2 and N_2 gases produced in the decomposition of urea are the reasons for the losses of N_2 from the fertilizer. Soils with low pH values are essential for this reaction (Allison and Doetsch, 1951).

Assimilatory Denitrification. Another type of reduction of NO_3^- is the so-called *assimilatory reduction*, by which NO_3^- is transformed into NH_4^+. The reaction takes place under anaerobic condition within the plant body for the biosynthesis of amino acids. In contrast to the denitrification process essential to the N_2 cycle, in assimilatory reduction, nitrogen is not lost in the air, but is accumulated in the plant body in the form of amino acids or proteins. The process of incorporating the NH_4 as an NH_2 group in the plant tissue is called *assimilation*. Assimilatory reduction is closely related with immobilization of NO_3^-, which is the topic of the next section.

3.2.8 Immobilization

Immobilization is the uptake of NO_3^- by plants, and its conversion from the inorganic into organic form. Nitrate is a source of food and energy for higher and lower plants, and will be consumed rapidly by these organisms. Because of the immobilization process some of the NO_3^- in soils will not be denitrified. Immobilization is the point where the overall N_2 cycle is bypassed and converges to become the so called *inner N_2 cycle* or *internal N_2 cycle*. Because of this process, N_2 is not returned to the atmosphere, but remains in the soil, as indicated earlier.

3.3 NONHUMIFIED ORGANIC MATTER

The nonhumified organic matter is composed of compounds released during decomposition in the original or slightly modified form. Although numerous organic compounds are present in the plant tissue, only a few exist in soils in detectable amounts after their release in soils. They are primarily (1) carbohydrates, (2) amino acids and proteins, (3) lipids, (4) nucleic acids, (5) lignins, and (6) organic acids.

3.3.1 Carbohydrates

Carbohydrates are important constituents of the plant body. Almost 75% of the plant's dry weight is composed of carbohydrates. Of the three major groups of food substances (carbohydrates, fats, and proteins) produced by plants, carbohydrates are formed first directly from CO_2 and water with the help of chlorophyll and sunlight, by a process called *photosynthesis*. They are, therefore, considered the immediate link between the energy of the sun and the energy displayed by living plants and other organisms on earth. Carbohydrates provide the source for the formation of fats, oils, amino acids, proteins, and other organic compounds needed in plant growth. Carbohydrates are also the ultimate source for formation of cellulose, chitin, pectin, and lignin, important structural components of the plant body. Ascorbic acid (vitamin C) and inositol are related carbohydrate compounds.

The carbohydrates range from simple sugars to polysaccharides or complex carbohydrates, and their properties consequently change with increasing molecular complexity. The sugars are usually crystalline compounds and sweet in taste. They form true solutions in water and are soluble in ethanol. The sugars are further subdivided into (1) monosaccharides or simple sugars, and (2) oligosaccharides, or compound sugars. Polysaccharides are usually amorphous and tasteless, and disperse in water to form colloidal suspensions. They are very complex in structure and have high molecular weights. Polysaccharides are sometimes distinguished into (1) *homopolysaccharides*, and (2) *heteropolysaccharides*. Homopolysaccharides are composed of a repeating monosaccharide, whereas heteropolysaccharides are made up of two (or more) different polysaccharides. For a more detailed classification of the carbohydrates, their structure and properties reference is made to Tan (1993).

Environmental Importance of Carbohydrates. Carbohydrates are the principal sources of food and energy for all organisms on earth, including humans, animals and especially soil microorganisms. Much has been said about the vital importance of complex carbohydrates in human nutrition and human health. Used in industry as raw materials for the production of pulp, paper, rayon, and starch, carbohydrates are also renewable resources of primary importance. As such, they are invaluable materials for the manufacture of alternative clean fuel and many other chemical compounds, such as butanol, ethanol, methyl alcohol, acetic acid, citric acid, and lactic acid.

As indicated above, carbohydrates serve as major sources of energy for many biological functions. Sugars are the first target of microbial attack, and are quickly subjected to aerobic and anaerobic decomposition. *Aerobic decomposition* is the complete oxidation of sugars into carbondioxide and water. Anaerobic decomposition is an incomplete breakdown of carbohydrates in the absence of oxygen. In pure biochemistry, the *anaerobic decomposition* of glucose is called *glycolysis* or *fermentation* of glucose. It is a non-oxidative breakdown and liberates only a small part of the energy of the glucose molecule. The ultimate end-products of glycolysis are methane, CH_4, and carbondioxide, CO_2. The reaction processes can be illustrated as follows:

$$\underset{\text{glucose}}{C_6H_{12}O_6} \rightarrow \underset{\text{methane}}{3CH_4} + 3CO_2 \qquad (3.12)$$

However, microorganisms vary greatly in their capacity for breaking down carbohydrates. In some fermentation processes, the end products can be alcohols, ketones, and various organic acids mixed with carbondioxide and/or hydrogen. The type of anaerobic decomposition of glucose leading to formation of ethanol and CO_2 is called *alcoholic fermentation*, and the reaction process can be illustrated as follows:

$$C_6H_{12}O_6 \rightarrow \underset{\text{ethanol}}{2C_2H_5OH} + 2CO_2 \qquad (3.13)$$

The formation of both ethyl alcohol and methyl alcohol or both, as depicted by reaction (3.13), form the basis for the production of alternative fuel sources. In practice, sugars from sugar cane or starches from corn or potato, $C_6H_{10}O_5)_5$, fermented with yeast are the least expensive sources. The production of methane and ethanol is always accompanied by the release of CO_2. The latter may create some concern about decreasing the quality of air in our atmosphere, since CO_2 is a *greenhouse gas*. However, in the presence of abundant plant growth, a natural production of CO_2 will be "filtered" from the atmosphere through absorption by green plants that use it in photosynthesis for the production of carbohydrates. Therefore, the chances of this CO_2 contributing to global warming due to the *greenhouse effect* are very small.

In contrast to simple sugars, polysaccharides, and especially soil polysaccharides, exhibit greater resistance to enzymatic degradation due to their size, more complex molecular structure, and their capacity to form complexes with soil inorganic constituents. The intimate association with soil clays particularly does not only slow down chemical decomposition, but also changes the electrochemical properties of clay surfaces important for adsorption of water. The polysaccharides compete with soil water for adsorption sites, and by expelling water reduce wetting and swelling of soil clays. They increase cementation of clay particles enhancing the development of soil aggregates. The soil structure formed is considered more stable than that produced by fungal mycelium.

3.3.2 Amino Acids and Protein

Amino acids are the building constituents of protein. These compounds contain N in the form of NH_2, called an amino group, attached to the C chain in their molecular structure. The acid part is composed of a terminal C in COOH form, called a carboxyl group. These are the reasons for the name *amino acids*. Twenty one amino acids are found as protein constituents. Both amino acids and proteins are major sources of nitrogen compounds in soils. They are more difficult to break down than carbohydrates because of their size and complexity in molecular structure. They are amphoteric in nature, and consequently react with acids and bases. At the isoelectric point, amino acids behave as *zwitter ions*, in other words, behave as cations and anions (Tan, 1993). In acid soils (soil pH > isoelectric point), the amino acids are positively charged and behave as cations, whereas in basic soils they are negatively charged and behave as anions.

Decomposition of Amino Acids and Protein. Amino acids and proteins are important sources of organic N in soils, and this N can become available again to plants upon decomposition of the amino acids and proteins. The main reaction process for the decomposition of these compounds is *hydrolysis*. Hydrolysis of proteins, brought about by proteinases and peptidases of soil microorganisms, results in cleavage of peptide bonds, releasing in this way the amino acids. The latter compounds are broken down further into NH_3 by the enzymes called amino acid dehydrogenases and oxidases. Schematically the main pathway of decomposition can be represented as follows:

$$\text{Proteins} \rightarrow \text{peptides} \rightarrow \text{amino acids} \rightarrow NH_3$$

The decomposition reaction of proteins as described above is frequently called *deamination* or *putrefaction* (Gortner, 1949; Stevenson, 1986). Deamination reactions can take place in aerobic or anaerobic conditions, and are, therefore, also called *oxidative*, and *non-oxidative* deamination, respectively. The reaction for oxidative deamination can be written as follows:

$$\underset{\text{amino acid}}{R\text{-}CH(NH_2)COOH} + O_2 \rightarrow RCOOH + CO_2 + NH_3 \quad (3.14)$$

Anaerobic deamination may result in (1) deamination or reduction, and (2) decarboxylation, as can be seen from the reactions below:

deamination or *reduction*:

$$\underset{\text{amino acid}}{R\text{-}CH(NH_2)COOH} + H_2 \rightarrow RCH_2COOH + NH_3 \quad (3.15)$$

decarboxylation:

$$R\text{-}CH(NH_2)COOH \rightarrow \underset{\text{amine}}{R\text{-}CH_2NH_2} + CO_2 \quad (3.16)$$

Reaction (3.15) above indicates that deamination is characterized by the destruction of the amino group and its transformation into NH_3. In contrast, decarboxylation (reaction 3.16) is distinguished by the decomposition of the COOH group into CO_2, and the subsequent transformation of the amino acid into an amine compound. The enzyme required for decarboxylation, called *amino acid decarboxylase*, is produced by *Clostridium* bacteria. When formed in animal bodies, some of the amines produced are reported to have important physiological effects. For example, *histidine decarboxylase* in animal tissue can produce *histamine*, an amine substance that can stimulate allergic effects and/or gastric secretion. Another enzyme, *tyrosine decarboxylase*, is an intermediate in the formation of *adrenalin*, an amine functioning as a *vasoconstrictor*. It is usually released in the bloodstream when a person or animal is startled or frightened (Conn and Stumpf, 1967).

3.3.3 Lipids

Lipids are heterogenous compounds of fatty acids, waxes, and oils. The basic component of lipids is glycerol, $C_3H_8O_3$, or other alcohols. They are classified into three groups: (1) simple lipids, (2) compound lipids, and (3) derived lipids. The simple lipids include the natural fats and oils, which can be divided into (a) nonvolatile fats and oils, and (b) volatile oils, such as turpentine and clove oil. The compound lipids are more fat-like in nature. They have been formed from fatty acids in combination with other organic compounds. For example, phospholipids are lipids in combination with organic phosphorus compounds, such as nucleic acids, phosphoproteins, and phytin. Glycolipid is a compound lipid, because the lipid is present in combination with a carbohydrate (galactose). The derived lipids are composed of fatty acids, alcohols and sterols. The fatty acids can be saturated fatty acids, such as palmitic acids, or unsaturated fatty acids, such as oleic acids. Palm oil and coconut oil are rich in palmitic acid. Cholesterol is an example of a sterol, which upon UV irradiation will form vitamin D.

Hydrolysis of fats by saponification with alkalies, yields glycerol and the salts of fatty acids. The metallic salts of the higher fatty acids are known as soap.

3.3.4 Nucleic Acids

All plant and animal cells contain discrete rounded or spherical bodies, called the *nucleus*, which contain nucleic acids. Nucleic acids, first isolated in 1869 by F. Miescher (Tan, 1993), are polymers with high molecular weights. Their repeating unit is a sugar attached to a mononucleotide, rather than an amino acid. Two types of nucleic acids are distinguished: (1) DNA, deoxyribonucleic acid, and (2) RNA, ribonucleic acid.

Currently it is known that nucleic acids can also be formed in other plant organelles: mitochondria and chloroplasts. However, the amount produced in the mitochondrion and chloroplast are much smaller than that produced in the nucleus. They are also smaller in size, and their genetic capabilities are less than the nucleic acids from the nucleus. When released in soils by decomposition of plant residue, nucleic acids are potential sources of P for plant growth.

3.3.5 Lignin

Lignin are highly aromatic polymers, and are produced by living plants from carbohydrates by a process called *lignification* (Tan, 1993). As indicated earlier, the ultimate source for formation of lignin is carbohydrates or intermediate products of photosynthesis related to carbohydrates. In the growth of plants, carbohydrates are synthesized first. The formation of lignin then begins. The process of conversion of nonaromatic carbohydrates into compounds containing phenolic (aromatic) groups, characteristic of lignin, is called *aromatization*. It is believed that dehydration of fructose contributes to the aromatization process. The end products of the aromatization process are pyrogallol, hydroxyhydroquinone, phloroglucinol, or a combination thereof. The spaces existing between the cellulose fibers in the plant body are then gradually filled with these lignified carbohydrates. This process is called *lignification* and serves a number of functions. Lignin cements and anchors polysaccharide fibers in the plant tissue, and gives resistance to the fibers against physical and chemical breakdown. The quantity of lignin increases with plant age, woody tissue, and stem content.

Plant lignin can be divided into three types of basic monomers: (1) coniferyl alcohol, derived mostly from softwood or coniferous plants, (2) sinapyl alcohol, derived from hardwood, and (3) coumaryl alcohol, derived from grasses and bamboo. For these reasons, lignin can perhaps be distinguished into softwood lignin, hardwood lignin and grass lignin. These basic monomers form large, complex polymers, and it is common to find a haphazard structure of lignin in many organic chemistry books. A hypothesis of a more systematic arrangement of the basic monomers into lignin is presented by Tan (1993).

Lignin, released in soils by decomposition of plant tissue, is highly resistant to microbial decomposition. Decay of plant material, especially of woody plants, results in an apparent increase in lignin content in soils owing to a preferential decomposition of carbohydrates. Certain fungi, e.g., *Tramitis pini*, have been reported to attack lignin. Depending upon the conditions, accumulation of lignin could result in the formation of peat, which in time can be converted into lignite, leonardite, and coal. Under the influence of high pressure and temperature for geologic time periods, these deposits can ultimately become fossil fuel (oil). In soil science, such a conversion process is called *metamorphosis*. In soils, lignin is an important source for the formation of soil humus or humic matter.

For a more detailed discussion on lignin and other soil organic substances reference is made to Tan (1993).

3.3.6 Organic Acids

The organic acids may range from simple aliphatic acids to complex aromatic and heterocyclic acids, e.g., formic acid, acetic acid, oxalic acid, amino acid, benzoic acid, and tannic acid. For a partial list of organic acids in soils, reference is made to Tan (1986). Many of them are present in such low concentrations that they can be detected only by thin layer or gas chromatography, and undoubtedly other organic acids may be present in the soils awaiting identification and isolation. The amount of formic acid is usually reported in the range of 0.5 to 0.9 mmol/100g soil, whereas that of acetic acid is between 0.7 and 1.0 mmol/100g soil (Tan, 1986). A large number of these organic acids are intermediate products of plant and microbial metabolism. Some may have been released into the soil as root exudates, whereas others are the result of oxidative degradation of organic matter.

The organic acids may have both favorable and unfavorable effects to plant growth. They play a significant role in the dissolution and mobilization of elements from rocks and minerals. Acetic acid and oxalic acid have been used in the study of mineral dissolution. They exhibit some metal complexing capacity.

3.4 HUMIFIED ORGANIC MATTER

Humified organic matter, or humic matter, is a group of compounds that includes humic acids, fulvic acids, hymatomelanic acids, and humins. This humified soil organic fraction is also known as *humus*, or currently as *humic compounds*. Today humic compounds are defined as amorphous, colloidal polydispersed substances with yellow to brown-black color and high molecular weights.

These humic compounds have been formed in soils by a process called *humification*. According to the lignoprotein theory, they are lignoprotein compounds produced by interpolymerization of phenolic compounds, peptides, amino acids and carbohydrates (Stevenson, 1982; Schnitzer and Khan, 1972; Tan, 1993). Lignin and lignin degradation products are the sources of the phenols. The polymers in humic compounds are relatively stable, being relatively resistant to microbial enzymatic attack, although they contain amino acids and amino sugar polymers in their structure.

The distinction into the different types of humic compounds is based on their solubility in alkali and acids or ethyl alcohol. *Fulvic acid* (FA) is soluble in alkali and acid, and is the low molecular weight fraction of humic matter. It is also soluble in water. *Humic acid* (HA), on the other hand, is soluble in alkali, but insoluble in acid and water. It is the high molecular weight fraction of humic matter. *Hymatomelanic acid* is the alcohol soluble part of HA, whereas *humin* is defined as the humic fraction insoluble in water, alkali and acid. However, it can be extracted by hot alkali solutions. In the German and Russian literature, they are collectively referred to as *humus acids* (Orlov, 1985; Tan, 1993), which is equivalent to the names humic matter or humic substances. Within the group, FA and HA are perhaps the most important fractions of humic matter. They are present in soils in relatively large amounts, although their contents may vary considerably from soil to soil (Tan, 1986). The terms humic and fulvic acids have been used for a long time, nevertheless a number of scientists still questions the correctness of the usage of these terms. They believe that the terms humic and fulvic acids are valid only as *operational terms* that relate the methods of extraction of these compounds (Aiken et al., 1985). Many other scientists, on the other hand, believe that the names refer to identifiable humic compounds, though complex in structure (Flaig, 1975; Kononova, 1975; Orlov, 1985; Stevenson, 1986).

3.4.1 Types of Humic Matter

Currently it is known that humic matter exists not only in soils, but also in streams, rivers, lakes, oceans, and their sediments. They can also be found as geologic deposits, e.g., lignite or leonardite, coal, and oilshale. These deposits are the source for the production of commercial humates, which are used as soil amendments (Lobartini et al., 1992). On the basis of present knowledge, humic matter can be classified into three broad groups:

(1) *Terrestrial* humic matter: humic matter in soils
(2) *Aquatic* humic matter: humic matter in streams, lakes, oceans, and their sediments
(3) *Geologic* humic matter: humic matter in lignite or leonardite, coal, and other geologic deposits.

Terrestrial humic matter can be subdivided again into three categories: softwood, hardwood, and grass humic matter (Tan, 1993). It is composed of humic and fulvic acids, although their contents may differ considerably from soil to soil. Aquatic humic matter is composed mainly of fulvic acid, and can be subdivided into *allochthonous*, and *autochthonous* humic matter. The allochthonous humic matter is believed to originate from soil humic matter, but after leaching into streams it has been subjected to further distinct changes (Jackson, 1975). The autochthonous humic matter originates from indigenous aquatic plant material, which has a different composition than terrestrial plants. Especially in the oceans, where plankton, kelp, and other seaweed are major forms of organisms, the nature of humic matter formed is quite different from soil humic matter. Aquatic humic matter consists of carbohydrate-protein complexes as opposed to terrestrial or soil humic matter which is mainly a ligno-protein complex.

3.4.2 Chemical Composition

In general, humic acid is higher in C and N, but lower in O and S contents than fulvic acid (Table 3.4). Comparison between terrestrial, aquatic, and geologic humic acids indicates that geologic humic acid tends to be higher in C, but lower in H, and especially N contents.

Table 3.4 Elemental Composition of Humic Matter

Origin	C	H	N	O+S
		--------------- % ---------------		
Humic Acid				
Terrestrial	50.6	5.6	4.3	38.5
Aquatic	51.7	4.8	2.3	41.1
Geologic	57.1	3.8	1.6	37.5
Fulvic Acid				
Terrestrial	48.1	4.5	1.7	45.7
Aquatic	47.4	5.0	1.5	46.1
Geologic	45.0	4.2	1.4	49.4

The total acidity also shows some variations because of origin (Table 3.5). These values are attributed to the sum of the carboxyl and phenolic-OH group contents, and indicate the cation exchange and complexing capacities of humic matter. A high total acidity value is indicative of a high CEC and complexing power. The data show that the lowest total acidity is exhibited by geologic humic acid, and the highest by geologic fulvic acid. The data in the literature often show that fulvic acids exhibit higher total acidity values than humic acids.

Geologic humic acid is also more aromatic, whereas aquatic humic acid tends to be more aliphatic in nature than terrestrial

Table 3.5 Aliphatic C, Aromatic C, COOH C Contents, Total Acidity, COOH and Phenolic-OH Group Contents

Origin	Aliphatic C	Aromatic C	COOH C	Total acidity	COOH	Phenolic OH
	------------%	-----------		---------mol/kg	---------	
Humic Acid						
Terrestrial	48.7	36.4	14.9	7.0	4.3	2.7
Aquatic	50.3	37.2	12.5	7.0	4.4	2.6
Geologic	45.1	43.0	11.9	5.8	3.8	2.0
Fulvic Acid						
Terrestrial	61.0	25.3	13.7	6.8	4.7	2.1
Aquatic	62.6	21.7	15.7	7.0	4.4	2.6
Geologic	—	—	—	9.4	8.2	0.8

humic acids. In the literature, the tendency can be noticed for fulvic acids to contain more aliphatic compounds than humic acids.

3.4.3 Chemical Reactions

The chemical reactivity of humic matter can be predicted from the total acidity value, which is defined as the sum of carboxyl and phenolic group content. The dissociation of protons from the carboxyl groups, which starts at pH 3.0, creates a negative charge. This negative charge increases in value, and becomes larger when at pH 9.0, the phenolic-OH group also dissociates its proton. The presence of such pH dependent, or variable, charges enable the humic molecule to perform many chemical reactions, e.g., adsorption of cations and water, complex formation or chelation of metals, and interaction with clays (Tan, 1993). These reactions will be discussed in more details in chapter 6.

3.4.4 Spectral Characteristics

Infrared spectroscopy produces different spectra for terrestrial humic and fulvic acids. The infrared spectra as a whole can be used as a fingerprint to distinguish humic from fulvic acid (Figure 3.6). NMR analysis indicates that terrestrial, aquatic and geologic humic matter are generally composed of aliphatic, aromatic, and carboxylic compounds (Tan, 1993). The NMR spectra demonstrate that humic acids are more aromatic in nature than fulvic acids.

3.4.5 Effect of Humic Matter on Soils and the Environment

Humic matter is an essential soil component, and is known to have a beneficial effect on soil physical, chemical, and biological properties. It may affect plant growth directly and indirectly. Directly, humic acid is capable of improving seed germination, root initiation, and elongation, respiration, uptake of plant nutrients, and development of green mass. Indirectly, humic acid can modify the properties of the medium in which plants grow. Humic acid is reported to enhance soil structure formation, increase soil water holding capacity, and cation exchange capacity. It can also reduce micronutrient toxicity in acid soils, especially Al toxicity (Tan and Binger, 1986; Ahmad and Tan, 1986). This is attributed to its capacity for complexing or chelating the metals. In addition, humic acid has also an important geologic and economic impact due to its occurrence as natural geologic deposits. These deposits are the main sources for the economical production of commercial humates used as soil amendments. Finally, it must be mentioned that humic matter may affect the environment. The presence of humic and

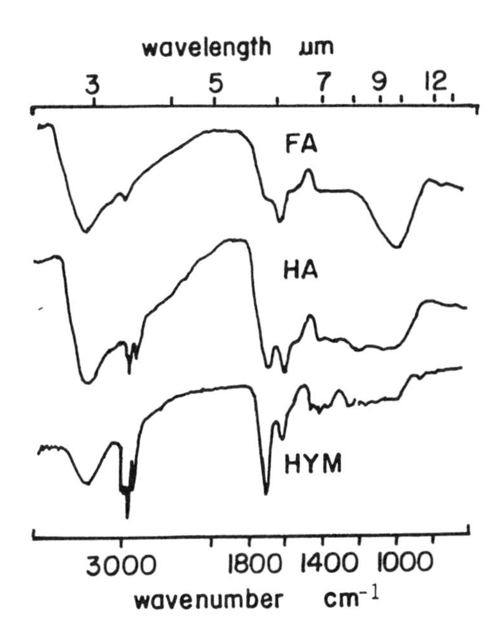

Figure 3.6 Characteristic infrared absorption spectra of fulvic acid (FA), humic acid (HA), and hymatomelanic acid (HYM), respectively. Absorption bands at approximately 2900 and between 1700 - 1600 cm^{-1} are attributed to aliphatic CH and carboxyl group vibrations, respectively.

fulvic acids in lakes and streams may stimulate the growth of phytoplankton. However, present in large concentrations, humic acids may reduce the photosynthesis of many aquatic green plants because of the dark brown color that they impart to the water. Due to its enormous chelation capacity, on the other hand, humic acid is capable in detoxifying lakes that are affected by metal pollution. Suggestions have also been made to use humic acid as a sink of radioactive metals polluting soils and streams. In the form of cations, these radioactive metals can be adsorbed and chelated by humic acids and rendered immobile.

CHAPTER 4

GAS PHASE IN SOILS

4.1 SOIL AIR

The gas phase in soils is called *soil air*. It is located in the pore space, which is defined as the space in soil that is occupied by the gas and liquid phases. This pore space is composed of *macro-* and *micropores*. The macropores are usually the spaces between the soil structural units and as such, they are the main channels for air movement. On the other hand, the micropores are the spaces within the structural units, and are the main spaces for water. The macropores will be filled first with water during a rainfall or by irrigation. This water then moves into the micropores, where it will be held for some time in the soil. The amount of total pore spaces, called soil *porosity*, differs from soil to soil and from soil horizon to soil horizon. The percentage of pore spaces may range from 25% or lower to 50% or higher. A soil with a loam texture and in optimum condition for plant growth has a total pore space of 50%, which is filled half with water and half with air (Brady, 1990).

Soil air is composed of the same type of gases commonly found in the atmosphere and differs from atmospheric air only in composition. The major gaseous components and their relative amounts in atmospheric air are listed in Table 4.1. Many other types of gases are present in minute amounts in soil air.

Table 4.1 Major Gaseous Components in Air Above the Soil

Gaseous Component	Volume %
Nitrogen, N_2	78.0
Oxygen, O_2	21.0
Carbon dioxide, CO_2	0.031
Argon, Ar	0.93
Helium, He	0.0005
Methane, CH_4	0.0002
Hydrogen, H_2	0.00005
Nitrous oxide, NO_2	0.00002

Sources: Taylor and Ashcroft (1972); Manahan (1975); Brady (1990).

For proper plant growth, the pore spaces must contain air in sufficient amounts and in the proper composition. The amount of soil air in the pore spaces is usually controlled by soil water. When the amount of soil water increases, air is pushed out of the pore spaces. When water content in the pore spaces decreases because of uptake by plants and/or evaporation, air content increases by mass flow and diffusion. As indicated earlier, for optimum plant growth, half of the pore space should be filled with air and half with water. The quality of this air is usually measured by its composition in O_2 and CO_2 content. Nitrogen is unavailable to most plants and, therefore, is not taken into consideration in this respect, though it is an important constituent in biological nitrogen fixation. Most biological reactions in soils consume O_2 and produce CO_2; hence, soil air is generally lower in O_2 ($<20\%$), but higher in CO_2 content ($>0.03\%$) than is atmospheric air above the ground. The CO_2 content shows a marked seasonal trend and usually increases with soil depth. Oxygen content in soil air appears to be low in soils saturated with water. It reaches a maximum level at *field capacity,* after which it remains almost constant with decreasing amounts of soil water (Brady, 1984). In general, oxygen deficiency is noted if O_2 content in soil air decreases to 15% or less (Taylor and Ashcroft, 1972). Several biochemical reactions, mediated by soil organisms, are responsible for the O_2-CO_2 balance in soil air, e.g., respiration of plant roots and microorganisms and aerobic decomposition of soil organic matter. Both reactions consume oxygen and produce carbon dioxide (see Tan, 1993). Respiration increases with the presence of abundant plant life; hence, soils under crops contain generally less O_2 and more CO_2 than bare or fallow soils. The application of manure or plant residues may also increase the consumption of O_2 and the production of CO_2. An additional source of CO_2 is the burning of crop residues. Biomass burning is a normal agricultural management process in sugar cane production. The amount of CO_2 generated and its effects on soil and fauna need further investigations.

Unfortunately, no biochemical reactions exist in soils that can reverse the process in favor of the oxygen content. Photosynthesis is the only biological reaction that absorbs CO_2 and produces O_2. However, photosynthesis takes place in green plant parts growing above the soil. Therefore, the O_2-CO_2 balance in soil air can only be corrected by exchange of soil air for atmospheric air, a process called *aeration.*

4.2 BIOCHEMICAL EFFECT OF AERATION

Aeration has a significant effect on many biochemical reactions. As discussed in Chapter 3, many of the decomposition reactions of soil organic matter are affected by the aeration status in soils. When adequate amounts of air (O_2) are present, aerobic reactions prevail. On the other hand, where aeration is poor (lack of O_2) anaerobic reactions predominate. In other words, aerobic reactions, e.g., oxidation, take place with adequate aeration, whereas anaerobic reactions, e.g., reduction, occur under poorly aerated conditions. As will be discussed in the next section, the properties of soils in an oxidized state are markedly different from those of soils in a reduced state. The solubility of many elements changes with a change in the oxidation-reduction state.

4.2.1 Biochemistry in Aerobic Conditions and Its Role in Environmental Quality

In well aerated soils, organic matter will decompose into CO_2 and H_2O, and the nutrient elements are released to the benefit of plant growth. In such soils, most of the nutrient elements are present in the oxidation state. For example, nitrogen is present as NO_3^-, manganese as Mn^{4+}, sulphur as SO_4^{2-}, and iron as Fe_3^+. Iron in the oxidized state (ferric iron) is more stable but less soluble than iron in the reduced state (Fe^{2+} or ferrous iron). Ferric iron has a red to reddish brown color, and soils rich in Fe^{3+} are, therefore, red to reddish brown in color. If pockets with anaerobic conditions are present in a well-aerated soil, the iron in these pockets are present in the reduced state. Ferrous iron is yellowish or greenish to grayish in color. Therefore, these pockets are yellowish or grayish in color, which produces in the soil pedon a color pattern called *mottling*. The presence of a mottled horizon indicates an inadequately drained soil horizon.

The carbon dioxide produced by aerobic decomposition of organic matter will react with soil water to form carbonic acid, which affects soil acidity. The increase in soil acidity increases the dissolution of soil minerals. Such a dissolution of primary minerals is important in soil formation, soil fertility and plant nutrition. For example, calcium carbonate, $CaCO_3$, the main component of limestone, is insoluble in pure H_2O. However, in water containing CO_2, calcium carbonate is made soluble by its conversion into calcium bicarbonate. The reaction, called *carbonation,* can be written as follows:

$$H_2O + CO_2 \rightarrow H_2CO_3 \quad (4.1)$$

$$H_2CO_3 + CaCO_3 \rightarrow \underset{\text{calcium bicarbonate}}{Ca(HCO_3)_2} \quad (4.2)$$

The calcium bicarbonate that is formed is soluble in water. Carbonation causes liming materials to react in soils. By releasing its Ca^{2+} in this way, lime reduces soil acidity. The rate of formation of calcium bicarbonate depends on the partial pressure of carbon dioxide. In other words, the solubility of calcium carbonate increases as the partial pressure of CO_2 increases (Taylor and Ashcroft, 1972). Dissolved carbon dioxide also increases the solubility of apatite, a natural phosphate mineral. In fact, almost any mineral in soils is affected by carbonic acid.

Other acids that are produced by aerobic decomposition of organic matter, such as humic acids and the inorganic acids, nitric and sulfuric acids, also contribute to the solubilization of soil minerals.

Soil acidity also increases by the oxidation of sulphur compounds, which produces sulfuric acid. The presence of extremely acid soils in the coastal regions are caused by these processes. These soils, frequently called *cat-clays*, are non-productive; fortunately, they occur only in limited areas. Of more practical significance is the increased acidity of soils contaminated with *acid mine spoil* due to oxidation of S-compounds. The residue from coal mines, called mine spoil, contains large amounts of pyrite, FeS_2, which upon bio-oxidation produces sulfuric acid, as can be noticed from the reaction

$$2FeS_2 + 2H_2O + 7O_2 \rightarrow 2Fe^{2+} + 4H^+ + 4SO_4 \quad (4.3)$$

Acid mine spoil is a harmful contaminant of soils and streams. The extremely high acidity created by acid mine spoil is toxic and has many undesirable effects on soils and the environment. The iron released remains soluble in the acid environment. Although many attempts have been made to solve the problem, the reclamation of soils containing acid mine spoil is facing many difficulties. One of the reclamation methods involves the application of lime, which neutralizes the acidity by converting the sulfuric acid into calcium sulfate. The reaction is written

$$CaCO_3 + H_2SO_4 \rightarrow CaSO_4 + H_2O + CO_2{\uparrow} \qquad (4.4)$$

The carbon dioxide formed is lost in the air. However, the decrease in soil acidity creates new problems. The large amounts of Fe^{2+} released in reaction (4.3) are rapidly oxidized into Fe^{3+}. In the slightly acid to neutral environment, as a result of liming, ferric iron precipitates as $Fe(OH)_3$. These processes can be illustrated by the following reactions:

$$3Fe^{2+} + O_2 + 4H^+ \rightarrow Fe^{3+} + 2H_2O + e^- \qquad (4.5)$$

$$Fe^{3+} + 3H_2O \rightarrow Fe(OH)_3 + 3H^+ \qquad (4.6)$$

The $Fe(OH)_3$ produced is often deposited as an amorphous colloidal material, or may form coatings around the liming particles. The latter occurrence inhibits any further reaction from taking place.

4.2.2 Biochemistry in Anaerobic Conditions and Its Role in Environmental Quality

Reduction processes prevailing in anaerobic conditions bring about the reduction of many nutrient elements in soils. Because of this, iron is reduced into Fe^{2+}, manganese to Mn^{2+}, sulphur to SO_3^{2-}, and nitrate to NH_4^+. Ferrous iron, Fe^{2+}, is usually gray or greenish gray in color; hence, a poorly drained soil exhibits gray colors. Pockets with aerobic conditions present in such a soil contain ferric iron, creating reddish to rusty colors. This also produces mottling in the pedon.

In anaerobic soil condition, nitrate tends to be reduced into nitrite, NO_2^-. The reaction, called *nitrate reduction*, can be illustrated as follows:

$$2NO_3^- + CH_2O \rightarrow 2NO_2^- + H_2O + CO_2 \tag{4.7}$$

This reaction indicates that nitrate acts as an electron acceptor. Such a process finds application in the reclamation of sewage sludge lagoons. The lagoons, which are typically deficient in O_2, are treated (fertilized) with $NaNO_3$, which provides an emergency source of O_2 for reaction (4.7) to take place. Such a treatment may re-establish normal bacterial growth (Manahan, 1975; Moore and Moore, 1976). The nitrite, NO_2^-, formed is, however, toxic, and when it is allowed to build up to sufficiently high concentrations, it may inhibit further bacterial growth.

Nitrate reduction may ultimately end up in a denitrification process, a process by which the nitrogen compound is reduced into N_2 gas, according to the reaction:

$$4NO_3^- + 5CH_2O + 4H^+ \rightarrow 2N_2 + 5CO_2 + H_2O \tag{4.8}$$

This reaction involves the transfer of five electrons. The denitrification reaction is often applied in water treatment procedures to remove nitrates, which are harmful pollutants. By treating water with small amounts of methanol, the nitrate is reduced under anaerobic condition into N_2 gas. The reaction is written

$$\underset{\text{methanol}}{5CH_3OH} + 6NO_3^- + 6H^+ \rightarrow 5CO_2 + 13H_2O + 3N_2\uparrow \tag{4.9}$$

The nitrogen gas is non-toxic and is lost in the air.

4.3 BIOLOGICAL EFFECT OF AERATION

4.3.1 Effect on Plant Growth

One of the most obvious biological effect of an imbalanced oxygen and carbon dioxide content in soil air is its impact on plant growth. It is an established fact that improper cultural practices, resulting in poor aeration, reduces plant growth. Water and nutrient uptake are inhibited. Under inundated or swampy conditions, toxic compounds, such as H_2S, are formed.

Aeration affects the growth and yield of crops as well as the growth of roots. However, roots are perhaps more affected by the aeration status of soils than the above-ground parts of plants. Root growth is inhibited by poor aeration in soils, and if roots are not growing adequately, the plant parts above the ground will also not grow well. Root growth of most plants usually ceases at a concentration of 1% O_2 in soil air. Only *hydrophytes*, plants growing in water (hydro = water), such as rice plants and aquatic plants, can grow roots in anaerobic conditions.

It appears that roots can grow and function at oxygen concentrations far below the normal O_2 concentration of atmospheric air. Root growth was recorded at oxygen concentrations as low as 2.2% (Taylor and Ashcroft, 1972). The term *critical value* was introduced to show the lowest limit of oxygen content required for growing roots, and growth is limited by aeration (Wiegand and Lemon, 1958). This critical value has no fixed limits, and seems to be a function of the soil moisture content as expressed in terms of the soil matric potential (ψ_m). The critical value decreases from 4 μg O_2/cm^3 to 1 μg O_2/cm^3 as soil matric potential increases from -30 Joules/kg to -10 Joules/kg (Wiegand and Lemon, 1958). The increase in matric potential means that soil moisture content increases. Plants are less affected by moisture stress at higher soil moisture content. Because of this, they can function with smaller amounts of oxygen. The definition and concept of soil matric potential are discussed in chapter 5 (see also Tan, 1993).

Plants grown in well-aerated soils usually develop long, well-branched fibrous roots. When aeration becomes restricted, these well-developed roots slowly deteriorate and a new root system is produced by undergoing morphological changes as an adaptation to poor aeration. In anaerobic conditions, the roots are frequently short and stubby, and often grow superficially to take advantage of the proximity of atmospheric air. A good example is the roots of cypress trees, called *cypress knees*, or roots of mangrove trees in swamps, that grow out of the water into the air.

Carbon Dioxide Toxicity and Oxygen Deficiency. As discussed before, when aeration is restricted, several of the processes in soils consume oxygen and produce carbon dioxide. The net effect is that the O_2 content in soil air decreases, whereas the CO_2 content simultaneously increases considerably. Two possible reasons have been suggested for the restricted root growth by the changing O_2-CO_2 composition in soil air. One hypothesis postulates that high amounts of CO_2 are toxic to plant roots, especially to root cell protoplasm. According to this theory, excessive amounts of CO_2 temporarily suppress the functional activity of root cells, inhibiting root growth (Hunter and Rich, 1925). However, the most accepted hypothesis is that O_2 deficiency in soil air reduces respiration of plant roots. An adequate supply of O_2 is necessary to maintain respiration and permeability of plant roots, factors that influence water and nutrient uptake.

Under normal field conditions, oxygen deficiency is considered more serious to root growth than excess CO_2 in soil air. At high oxygen concentrations, root performance, e.g., water uptake, is not affected by the presence of high CO_2 concentrations (Taylor and Ashcroft, 1972).

However, no definite answers have been given yet as to the harmful effect of poor aeration on root growth. Is it because of the reduced concentration of O_2 or is it attributed to increased concentrations of CO_2? Perhaps it is the result of the interaction of decreased O_2 and increased CO_2 content.

Plant Species. The problem discussed above is complicated by the fact that different plants may react differently to the variation in O_2 and CO_2 concentration in soil air. The factor of plant species can be illustrated by the following examples. Tomato plants are very sensitive to the aeration status of soils. Maximum growth of tomato plants is reported to occur only when the O_2 concentration of the air is at 21%. Sugar beets require proper aeration, in contrast to ladino clover, which can grow in poorly aerated soils. Barley is another plant which will grow at low concentrations of oxygen. Red pines also grow well in poorly drained soils, but root crops are affected harmfully by poor aeration. Abnormally shaped carrots and sugar beets develop when these plants are grown in compacted, poorly aerated soils (Taylor and Ashcroft, 1972; Brady, 1984).

In addition to respiration and aerobic decomposition, the aeration status in soils is affected by many other factors, such as *soil compaction, soil moisture content,* and *soil temperature.*

Soil Compaction affects the pore spaces, which constitute the main venues for air movement and storage. When the pores, especially macropores, are destroyed due to compaction of soils, not only will air be deficient, but also the soil becomes dense and hard. A compacted soil has an adverse effect on root growth by (1) increasing the mechanical impedance to root growth, and (2) decreasing and altering the configuration of pore spaces (Taylor and Ashcroft, 1972). It is believed that the amount of O_2 needed by roots depends on the amount of work that a root must do in expanding against the mechanical impedance present in soils. In a loose and friable soil, only a small amount of energy will be used by roots to penetrate the soil, hence low concentrations of O_2 will give satisfactory growth. On the other hand, in a compacted soil, the root has to use more energy to grow in the soil, and as the amount of energy required for growth increases, the amount of O_2 necessary for growing also increases. In simulated conditions, it was noted that at an oxygen concentration of 20%, root growth was normal in a sand medium at normal pressure (no pressure applied). However, the growth rate of these roots was only one-half as fast when a pressure of 69.0×10^3 Pascal (10 lbs/in^2) was applied to the medium (Gill and Miller, 1956).

Soil Moisture Content is another factor that affects soil aeration. As discussed in chapter 5, water is held in the pore spaces by varying forces of attraction. These forces can be expressed in various ways, e.g., in terms of *water potential* (ψ_w) or soil moisture tension (see chapter 5). When the soil is saturated with water, the water potential has the highest value (0 Joules/kg), The value of the water potential becomes increasingly smaller (becomes more negative in value) with decreasing amounts of water. At *field capacity* the water potential equals -30 J/kg, whereas at wilting point the water potential is -1500 J/kg. At high soil water potentials, there is less or no tension in soils, hence the soil moisture tension is low. Similarly at low water potentials, the tension in soils increases, consequently the soil moisture tension is high. These conditions affect root growth.

Since the amount of water in the pore spaces usually determines the air content in soils, low soil moisture tension corresponds to low amounts of air or, in other words, translates to poor aeration status. In temperate region soils, this condition occurs in winter and spring when soil moisture content is generally highest. The air content, hence O_2 content, reaches a maximum at *field capacity* (0.3 bars or -3 x 10^5 ergs/g), after which it remains constant with increased drying of the soil (Figure 4.1). The curve indicates that at field capacity, the O_2 content in soil air is approximately 15%, which is rather low. However, when soil moisture content is not a limiting factor, this amount of oxygen still appears to be sufficient for normal root growth. Root growth will be inhibited when the O_2 concentration in soil air decreases to 10.5% (Gingrich and Russell, 1956). In the presence of adequate amounts of O_2, root growth is generally better at low moisture tension than at high soil moisture tension. At high soil moisture tension, the soil is too dry for plants to grow although the oxygen content may be adequate.

Soil Temperature is also a factor on oxygen content in soil air. Cooler temperatures usually decrease the O_2 concentration in air. Consequently, decreasing temperatures may be harmful for root growth. Maximum rate of root growth at 21% oxygen was reported to occur at 30°C. However, this growth rate was noted to decrease almost 50-60% when plants were grown at temperatures of 15° to 20°C. In the presence of 2.2% O_2 the growth rate appears to be 50-70% less than that at 21% O_2 over the range of 15° to 30°C (Taylor and Ashcroft, 1972).

4.3.2 Water Uptake

Root cells consist of (1) cell walls, which are rigid, but exhibit some elasticity; (2) protoplasm, which acts as a semipermeable

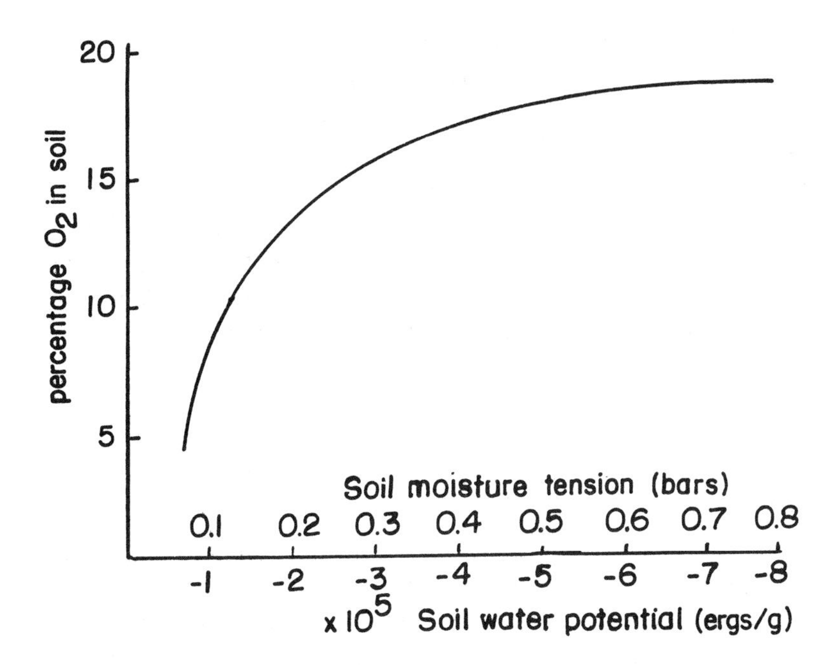

Figure 4.1 The relationship between soil water potential and oxygen content in soil air (adapted from Meek et al., 1980; Brady, 1984).

membrane through which water and ions move; and (3) vacuoles that contain cell sap, which is rich in solutes and colloids. The high solute and colloid concentration in the cell sap attracts water from the soil into the plant cell. The forces responsible for the movement of water into the root cells are called *osmotic forces,* and the energy related to these forces is called *osmotic potential* (Tan, 1993). Such a movement, considered a *passive movement*, requires good permeability of the root cells. Permeability of cell protoplasm is reported to increase by an adequate oxygen supply (Taylor and Ashcroft, 1972). Water can also be transported by *active movement*, especially in the transport of water upwards from cell to cell in the plant body. The energy required for such an active transport is provided by respiration. Active movement is responsible for *exudation* of water from a root or stem cut (Taylor and Ashcroft, 1972). Since adequate O_2 supply is required for respiration, proper aeration is essential for active water transport.

4.3.3 Nutrient Uptake

Movement of plant nutrients from soils into root cells also occurs by *passive* and *active* transport. The passive transport, e.g., mass flow and diffusion, obeys physico-chemical laws (Tan, 1993), whereas active transport requires the expenditure of energy, which is provided by the respiration process. However, the production of CO_2 by respiration and its consequent increase in soil air is reported to decrease nutrient uptake by roots in the following order (Chang and Loomis, 1945):

$$K > N > P > Ca > Mg$$

The lyotropic series above indicates that the decrease in ion uptake decreases in the direction of Mg. The decrease in K uptake is larger than the decrease in N uptake, and so on, and the smallest decrease in uptake is noticed with Mg.

The decrease in K and Fe uptake may result in K and Fe deficiency in plants. The deficiency symptoms disappear after the O_2 content in soil air is replenished artificially. The latter is reported to increase absorption of N, P, Ca, and Mg at the same time (Lawton, 1945).

4.3.4 Microorganisms

In most soils, respiration by microorganisms is more important than that by higher plants. As indicated in chapter 2, microorganisms are numerically the most abundant of all soil organisms. They are even more numerous than plant roots. Therefore, their respiration process requires more O_2 than that needed by plant roots, and a deficiency of O_2 in soil air significantly affects all microbial activity. In anaerobic conditions, where aeration is very poor, microbial decomposition of organic matter is very slow or inhibited, and organic residue tends to accumulate. Different redox conditions also affect the development of different types of microorganisms, e.g., aerobic and anaerobic bacteria. *Aerobic bacteria* need oxygen from soil air, whereas *anaerobic bacteria* supply their oxygen need from bonded oxygen. When O_2 is deficient in soil air, the anaerobic bacteria use the O_2 in nitrate, sulfate and carbon dioxide. Between the aerobic and anaerobic bacteria is another bacterial group, called *facultative bacteria*. Facultative bacteria use O_2 when it is available, or bonded O_2 when O_2 is deficient in soil air. Soils in an oxidized state contain predominantly aerobic bacteria, whereas soils in reduced conditions contain mostly anaerobic bacteria. Aerobic bacteria are responsible for the oxidation of Fe, S, and N. The oxidation reactions for these elements into ferric, sulfate, and nitrate compounds have been presented above. The basic metabolism of aerobic bacteria differs from that of anaerobic bacteria; the first produces CO_2, whereas the second yields H_2, H_2S, and CH_4 as ultimate end products. In addition, biological oxidation yields hydrogen or electrons, with O_2 acting as the electron acceptor. In anaerobic reactions, other compounds become electron acceptors, e.g., CO_2, NO_3^-, and SO_4^{2-} (Stevenson, 1986).

4.3.5 Decomposition of Organic Matter and Its Effect on Environmental Quality

In the absence of air, organic matter decomposition follows a different pathway. Anaerobic decomposition results in an incomplete breakdown of organic matter, yielding hydrogen, methane, and other foul-smelling intermediate organic compounds, such as H_2S, indoles, and mercaptans.

The formation of methane, CH_4, is mediated by methane bacteria that use oxygen from carbon dioxide. Expressed in scientific terms, methane bacteria utilize CO_2 as an electron acceptor. The organic compounds attacked by the bacteria are usually organic acids and alcohols (Manahan, 1975; Moore and Moore, 1976; Stevenson, 1986). The reactions can be illustrated as follows:

$$\underset{\text{acetic acid}}{CH_3COOH} + 2H_2O \rightarrow 2CO_2 + 8H^+ + 8e^- \qquad (4.10)$$

$$CO_2 + 8H^+ + 8e^- \rightarrow \underset{\text{methane}}{CH_4} + 2H_2O \qquad (4.11)$$

The production of methane is important in the decomposition of organic matter in an anaerobic environment. It usually occurs at the bottom of lakes and swamps and in coastal regions affected by the tide. It also takes place in landfills and old garbage dumps, where the methane by-product becomes a hazardous pollutant. Methane is a good fuel source, and its presence increases the chances of fire and explosions. It is considered hazardous to human health, and a pollutant gas that contributes to the greenhouse effect responsible for the global warming process. Because methane production is a biological reaction under anaerobic conditions, proper aeration of landfills may inhibit the anaerobic bacteria activity and hence stop the production of methane.

Today, attempts have been made to apply the process of methane production to the biological destruction of municipal waste and sewage sludge, using the methane produced as fuel. Unconfirmed reports indicate that the amount of methane produced is more than sufficient to power the treatment plants.

In another process, bonded O_2 is used in the anaerobic decomposition of organic matter for the reduction of sulfate into H_2S. Sulfur bacteria are capable of decomposing organic matter in anaerobic condition by using the oxygen obtained from sulfate. The reaction can be illustrated as follows:

$$2CH_2O + SO_4^{2-} + 2H^+ \rightarrow H_2S + 2CO_2 + 2H_2O \qquad (4.12)$$

Formation of H_2S occurs especially in swamps and coastal plain soils affected by sea water. Sea water contains high amounts of sulfates, which are retained by the soils and coastal sediments. The reduction of this residual sulfate into large amounts of H_2S creates a potential hazard for pollution in coastal regions. Because of the presence of FeS, formed by the reaction of H_2S with ferrous iron, soil and coastal sediments are frequently black.

The H_2S, CH_4, and other organic compounds produced during anaerobic decomposition will be oxidized by adequate aeration of the soil. The oxidation products are often beneficial, but can sometimes be harmful to the environment, soil conditions and plant growth. A beneficial effect is the oxidation of H_2S. When hydrogen sulfide, H_2S, is allowed to accumulate, it is not only toxic to soil organisms, but it also creates pollution problems. Fortunately, a group of bacteria present in soils is capable of oxidizing the H_2S into elemental S and SO_4 compounds. The reactions can be written

$$2H_2S + O_2 \rightarrow 2S + 2H_2O \tag{4.13}$$

$$2S + 2H_2O + 3O_2 \rightarrow 2H_2SO_4 \tag{4.14}$$

This process is applied in the development of acid conditions for growing *acid loving* plants and in the reclamation of alkaline soils. Azaleas and tea plants require acid soils, and powdered S is frequently supplied to the soil in which they are grown. In alkaline soils, the soil pH is usually too high for adequate crop growth and needs to be decreased to a suitable level. The latter result is also attained by applying adequate amounts of powdered S to the soil. The sulfuric acid produced by the oxidation by sulfur bacteria increases soil acidity.

4.4 CHEMICAL EFFECT OF AERATION

As discussed previously, in the presence of sufficient amounts of air (O_2) oxidation processes prevail over reduction reactions. Such a condition will generally be found in well-drained or well-aerated soils. In well-aerated soils, most of the soil constituents are in an oxidized state, which usually provides a physical and chemical environment suitable for plant growth. Under poor aeration, the soil constituents are in a reduced state, which creates a less favorable condition for plant growth.

Biological reactions in aerobic conditions produce CO_2 and, as discussed before, this reacts with soil water to form H_2CO_3. Other acids are also produced by the aerobic decomposition of soil organic matter, e.g., nitric acid, sulfuric acid, and oxalic acid. All these acids increase the dissolution power of soil water, and play an important role in the weathering and dissolution of rocks and minerals. Most of the soil minerals are attacked by these inorganic and organic acids and especially by carbonic acid. The presence of H_2CO_3 is considered essential in the weathering of limestone. $CaCO_3$, the major component of limestone, is insoluble in water, but will dissolve in water containing H_2CO_3 (see reaction 4.2). The stable solid phase of Ca in a soil system of CaO-H_2O-CO_2 is either $Ca(OH)_2$, $CaCO_3$, $Ca(HCO_3)_2$, or a combination of these. At CO_2 pressures normally present in soils, the stable solid phase is $CaCO_3$. However, the solubility of $CaCO_3$ increases as the partial pressure of CO_2 increases from 0.01 to 0.1 bars (Frear and Johnston, 1929).

Carbon dioxide in water will also affect the solubility of natural phosphate minerals in soils. These minerals are converted into various forms of calcium phosphates, e.g., apatites. The redox state of several elements, serving as plant nutrients, has been discussed earlier in relation to aerobic and anaerobic conditions in soils. In an anaerobic environment, nitrogen exists in ammonium, NH_4^+, form. Under these conditions, ammonium nitrogen is taken up by plants more readily than nitrate, NO_3^-, nitrogen. Nitrate, when present and absorbed, is apparently broken down by *anaerobic respiration*, to supply part of the oxygen requirement of plants (Taylor and Ashcroft, 1972). Iron exists as ferrous ions in poorly aerated soils, whereas Mn is present as manganous ions. Because these forms of Fe and Mn are the most soluble forms of iron and manganese, respectively, their accumulation may increase their concentrations and create Fe and/or Mn toxicity to plants.

CHAPTER 5

LIQUID PHASE

5.1 SOIL SOLUTION

The liquid phase, also called *soil water* or *soil solution*, is composed of water, dissolved substances, and colloidal materials. The dissolved substances are both solids and gases. The water itself is a renewable resource and is part of the global hydrologic cycle. When this water is present in the soil, it can be distinguished into (1) *surface water*, water above the soil, such as in streams, runoff, lakes, and ponds; (2) *ground water*, which is water present underground; and (3) *soil water*. The chemistry of surface water differs from that of ground or soil water. Surface water may contain high amounts of nutrients, resulting in excessive growth of algae. It may also have high levels of dissolved organic material, which promote bacterial growth. These factors affecting the quality of water are less serious in ground and soil water. Ground water, which percolates through deposits, may contain dissolved substances. It may also accumulate such substances through leaching, but most dissolved inorganic and organic compounds are gradually filtered as ground water moves through the soil. Therefore, chemically, ground water is generally of better quality than surface water. Soil water is usually in between the two in chemical characteristics and water quality.

Many of the chemical properties of water are attributed to its dipolar molecular structure. Water exhibits a high dielectric constant, which affects the dissociation of many compounds in water. Because of these two factors, water is an excellent solvent for a number of compounds. It is the most important transporting agent for nutrient elements and waste products in soils. Water stabilizes the body temperature of organisms, and is also known to stabilize the climate. This is due to the fact that a large amount of energy is required to increase the temperature of a unit mass of water. One calory of energy is needed to raise the temperature of 1 g of water 1°C, whereas more energy is required to evaporate water. On the average, 585 calories are needed to evaporate 1 g of water. These factors prevent sudden and large fluctuations in temperature from taking place in water, and their stabilizing effect protects aquatic organisms in lakes from the shock of abrupt temperature changes.

5.1.1 Forces Attracting Water in Soils

The term *soil moisture* is frequently used instead of soil water or soil solution. Soil moisture is located in the macro- and micropore. When the soil is saturated with water, all the pores are filled with water. After excess water has drained by gravity, water is present in the macropores in the form of a thin film around solid particles, whereas the micropores are still filled with water. Evaporation and consumption of water by soil organisms causes the water content in soils to decrease. At low water content, water exists as thin films and as wedges on the contact points of soil particles.

Water is held in the pore spaces by forces of attraction exerted by the soil matrix, by attraction to the ions, and by surface tension in the capillaries. The water retained in the soil by these forces constitutes the reserve water supply for plant use. These forces, expressed in terms of matric (ψ_m), osmotic

(ψ_o), and pressure potential (ψ_p), are collectively called the *water potential* (ψ_w) (Tan, 1993). The definition of the water potential can thus be written as follows:

$$\psi_w = \psi_m + \psi_o + \psi_p \tag{5.1}$$

The matric potential is the force by which soil water is retained by the soil matrix (soil solids). The osmotic potential is the force by which water is attracted by osmotic forces exerted by soil solutes. The pressure potential results from pressure differences in soils, and is a reflection of the total effect caused by retention of water in soil pores (capillary forces) and on the surfaces of soil particles (adsorption).

The water potential (ψ_w) has a negative value because the attraction by matrix and osmotic forces reduces the free energy level of soil water. In simple terms, soil water cannot move freely. The larger the negative the value of ψ_w, the smaller the amount of water present in soils. At field capacity (the maximum amount of water available for plants) ψ_w = - 30 Joules/kg, whereas at wilting points ψ_w = -1500 Joules/kg. Many plants can live below the wilting point by adjusting in a number of ways. The most common method is by shedding their leaves during periods of moisture stress, thereby decreasing the intake of moisture. Plants may also adjust to water stress by decreasing their intake of CO_2 through closing or regulating their stomata openings. The latter will reduce their rate of metabolism to the minimum required to stay alive. Intake of moisture is then also reduced to a minimum. These processes are called *osmotic adjustments*, adjustments of the osmotic potential so that only the minimum amount of water to sustain the life functions is adsorbed.

These water potentials can also be expressed in terms of positive values. The latter represents the opposite force, or suction force, which is called *soil moisture tension*. The tensional force can be expressed in a variety of ways, pounds/square inch, cm of water, cm of Hg, atmospheres, bars, or pF. The units *cm of water, bars*, and *pF* are the most common units used in soil science. The basic unit is the cm of water, which is defined as the force equal to the weight of the height of a water column in cm. It is interpreted in the same way that the cm Hg for barometric pressures is interpreted. The values for soil moisture tension in cm of water range from 0 to 10 000 000 cm. A moisture tension of 0 cm water indicates that there is no tension, which is attributed to the presence of excessive amounts of water in soil. A soil moisture tension of 10 000 000 cm means that water is held in soils with a very large force, in other words there is not much water in the soil (the soil is dry). The unit cm H_2O can be converted into bars by dividing by 1000. Hence,

$$0 \text{ cm } H_2O = 0/1000 \text{ bar} = 0 \text{ bar}$$
$$10\,000\,000 \text{ cm } H_2O = 10\,000\,000/1000 = 10\,000 \text{ bars}$$

The pF unit is also derived from the soil moisture tension in cm H_2O by taking the logarithm as follows:

$$pF = \log \text{cm } H_2O \tag{5.2}$$

The minimum value for cm H_2O to be used in the log equation is then a soil moisture tension of 1: pF = log 1 = 0. The maximum value is pF = log 10 000 000 = 7.

The pF is unique to soil moisture expression, although atmospheres or bars are also used. As indicated above, water can exist in soil under a tension varying from pF = 0 (no tension) to pF = 7.0 (very high tension). The pF is zero when the soil is saturated with water. At field capacity, the soil moisture tension equals 0.3 bars, which equals a pF of 2.54. This is the point at which the soil contains the maximum amount of water readily available to plants. Plants use little gravitational water since this water drains quickly to a depth below the root zone. As the soil dries and the water content decreases, the remaining water is present as thin films around the soil particles. These films become increasingly thinner upon continued drying of the soil. The forces holding the remaining water then become increasingly larger (pF value increases). Consequently, the force that the plant has to exert to remove the remaining water increases as the soil dries. Eventually a point is reached at which the force exerted by plants is not sufficient for sustaining growth. At this point, known as the wilting point, the plant starts to wilt. At wilting point the soil moisture tension equals 15 bars, which is proportional to a pF of 4.2. The amount of water held between the field capacity and the wilting point is called *available water.*

5.1.2 Classification of Soil Water

Over the years several soil moisture values, frequently called *soil moisture constants*, have been distinguished on the relative degree of soil moisture tension. The soil moisture constants range from saturation to oven dry condition (Table 5.1). These moisture constants are defined as follows.

Maximum retentive capacity: The amount of water held by soils at saturation. All pore spaces are filled with water.

Field capacity: The amount of water held by soils after excess water has drained by gravity and the downward movement has materially ceased.

Table 5.1. Soil Moisture Constants

Soil moisture constant	cm H_2O	bars	pF
Maximum retentive capacity	0	0	0
Field capacity	346	0.3	2.54
Moisture equivalent	1 000	1	3.0
Wilting point	15 849	15	4.2
Hygroscopic coefficient	31 623	31	4.5
Air dry soil	1×10^6	1 000	6.0
Oven dry soil	1×10^7	10 000	7.0

Moisture equivalent: The amount of water held in soils after excess water has been removed by centrifugation.

Wilting point: The amount of water held in soils at which plants start to wilt. The moisture content is not sufficient for plants to maintain their turgor.

Hygroscopic coefficient: The amount of water adsorbed by soils from an atmosphere of known relative humidity. The exact amounts of water are variable depending upon the method and relative humidity at which it is determined. Most scientists in the United States use 3.3% H_2SO_4 which gives about 98% relative humidity.

Air dry: The moisture content of an air dry soil or a soil at equilibrium with the atmosphere.

Oven dry: The moisture content remaining in the soil after the soil has been dried at 105-110°C until no more water is lost.

Physical Classification of Soil Moisture. These soil moisture constants and the relative degree of tension have been used to classify soil water. Such a classification of the many forms of soil water may be undertaken from a purely physical standpoint relating it to the degree of tension only, or from a biological standpoint relating it also to plant response. The following three types of soil water are distinguished in the physical classification:

Free water: Water held between pF 0 and 2.54. A saturated soil contains free water.

Capillary water: Water held between pF 2.54 and 4.5, or water held between the field capacity and the hygroscopic coefficient.

Hygroscopic water: Water held at the hygroscopic coefficient (pF = 4.5).

Biological Classification of Soil Moisture. The biological classification defines the types of soil water somewhat differently. The distinctions are similar in some respects to those listed in the physical classification. Three types of soil water are also recognized in the biological classification:

Superfluous water: Water in a saturated soil that is of no benefit to ordinary plants. It is related to free water.

Available water: The total amount of water present in soils between the field capacity and wilting point (or between pF 2.45 and 4.2). This amount is available to plants.

Unavailable water: Water held above a pF of 4.2, or the amount of water below the wilting point. This water is unnavailable to most ordinary plants.

5.2 DISSOLVED SOLID SUBSTANCES

Water is the main solvent in soil for a variety of compounds, and contains, therefore, an assortment of dissolved materials. Many of the dissolved materials are in ionic forms. If a compound with a general formula B_nA_x is in contact with soil water, it dissociates into its ionic components B^{n+} and A^{x-}, in which B is a metal cation with charge n, and A is the anion with charge x. As is the case with protons (H^+), which exist as H_3O^+, a metal ion cannot exist by itself. In soil water the metal reacts with water molecules, which form a hydration shell. The number of water molecules attracted to the metal ion depends on the coordination number of the cation. The hydrated cation carries the original number of positive charges. Hence, the symbol for such a hydrated ion is then $B(H_2O)_x^{n+}$. This concept will be illustrated below.

5.2.1 Aluminum

Aluminum is an important constituent of soils. It is the second most abundant element in rocks and minerals (Hunt, 1972), and is released in soils upon weathering of these rocks and minerals. It is chemically very active, hence the element will seldom occur free in nature, and will usually be present as oxides or as a constituent of alumino-silicate minerals and sesquioxide clays.

The most important form of aluminum oxide is *bauxite*, $Al_2O_3.2H_2O$, and *gibbsite*, $Al(OH)_3$, a sesquioxide clay. More exotic forms of aluminum oxides are *corundum*, Al_2O_3, *ruby* and *sapphire*. Ruby is in fact a red colored variety of corundum, whereas sapphire is a blue colored species of corundum. All three varieties belong to the hematite group of minerals, characterized by the formula X_2O_3 (Hurlbut and Klein, 1977), in which X represents Al or Fe. If X is Fe, the mineral is hematite, Fe_2O_3. Corundum is usually present as an accessory mineral in metamorphic and silica deficient igneous rocks, such as syenite.

The mineral occurs in the USA in the eastern part of the Appalachian Mountains of North Carolina and Georgia. Rubies are found in limestone affected by metamorphism in Burma, Thailand, and Cambodia, whereas most sapphires come from alluvial deposits of Sri Lanka, Thailand and Cambodia. Kashmir, India, central Queensland, Australia, and Montana, USA, are additional regions where sapphires have been discovered. Corundum is usually used as an abrasive or polishing material, whereas rubies and sapphires are valuable as gem stones. Stones of gem quality also have applications in the watch industry and as bearings in scientific instruments.

The concentration of soluble Al in soil water is very small and amounts to only 1.0 mg/L (Manahan, 1975). When an Al compound dissolves in soil water, the Al^{3+} ion is quickly surrounded by 6 molecules of H_2O in octahedral coordination, forming $Al(H_2O)_6^{3+}$. This ion is called an *aluminum hexahydronium* ion, and is subject to hydrolysis, especially as soil pH increases. Protons are dissociated from the coordinated water by the hydrolysis reaction, yielding a series of dissociation products:

$$
\begin{aligned}
Al(H_2O)_6^{3+} &\leftrightarrow Al(H_2O)_5(OH)^{2+} + H^+ \\
&\leftrightarrow Al(H_2O)_4(OH)_2^{+} + 2H^+ \\
&\leftrightarrow Al(H_2O)_3(OH)_3^{o} + 3H^+ \\
&\leftrightarrow Al(H_2O)_2(OH)_4^{-} + 4H^+ \\
&\leftrightarrow Al(H_2O)(OH)_5^{2-} + 5H^+
\end{aligned}
$$

For simplicity, the aluminum hydroxide monomers above are usually written without the coordinated water:

$$
\begin{aligned}
Al^{3+} + H_2O &\leftrightarrow Al(OH)^{2+} + H^+ \\
Al^{3+} + 2H_2O &\leftrightarrow Al(OH)_2^{+} + 2H^+
\end{aligned}
$$

$$Al^{3+} + 3H_2O \leftrightarrow Al(OH)_3^{o} + 3H^+$$
$$Al^{3+} + 4H_2O \leftrightarrow Al(OH)_4^{-} + 4H^+$$
$$Al^{3+} + 5H_2O \leftrightarrow Al(OH)_5^{2-} + 5H^+$$

The reactions above show that hydrated metal ions with a charge of 3 or more are proton donors and may affect soil acidity. The charges of the aluminum products change from positive through zero to negative. As the degree of hydrolysis increases from 1 to $5H_2O$, the solubility of the aluminum hydrates decreases.

The aluminum hydroxide monomers formed tend to form polymers according to the reaction in Figure 5.1. These polymers are also capable of donating protons, and hence they behave as acids. The reaction is represented in Figure 5.2.

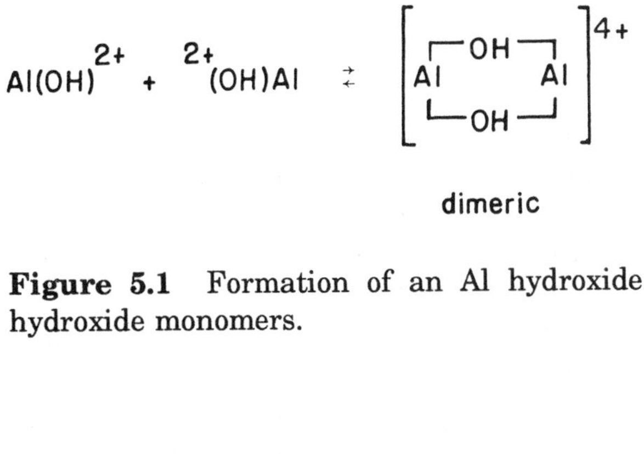

$$Al(OH)^{2+} + {}^{2+}(OH)Al \rightleftarrows \left[Al \begin{matrix} OH \\ OH \end{matrix} Al \right]^{4+}$$

dimeric

Figure 5.1 Formation of an Al hydroxide dimer from two Al hydroxide monomers.

Free Al or hydrated Al ions are usually present in large amounts in acid soils. Large amounts of these Al ions may cause

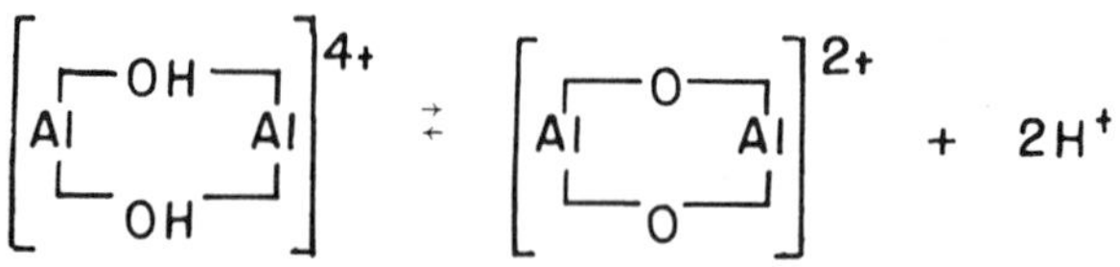

Figure 5.2 Dissociation of H^+ from an Al hydroxide dimer.

Al toxicity to plants. They also react with phosphates to form insoluble Al phosphate compounds, which may cause P deficiency in plants. The reaction between Al and phosphate that results in the formation of an insoluble Al phosphate compound is called *phosphate fixation*.

5.2.2 Iron

Iron is another important element in soils. It is the third most abundant element in rocks and minerals. The central core of the earth is made up mostly of iron. All rocks, minerals, soils, and plants contain iron. In animals, it is present in the blood hemoglobin, which acts as a carrier of oxygen.

The most important iron mineral is *hematite*, Fe_2O_3, and *magnetite*, Fe_3O_4. The hydrated form of hematite is often called *limonite*, $2Fe_2O_3.3H_2O$. Hematite is red in color and its presence gives to the soils a red color. Magnetite is black in color and crystalline in nature. It has strong magnetic properties. Another iron mineral is *pyrite*, FeS_2, which occurs in soils as yellowish crystals with a metallic luster similar to gold, hence the name *fool's gold* is used for this mineral. *Ilmenite*, $FeTiO_3$, is also an important iron mineral. The name is derived from the *Ilmen*

Mountains, Russia, where ilmenite has been discovered in large quantities. It is a common accessory mineral of igneous rocks, such as gabbros and diorites. It is found in the USA in several locations in the Adirondack Mountains and in the humic acid deposits in Florida and southern Georgia. In Western Australia, ilmenite is currently mined from beach sands near Perth. This mineral is the major source of *titanium*, used in the plastic and paint industries as pigment, replacing older pigments such as lead, Pb. Metallic titanium is currently very valuable in the aerospace industry because of its high strength/weight ratio. It is the most desirable lightweight-but-strong metal for the production of aircrafts and supersonic spacecrafts.

When released in soil water, iron can exist in two different forms. The redox condition in soils determines the ionic form of iron in soil water. In anaerobic conditions, iron may be present as ferrous iron, Fe^{2+}. It is the dominant iron species in ground water, where its concentration may range from 1.0 to 10 mg/L. In aerobic conditions, iron is generally present as ferric iron, Fe^{3+}. In aerobic conditions, ferrous iron is unstable and will be oxidized into Fe^{3+}:

$$Fe^{2+} \leftrightarrow Fe^{3+} + e^- \tag{5.3}$$

Ferric iron behaves similarly as Al^{3+} ions and will be quickly surrounded by 6 molecules of H_2O in octahedral coordination, yielding $Fe(H_2O)_6^{3+}$. The latter is also subject to hydrolysis, which produces Fe hydroxide monomers and protons. Upon polymerization, the monomers yield Fe hydroxide polymers, which disperse in water and cause turbidity. With increased formation of ferric hydrates, the color of soil water becomes brown. This is perhaps the reason why too much iron in water is considered harmful for agricultural, engineering, and domestic purposes. In engineering, the use of water that contains iron, may cause corrosion and the formation of unsightly deposits of Fe hydroxides. Dissolved iron at levels >0.31 mg/L produces an unpleasant taste in drinking water. It will also stain laundry and porcelain. Iron is needed only in trace amounts by plants, and too much iron can cause Fe toxicity. When phosphate is present, Fe may react with phosphate to form insoluble Fe phosphate, a process called *phosphate fixation*. This may cause P deficiency in plants.

5.2.3 Silicon

Silicon is perhaps next to oxygen in abundance in the earth's crust. It occurs in the soil as six distinct crystalline minerals: quartz, tridymite, crystobalite, coesite, strishovite, and opal, which are classified today in the SiO_2 group of *Tecto-silicates*. The minerals quartz, tridymite, crystobalite, coesite, and strishovite are all characterized by the formula SiO_2, but differ from each other in their framework of geometric arrangements of the silica tetrahedrons. Opal, on the other hand, is characterized by a formula of $SiO_2.nH_2O$. Flint is also a silica mineral, and a number of amorphous or noncrystalline and paracrystalline species can also be found.

Quartz is a common mineral of acid igneous rocks, such as granite and rhyolite. The mineral is used for a wide variety of purposes. It is used as sand in mortar and concrete and as an abrasive in the production of sandpaper. In powdered form, it is an important ingredient in the production of porcelain and crystal glass. Quartz also finds application in optical instruments because of its capacity to be ground into lenses and prisms. Because of its optical activity, its ability to rotate the plane of polarization of light, quartz is valuable for instruments used in the generation of *monochromatic* light of different wavelengths. Tiny quartz plates, serving as oscillators, are used in digital watches and clocks. Quartz oscillators are useful today in the measurement of instant high pressures resulting from atomic explosions and the firing of firearms. Quartz varieties, that are of gem quality are very valuable ornaments. These include amethyst, rose quartz, agate, and onyx. Today, yellow, brown, blue and violet quartz are produced artificially by hydrothermal methods for gemstones and lenses. Tridymite is also a mineral of many acidic igneous rocks, whereas crystobalite is usually volcanic of origin. Volcanic ash often contains the mineral crystobalite. Opal, on the other hand, is considered biogenic in origin. The original materials are petrified plant materials or diatomites. For instance, *wood opal* is in fact fossilized wood with opal as the petrifying substance. The major colors of opal are white, yellow, or milky-white, in which a variety of blue, yellow, red, or black reflections can be seen. Opal with red reflections, called *fire opal*, is a very valuable gem stone. *Black opal* is another example of a precious gem.

Of the minerals discussed above, quartz is the most common SiO_2 mineral. The silicon in quartz is surrounded by 4 oxygen atoms in tetrahedral coordination. These silica tetrahedrons are linked together by sharing oxygen atoms. The Si-O-Si bonds, called the *siloxane bonds*, are the strongest bonds in nature, and are of primary importance in crystalline minerals (Tan, 1993). Quartz minerals are, therefore, very resistant to weathering and, hence, very difficult to dissolve. Most of the soluble silica originate from amorphous silica and from primary minerals, such as anorthite ($CaAl_2Si_2O_8$) and albite ($NaAlSi_3O_8$), both plagioclase minerals, which are the least stable minerals to weathering. Soluble silica can also be introduced to the soil through artificial compounds. Silicates are used in detergents and as anticorrosive agents in antifreeze. In silicon chemistry, the term silica is used for Si compounds, whereas the term silicon is reserved for the element Si. The element Si itself is inactive at low temperatures and is very resistant to chemical attack. Si crystals are used today for the production of computer chips, semiconductors, and transistor devices in solar batteries.

Elemental Si also finds application as a deoxidant in the manufacture of steel, copper, and highly acid-resistant alloys, such as *duriron*.

The concentration of dissolved silica in natural water is usually very small, ranging from 1 - 30 mg SiO_2/L, but concentrations of 100 mg SiO_2/L are also common (Garrels and Christ, 1965; Manahan, 1975; Moore and Moore, 1976). Seawater is usually low in silica content because Si is used by marine organisms in the formation of their skeletons and shells. Present in amounts below 140 mg SiO_2/L (25°C), soluble silica is found mainly as monosilicic acid, which is a true solution. Its formula can be written as H_4SiO_4, $Si(OH)_4$, or $SiO_2(OH)_2$ (Figure 5.3). This type of silicic acid is also known as *orthosilicic*

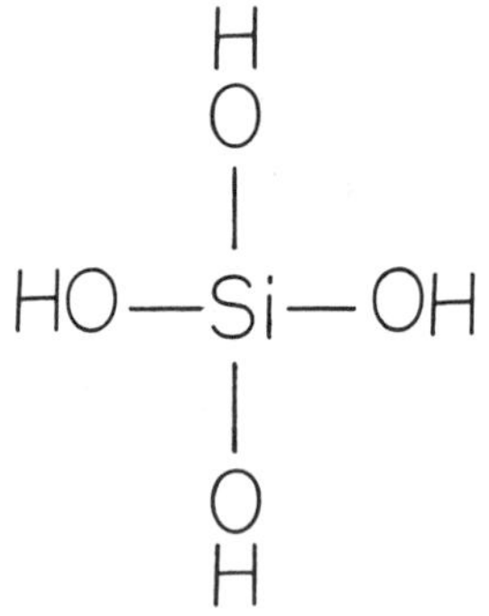

```
      H
      O
      |
HO—Si—OH
      |
      O
      H
```

Figure 5.3 Schematic structure of monosilicic or orthosilicic acid, H_4SiO_4.

acid. Monosilicic acid forms *silica gel* by dehydration until the proper percentage of moisture is reached. The dehydration process, assumed to take place stepwise through formation of *metasilicic acid*, H_2SiO_3, *disilicic acid*, H_6SiO_7, *trisilicic acid*,

$H_4Si_3O_8$, etc., is a type of polymerization.

The silica minerals are insoluble at low pH, and their solubility does not increase if pH is increased from 2 to 9. Only above pH 9.0 will silica minerals dissolve. In the range of pH 2 to 9, the solubility of silica remains constant at 140 mg/L (Tan, 1993; Krauskopf, 1956), and this solubility is generally determined by the law of polymerization. If the concentration of dissolved silica in the soil solution exceeds 140 mg/L, polymerization of silica usually occurs (Figure 5.4), and a mixture of

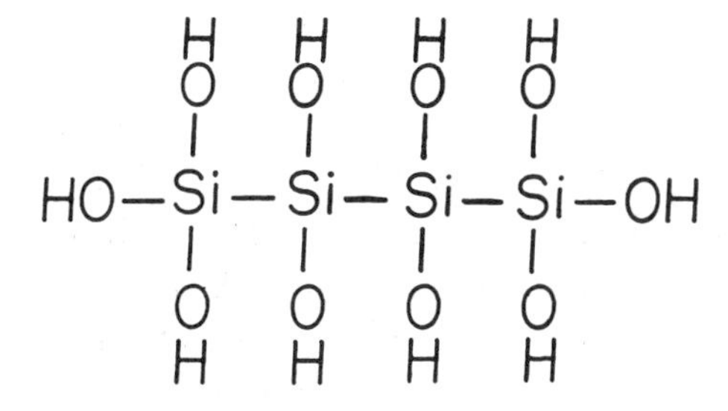

Figure 5.4 Polysilicic acid or polymeric silicic acid with linear structure. Cyclic structures and cross-linked polymeric structures are also possible.

polymers and monomers of $Si(OH)_4$ is found in the soil solution. Two or more monosilicic acids can react linearly or can form cyclic combinations with endless variations. Although not clearly understood, the formula of a polynuclear silicate ion is frequently written as $Si_4O_6(OH)_6^{2-}$, which differs somewhat from the one indicated in Figure 5.4.

Silica in the form of monosilicic acid can be adsorbed by sesquioxides. This reaction forms the basis for the formation of silicate clays. It can be illustrated as follows:

$$H_4SiO_4 \leftrightarrow H^+ + H_3SiO_4^-$$
$$H_3SiO_4^- + Al(OH)_3 \leftrightarrow Al(OH)_2OSi(OH)_3 + OH^-$$

The monosilicic acid must first be converted into an anion by dissociating a proton. Only when it is negatively charged, can it react with positively charged sesquioxides.

In addition to the above reaction, monosilicic acid is able to form complexes with metal ions. Such a complexation reaction, as illustrated in Figure 5.5, is of importance in the weathering of primary minerals. The resulting metal-silicate complex is present in ionic form, hence remains in solution. This is perhaps one of the mechanisms in podzolization, by which Al and Fe may be transported as inorganic complexes to form Bs horizons, which are B horizons rich in Al and Fe compounds (s = sesquioxides). Such complex reactions and transport phenomena have received little research attention. The most commonly accepted version of podzolization is that Al and Fe move down the profile in the form of Al- and/or Fe-humic acid chelates (De Coninck, 1980; Tan, 1986).

Monosilicic acid is also known to form complexes with soil organic compounds, especially with humic and fulvic acids. The complexation process can be represented by the reactions in Figure 5.6. These reactions play a significant role in the weathering of rocks and minerals. The high affinity of humic acids for Si and metal ions bring about the degradation of many rocks and minerals (Tan, 1986). The subsequent release of Si in the form of complexes or chelates has an important bearing in soil formation and movement of Si in the pedon. Today this type

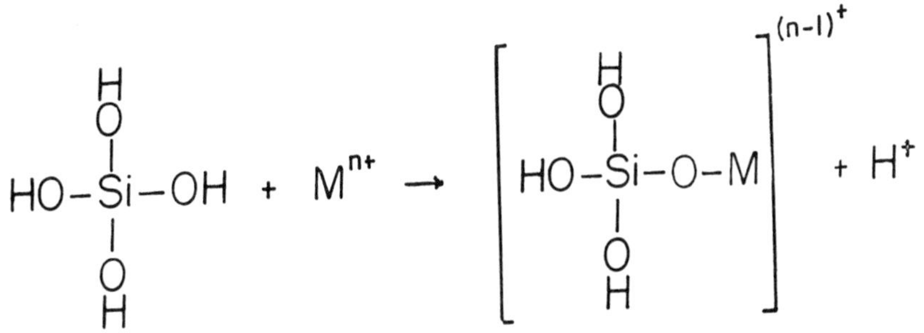

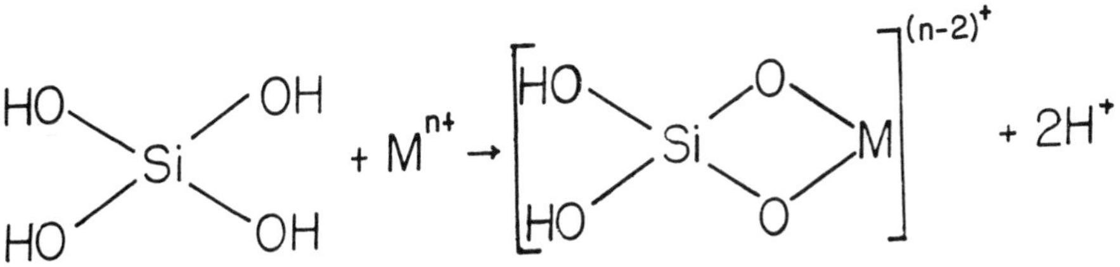

$$HO{-}\overset{\overset{H}{O}}{\underset{\underset{H}{O}}{Si}}{-}OH + M^{n+} \rightarrow \left[HO{-}\overset{\overset{H}{O}}{\underset{\underset{H}{O}}{Si}}{-}O{-}M\right]^{(n-1)^{+}} + H^{+}$$

$$(HO)_2Si(OH)_2 + M^{n+} \rightarrow \left[(HO)_2Si{<}^{O}_{O}{>}M\right]^{(n-2)^{+}} + 2H^{+}$$

Figure 5.5 Top: Complex formation between monosilicic acid and a cation, M^{n+}, in which n^{+} = the number of positive charges. Bottom: Chelation reaction between monosilicic acid and a cation, M^{n+}.

of complex formation between silicic acid and organic compounds finds application in industry in the production of *silicones*. The general formula of silicone is R_2SiO_2, in which R is an organic radical. This could be a simple organic compound, such as a methyl group, CH_3, an ethyl group, C_2H_5, or a complex humic molecule. These silicones can be linear or cyclic in structure (Figure 5.6). Silicones composed of cross-linked silica

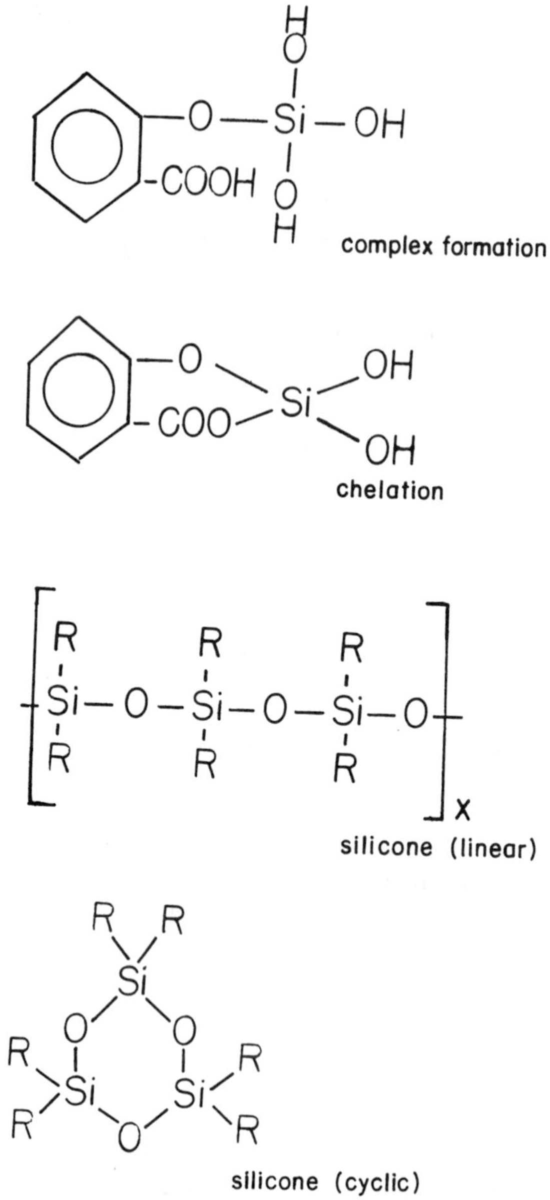

complex formation

chelation

silicone (linear)

silicone (cyclic)

Figure 5.6 Top two: Complex formation and chelation between monosilicic acid and a humic acid molecule. Bottom two: Formation of linear and cyclic silicones.

polymers are also possible. Depending on their molecular complexity, silicones have the appearance of oily, greasy, or rubberlike substances. Consequently, they are used as lubricants, hydraulic fluids, and electrical insulators. Antifreeze for automobiles contains silicone for lubricating the water pump. In medical science, silicone finds application as filling material and implants in human bodies. The controversial use of silicone for breast implants has currently received a lot of attention in the media.

5.2.4 Nitrogen

Nitrogen, discovered as an element in 1772 by Rutherford, is an inert gas that does not support life and that can not burn. However, it is an essential constituent of proteins and amino acids in plants and animals. Natural gas may contain some nitrogen. Its formula is N_2, and this diatomic molecule is known to have the most stable structure in nature. This high structural stability is the reason for its inert property and its lack of chemical reactivity. Inorganic sources of nitrogen include *saltpeter*, KNO_3, deposits in India, and *Chile saltpeter*, $NaNO_3$, deposits in Chile, South America.

Because of its inert property, gaseous nitrogen is used in chemical reactions that need to take place in an inert atmosphere. It is used in electric light bulbs to inhibit rapid oxidation of the filament. The more modern light bulbs of today contain argon gas, which is even more inert than nitrogen. Nitrogen finds extensive application in the food industry to reduce rapid deterioration of canned products. Canned foods, sliced meats and hydrogenated vegetable oils are frequently sealed with nitrogen gas to prevent spoiling.

Nitrogen exists in soils in organic and inorganic forms, and is present in several oxidation states, e.g., from -3 to +6. The total soil N content varies considerably — from 0.05% in the desert soils and in warm humid region soils to 0.3% or higher in the soils of semi-humid regions, e.g. mollisols. In soil water, the concentration of nitrogen is even lower, constituting only a very small fraction of the amount present in soils. Under normal conditions, 2.4 mL nitrogen will dissolve in 100 mL water. Most of the nitrogen in soils (98%) is in organic form (Bremner, 1965). It is present in plant residue, barnyard manure, and industrial and domestic waste. Some of these organic nitrogen compounds, such as amino acids are soluble in soil water. However, most of the nitrogen in soil water are in inorganic form, e.g., NH_4^+, NO_3^-, and NO_2^-. The latter is released in soil water by decomposition of soil organic matter. Inorganic nitrogen can also be added to soils by the application of fertilizers.

Ammonia. One of the most common inorganic nitrogen species in soils is ammonia, NH_3, a product of ammonification. Ammonia, a gas, dissolves in soil water and becomes ammonium, NH_4^+. Gaseous ammonia is colorless, and has a strong odor. It is used as a heart stimulant and people who have fainted are often revived by letting them inhale ammonia gas. However, some people may be allergic to the gas and some may even die by inhaling it.

Ammonia gas can be liquified by compression and/or by cooling. This property is used in the manufacture of liquid N fertilizers, such as *anhydrous ammonia*, or NH_3. This fertilizer is soluble in water, since 1.2 L of gaseous ammonia can dissolve in 1 L of water (O°C). Other nitrogen fertilizers are also produced from ammonia, e.g., sulfate of ammonia. In addition, ammonia gas is used in industry as a refrigerant and in the production of ice because its *heat of vaporization* (328 calories/g) is the highest among many liquids, except water. It also finds application in domestic chemicals in the form of *household ammonia* for cleansing and washing.

Ammonium is generally stable only in anaerobic conditions, whereas nitrate prevails in aerobic conditions. Ammonium ions are chemically more reactive than nitrate ions. They react quickly with negatively charged clay minerals and form complexes with metals and organic compounds. The cationic nature of NH_4^+ is the reason for its adsorption and retention by soil clays. This process prevents NH_4^+ from being leached to deeper layers of the pedon. When NH_4^+ is adsorbed in intermicellar spaces of expanding types of clays, such as smectite, entrapment of NH_4^+ occurs, a process called *ammonium fixation*.

Ammonium is believed to dissociate according to the following reaction (Manahan, 1975; Moore and Moore, 1976):

$$NH_4^+ \leftrightarrow H^+ + NH_3 \qquad (5.4)$$

The pK_a value of the dissociation reaction is 9.26, which means that at pH 9.26 this dissociation produces equal concentrations of NH_3 and NH_4^+. In soils with a pH value above 9.26, reaction (5.4) proceeds to the right. However, most soils and waters in lakes and streams have pH values below 9.26; hence, the reaction goes to the left. In other words, the dissociation does not take place, and NH_4^+ is stable.

Nitrates and Nitrites. Other species of inorganic nitrogen compounds are nitrite, NO_2^-, and nitrate, NO_3^-, which are the products of nitrification of NH_4^+. Nitrate is used in industry for the manufacture of drugs, plastics, rayon, dyes and for curing meat products. Ham and bacon are cured with $NaNO_3$. Nitrate is also an important ingredient for the production of explosives, e.g., *TNT* (trinitrotoluene) and gunpowder. An explosive, composed of ammonium nitrate and aluminum powder, is called *ammonal*. The acid form of nitrate is called *nitric acid*, HNO_3, whereas the acid of nitrite is called *nitrous acid*, HNO_2. When nitric acid reacts with human skin, it may yellow the skin. The reaction is called a *xanthoprotein reaction*, and is the reason for the development of yellow fingers in people using nitric acids in the laboratory.

As indicated earlier, nitrite is usually quickly converted into nitrate, so that the most important inorganic species of N in soil water are the ammonium and nitrate forms. In contrast to ammonium, nitrate ions are anionic in nature, and consequently will not be attracted by negatively charged clay minerals. Therefore, NO_3^- tends to be leached into the ground water. The presence of nitrate in amounts above 30 mg/L is considered hazardous to human health by EPA standards and is particularly harmful to babies. When consumed, NO_3^- may not only be carcinogenic, it will also be reduced into NO_2^- in the anaerobic environment of the digestive system. The nitrite reacts with hemoglobin and interferes with its function as an oxygen carrier, causing blue coloring in babies. A similar reduction process can also take place in the digestive system of ruminants.

In soil water, nitrate is stable in the absence of organic compounds. Several of these organic compounds may act as biological catalysts, which induces the reduction of nitrates. This process finds application in sewage treatments, as discussed before in the denitrification process.

5.2.5 Phosphorus

Phosphorus is a nonmetallic element and exists in two allotropic varieties, called *white phosphorus* and *red phosphorus*. White phosphorus is a white, soft, waxlike solid, but its color will turn yellow when it is exposed to light. Red phosphorus has a red color, and vaporizes when heated. White phosphorus is very poisonous, and inhaling the fumes of white phosphorus may cause necrosis of the bones in the jaw and nose, and may also cause death. It has been used in the past for making matches, but since the fumes are very toxic, the match heads today contain *tetraphosphorus trisulfide*, P_4S_3, a less toxic substance. Those matches were the once-famous *strike-anywhere* matches. Phosphorus is still used today as rat poison and in making explosives, fireworks, chemicals, fertilizers, and as spoil retardants in food substances.

Phosphorus in soils exists as organic and inorganic compounds. Humus, manure, and other types of nonhumified organic matter are the major sources of organic phosphorus in soils. Some of the compounds in the soil organic fraction considered potential sources of phosphorus are phospholipids, nucleic acids and inositol phosphates. Bones, teeth, and muscle tissue in animals are rich in phosphorus. Inorganic phosphorus is derived mostly from the apatite minerals, which are accessory minerals in all types of rocks. The most important minerals in the apatite group are fluorapatite, $Ca_5(PO_4)_3F$, chlorapatite, $Ca_5(PO_4)_3Cl$, and hydroxyapatite, $Ca_5(PO_4)_3(OH)$. Apatite is an accessory constituent in igneous, sedimentary, and metamorphic rocks. Large deposits have been detected in the Kola Peninsula near Kirovsk, Russia, the southern coast of Norway, in Kiruna, Sweden, and Tahawus, New York. Large amounts of apatite have also been found in Ontario and Quebec, Canada. Present as large deposits, apatite is valuable in the manufacture of phosphate fertilizers. By treatment with sulfuric acid, the apatite is converted into *superphosphate*. A by-product of this process is *gypsum*, $CaSO_4$, a liming material. Phosphoric acid can also be used for treatment of apatite, and the product is then called *double-* or *triple-superphosphate*.

In general, the inorganic P content in soils is higher than the organic P content (Tisdale and Nelson, 1975, 1993). The total phosphorus content in surface soils of the USA may range from 0.04% to 0.3% P_2O_5 or higher. High phosphorus contents are found in soils of the northwestern region, whereas low phosphorus contents are usually detected in soils of the southeastern region of the United States.

In solution, phosphorus is present only in the inorganic form, as either the primary, $H_3PO_4^-$, or the secondary, HPO_4^{2-} orthophosphate ion. The concentration of these ions in the soil solution depends on the pH. In acid soils, $H_2PO_4^-$ will be more dominant than HPO_4^{2-}. At pH 6—7, both forms are equally represented in the soil solution, whereas at pH >7.0, HPO_4^{2-} will be dominant together with some PO_4^{3-} ions. Scientifically the stability of these ions can be explained by the pK_a values of orthophosphoric acid, H_3PO_4. Orthophosphoric acid exhibits three steps of dissociation reactions, each characterized by a specific pK_a:

$$H_3PO_4 \leftrightarrow H^+ + H_2PO_4^- \qquad pK_{a1} = 2.17$$
$$H_2PO_4^- \leftrightarrow H^+ + HPO_4^{2-} \qquad pK_{a2} = 7.31$$
$$HPO_4^{2-} \leftrightarrow H^+ + PO_4^{3-} \qquad pK_{a3} = 12.36$$

As defined previously, the pK_a value is the pH at which the compound dissociates producing equal concentrations of anions and original material. The soil pH or water pH is usually above pH (pK_{a1}) 2.17, but below pH (pK_{a3}) 12.36. Therefore, the first and second step of dissociation will occur in soils and natural waters. The final step of dissociation, characterized by pK_{a3} 12.36, will occur only if the soil pH is above 12.36. These chemical considerations support the idea above indicating that under normal conditions $H_2PO_4^-$ and HPO_4^{2-} are the dominant species of phosphorus in the soil solution.

The concentration of these ions is very small and is estimated to be 1 mg/L or less. Maximum availability of these phosphate ions for plant growth occurs within the pH range of 5.5-6.5 (Tisdale and Nelson, 1975, 1993). Large amounts of phosphorus ions are detrimental to the environment. The use of household detergents, and the overuse of phosphate fertilizers are the main reasons for accumulation of phosphate in soil water. In lake water, excessive amounts of phosphorus result in excessive growth of unwanted aquatic plants. This phenomenon is called *eutrophication*.

Phosphate reacts readily with metals present in soils. Acid soils contain large amounts of Al, Fe and Mn, which form complexes or insoluble metal-phosphate compounds. The reaction was previously called *phosphate fixation*. The ultimate end product of the reaction between Al and phosphate is *variscite* ($AlPO_4.2H_2O$), and that of Fe and phosphate is *strengite* ($FePO_4.2H_2O$). A series of intergrade compounds between variscite and strengite is usually present in soils, which is called the *variscite-strengite isomorphous series* (Lindsay *et al.*, 1959). Phosphate fixation can also occur at high pH values. Many aridisols with high pH contain large amounts of Ca, which can form insoluble $Ca_3(PO_4)_2$, and/or other Ca phosphate compounds in the apatite group.

5.2.6 Sodium and Potassium

Sodium, Na, and potassium, K, are alkali metals. They are very reactive, and react vigorously with water, releasing hydrogen gas while producing at the same time the strong bases NaOH and KOH, respectively. The heat of reaction may cause the evolved hydrogen to ignite, hence sodium and potassium elements should never be touched with bare hands. The amount of moisture on the skin is sufficient to cause the exothermic reaction. The Na and K elements are usually stored under kerosene in sealed containers. Sodium is used in industry as a reducing agent in the production of drugs, perfumes, and dyes. It is used for making *sodium lights*, which produce yellow light that penetrates dense fog. These lights are frequently used for automobile headlights and streetlights. Potassium is generally more reactive than sodium. However, it is not used much in industry, because it can be easily replaced by sodium.

Sodium and potassium compounds are widely distributed in nature. The sodium content of normal soils is on the average

0.63%, whereas that of potassium is approximately 0.83%. The mineral sources for Na and K are Na aluminum silicates, e.g., albite, and K aluminum silicates, e.g., orthoclase, respectively. They can also occur in nature as chloride, sulfate and borate minerals. The dissolution of Na and K from the aluminum silicates is attributed to hydrolysis reactions, which are weathering processes. The chemical reactions can be represented as follows:

$$\underset{\text{albite}}{NaAlSi_3O_8} + H_2O \rightarrow HAlSi_3O_8 + \underset{\text{soluble}}{NaOH} \tag{5.9}$$

$$\underset{\text{orthoclase}}{KAlSi_3O_8} + H_2O \rightarrow HAlSi_3O_8 + \underset{\text{soluble}}{KOH} \tag{5.10}$$

The NaOH and KOH dissolve in soil water and release their sodium and potassium in the form of Na^+ and K^+ ions, respectively. The concentrations of these ions in soil water are relatively low if compared with their contents in soils. On the average, the K concentration in the soil solution is 5 mg/L, whereas that of Na is 10 mg/L or larger. Both ions are stable in soil water and are very difficult to precipitate. Only by complex formation can K ions be precipitated. In soils, these ions exist mostly as exchangeable cations. Sodium reacts rapidly with Cl^- to form NaCl, which can accumulate in arid regions or where drainage is inhibited. Accumulation of sodium salts in aridisols gives rise to crust formation on the surface soil and/or the development B_n horizons (see chapter 1). In other soils, such an accumulation of NaCl contributes toward development of salinity, resulting in a decrease in the quality of soil and water.

5.2.7 Calcium

Calcium, Ca, is an element that belongs to the *alkaline earth metal* group. The primary sources of Ca are calcite, aragonite, dolomite and gypsum. Calcite, $CaCO_3$, is the major constituent of limestone, calcareous marls, and calcareous sandstone (see chapter 2). It comes in many varieties, and Mexican onyx is a common variety of calcite. The mineral calcite possesses an optical property called *birefringence* or *double breaking* or *double refraction*. This is a property by which a light beam entering the crystal is broken up into two beams. Hence, calcite crystals find useful application as lenses in petrographic or polarizing microscopes. However, the most important use of calcite is in the production of cements. Aragonite is another $CaCO_3$ mineral. Under normal atmospheric condition, it is less stable than calcite. The pearly layer of seashells is composed of aragonite. Pearl itself is built up of concentric layers of aragonite formed around a nucleus of a foreign particle, which can be a small grain of sand. The name aragonite is derived from the town Aragon, Spain, where the mineral was first discovered. Dolomite is a calcium-magnesium carbonate mineral, $CaMg(CO_3)_2$, belonging to the dolomite group. In addition to being a source for Ca, it is also a common source of Mg. The name is derived from the name of the French chemist *Dolomieu*. This mineral is a potential source of metallic Mg. Gypsum is a calcium sulfate mineral with a composition of $CaSO_4.2H_2O$. It is a common mineral of sedimentary rocks and has been found in large amounts in the USA, Canada, England, France, and Russia. Gypsum is usually used for the production of *plaster of Paris* and gypsum boards used for walls in the housing industry. In agricultural operation it is a liming material.

The element calcium itself finds application as a dehydrating agent for organic chemicals. It is also used as an adsorbent of gases in metallurgy and in the steel industry for making alloys with silicon. Ca is often applied as a hardening material in cables and for the production of storage battery grids and bearings.

Calcium is a very important cation in soils, soil water, and waters in lakes and streams. The average Ca content in soils is estimated to be 1.4%. Depending on climatic conditions and parent materials, the Ca content may vary considerably from soil to soil. Soils in desert climates may be high in Ca, often containing $CaCO_3$ in the B horizon, which is then called a B_k horizon (see chapter 1). This B_k horizon is thick and close to the surface in aridisols, but is relatively thinner and located deeper in the pedon of mollisols. In humid regions, drastic leaching has removed most of the Ca minerals from the soils. Therefore, the soils in humid regions, e.g., alfisols and ultisols, do not exhibit B_k horizons and are low in Ca. They are often acidic in reaction.

Calcium carbonate is insoluble in water, but will dissolve in water containing CO_2, a process called previously *carbonation* (chapter 4). The partial pressure of CO_2 in soil air controls the amount of CO_2 gas dissolved in soil water, and therefore determines the rate of dissolution of $CaCO_3$. The main source of CO_2 is the respiration process of plant roots and microorganisms, which accounts for high CO_2 partial pressures in soil air.

In soil water Ca occurs as a Ca^{2+} ion or as ion pairs with HCO_3^-, SO_4^{2-}, or Cl^-. It contributes to the hardness of water, which may prevent soap from producing foam, and may cause a white crust to form on glass and on pots and pans. In agricultural operations, it is common practice to lime acid soils to a pH of 6.0. Four major benefits of liming are (1) decreasing soil acidity, (2) replenishing Ca, (3) making nutrients more available to plants, and (4) decreasing micronutrient toxicity. The lime reaction, showing the decrease in soil acidity, can be illustrated as follows:

$$CaCO_3 + 2H\text{-clay} \leftrightarrow Ca\text{-clay} + CO_2 + H_2O \qquad (5.5)$$

Aluminum toxicity is reduced by liming because the Al^{3+} is converted into $Al(OH)_3$, which is a solid compound and chemically inactive. The reaction can be represented as follows:

$$3Ca(OH)_2 + 2Al\text{-clay} \leftrightarrow 3Ca\text{-clay} + 2Al(OH)_3 \qquad (5.6)$$

5.2.8 Magnesium

The minerals containing Mg are dolomite, Mg silicates, Mg phosphates, Mg sulfides and Mg molybdates. As indicated previously, dolomite, $CaMg(CO_3)_2$, the major constituent of dolomitic limestone, is the most common source of Mg in soils. It is a mineral found usually in sedimentary rocks. Large deposits of dolomite are detected in the dolomite region of southern Tyrol, Switzerland. In the United States, dolomite is found in sedimentary rocks of the midwestern states. Dolomite is used as building stones and ornaments and in the production of certain types of cements. The element Mg itself does not occur as a free element in nature, although it is widely distributed on earth as minerals and/or other types of compounds. Seawater contains abundant amounts of Mg in the form of $MgCl_2$ and $MgSO_4$. The element Mg, a white-silvery metal, is chemically very active, and will react rapidly with air, water and most nonmetal compounds. It is used for the production of lightweight alloys, flares, and flashlight powders. These powders produce an intense white light upon burning.

The average Mg content in soils is approximately 0.5%, whereas its concentration in soil water is estimated to be 10 mg/L. In soil water, Mg exists as the cation Mg^{2-}, or as ion pairs with HCO_3^-, SO_4^{2-}, and Cl^-. The dissolution of dolomitic limestone is also affected by the CO_2 content in soil water and can be illustrated by the following reaction:

$$CaMg(CO_3)_2 + H_2CO_3 \leftrightarrow Ca^{2+} + Mg^{2+} + 4HCO_3^- \quad (5.7)$$
dolomite

5.2.9 Sulfur

Sulfur has been known for a long time since it can occur free in nature. Yellow crystals of pure sulfur are deposited on the walls of active volcano craters by the gases coming out from the craters, loaded with sulfur particles. Sulfur gives these gases their pungent smell.

Sulfur is present in soils in organic and inorganic form. Organically, sulfur is an important constituent of proteins and amino acids. Inorganic sulfur comes from a number of different sources. It comes from the dissolution of gypsum, $CaSO_4$, and from the microbial oxidation of pyrite, FeS_2, as discussed previously. Gypsum is the most common source of S in soils. It is widely distributed in the world. Gypsum has been discovered in Canada, England, France, and Russia. Large amounts of gypsum in the United States occur in Arizona and New Mexico in aeolian sand deposits. As indicated previously, it is used primarily in the production of plaster, wallboard, fertilizers, and all kinds of casts. In medicine, gypsum is used for setting casts around broken bones. Sulfur can also be added to soils by the use of powdered S in agricultural operations, by industrial pollution causing acid rain, and by the use of chemicals containing S, such as insecticides and detergents.

Sulfur exists in soils and soil water as a SO_4^{2-} ion in combination with the cations, Ca, Mg, K, Na or NH_4^+. Present in the form of elemental sulfur, S, it will be oxidized in aerobic condition and converted quickly into SO_4^{2-}. Under anaerobic condition, SO_4^{2+} may be reduced by microorganisms into SO_3^{2-}, or H_2S. Hydrogen sulfide is formed especially in swamps and other areas with stagnant water. Waterlogging in coastal regions and paddy soils provide a suitable environment for formation of H_2S. The presence of hydrogen sulfide in paddy soils in Japan causes the development of the so-called *Akiochi disease*. These paddy soils are reportedly low in Fe (Tisdale and Nelson, 1975, 1993). In soils rich in Fe, H_2S is usually precipitated as Fe_2S, which imparts to soils a black color, as is frequently noted in soils of the coastal regions and tidal marshes.

Because most of the sulphur salts are soluble, sulfate is expected to be lost rapidly by leaching. The anionic nature of the sulfate ion prevents its attraction by clay colloids. However, soils containing hydrous oxide clays or sesquioxides have been reported to adsorb considerable amounts of sulfate (Tisdale and Nelson, 1975, 1993). The positively charged surfaces of these sesquioxide clays may cause electrostatic attraction of the negatively charged sulfate ions.

5.2.10 Manganese

Manganese is present in small quantities in many crystalline rocks. It is released into the soil by rock weathering and is redeposited in various forms of Mn oxides, e.g., *pyrolusite*, MnO_2, *braunite*, Mn_2O_3, and *manganite*, $MnO(OH)$ or $Mn_2O_3.H_2O$. Pyrolusite is a mineral that belongs to the *rutile* group, which is characterized by the formula XO_2. If the X is Ti, the mineral is rutile, but when X is Mn, the mineral is pyrolusite. Uranium oxide also belongs to this group. Pyrolusite occurs as an accessory mineral in crystalline rocks. Commercial deposits of pyrolusite are found in Russia, Gabon, South Africa, India, Australia, and Cuba. Small deposits have been discovered in the United States in Virginia, Tennessee, Georgia, Arkansas, California, and in the region of Lake Superior. This mineral is the most important source of Mn. The element Mn is used in the production of hard steel, chemicals, and disinfectants ($KMnO_4$). It is an important element for the production of batteries, and dry cells. Often it is also used in the glass industry as a decolorizer of glass, or as a coloring material in glass, pottery, and bricks.

Manganese can exist in three oxidation states: Mn^{2+}, Mn^{3+}, and Mn^{4+}. The divalent manganese ion is the main form of manganese in soil and soil water. Because it is a cation, Mn^{2+} is usually adsorbed on the negatively charged clay surfaces. The trivalent form usually exists as Mn_2O_3, which can be found in substantial amounts in acid soils. The tetravalent form, MnO_2, is perhaps the most stable and inert form of manganese.

The concentration of Mn^{2+} in soil water is very low, seldom exceeding 0.05 mg/L. Large amounts of soluble Mn in water cause Mn toxicity in plants, since it is needed only as a micronutrient. If it is used for household purposes, water containing Mn may stain clothes and bathroom fixtures. The stability of Mn^{2+} in solution depends on pH. At high pH values, Mn^{2+} precipitates as $Mn(OH)_2$ or is converted into MnO_2, or Mn_3O_4. Therefore, liming acid soils may frequently result in Mn deficiency in crops (Tisdale and Nelson, 1975, 1993). However, in the presence of high amounts of CO_2, manganese may exist as $MnHCO_3^+$. The concentration is, however, very low, and Mn is more likely to precipitate as hydroxides and oxides than to form $MnHCO_3^+$, especially when CO_2 partial pressures fluctuate suddenly.

5.2.11 Soil Colloids

A colloid is a state of matter consisting of very fine particles that approach but never reach molecular size. The upper size limit of colloids is 0.2 μm, and the lower size limit is approximately 50 Å or 5 nm, the size of a molecule. Colloids can be organic or inorganic in nature. On the basis of their interaction with water, colloids can be divided into hydrophobic and hydrophilic colloids. *Hydrophobic* colloids will not interact with water; in other words they repel water, whereas hydrophi-*lic* colloids will interact with water. Several organic colloids exhibit both hydrophobic and hydrophilic properties in one molecule. Such colloids are called *amphiphilic*, and include phospholipids and many amino acids. Detergents are examples of synthetic amphiphilics. Plant and soils contain large amounts of colloidal particles. Most plant colloids are hydrophilic, whereas soil inorganic colloids are hydrophobic. The inorganic fraction of soils consists of sand silt and clay. Clay comprises all inorganic solids with a diameter of <0.002 mm (<2 µm) in effective diameter and exhibits colloidal behavior.

Many of these inorganic and organic colloids, such as clay, carbohydrates, amino acids, protein, bacteria, and algae, are present in soil water. However, the amount dispersed in soil water is smaller than the amount present in the solid phase. When clay is added to water, it forms a suspension. The clay is then dispersed and exists as single, individual particles. Since clay usually carries negative charges, it attracts cations. This is necessary to maintain electroneutrality in the soil system. The cations are held on the clay surfaces by electrostatic bonds, which are weak bonds. Consequently, the adsorbed cations can be replaced or exchanged by other cations from the soil solution. The process of exchange is called *cation exchange*. The ions involved in the exchange reaction are referred to as *exchangeable cations*, and the clay particles that adsorb these ions are frequently called the *exchange complex*. Under natural conditions, H^+, Ca^{2+}, Mg^{2+}, K^+, and Na^+ are the most common cations in soils, and they can replace each other. When Ca, Mg, K, and Na are exchanged by H^+, the exchange complex is then saturated with H^+. This produces an acid reaction in soils.

Because of the high surface area of clays and because of their electrochemical properties, colloids may adsorb a variety of chemical compounds dissolved in soil water, e.g., products from microbial reactions, organic waste, gases, heavy metals and other pollutants. By adsorption to clay surfaces, many toxic metals can be immobilized or precipitated. The clay fraction, especially in the solid phase of soils, also provides for a buffer and intercepts pollutants. For example, heavy metals carried by soil water trickling through the pedon are removed because of the cation exchange capacity of clays. Consequently, clay acts as a purifying agent in nature, improving in this way the quality of soil water. However, this property of clay depends on its *cation exchange capacity* (CEC), which may vary with the different types of clay. Exchange reactions and their importance in plant growth and the environment are discussed in more detail in chapter 6.

5.3 DISSOLVED GAS

The two most important gases in soil air that affect soil properties and plant growth are CO_2 and O_2. As indicated in chapter 4, these gases may dissolve in soil water. The amount dissolved is usually very small and is controlled by the partial pressure of the gas in contact with soil water. *Henry's law* dictates that the solubility of a gas in a liquid is proportional to the partial pressure of that gas in contact with the liquid, as expressed by the equation:

$$C_{aq} = k\, P_t \qquad (5.8)$$

In this equation, C = concentration of gas dissolved in moles/L, k = Henry's law constant, and P = partial pressure of gas at temperature = t, in atm. The k values for the most important gases in soil air are very small:

	k (moles/L/atm)
CO_2	3.38×10^{-2}
O_2	1.28×10^{-3}
N_2	6.48×10^{-4}

Since the medium, water, in which the gas dissolves also exhibits a vapor pressure, both the water vapor pressure and partial pressure of the gas then determine the amount of gas dissolved. The vapor pressure (or partial pressure) of water at 25°C is 0.0313 atm. Using these parameters, the amount of gas dissolved can be easily determined. An example of the calculation of the amount of oxygen dissolved is given below. Soil air in equilibrium with atmospheric air has a pressure of 1 atm, and since atmospheric air contains 21% O_2, at 25^{oC} the following is valid:

$$P_{oxygen} = (\text{atmospheric pressure - water vapor pressure}) \times 0.21$$
$$= (1 - 0.0313) \times 0.21 = 0.2034 \text{ atm}$$

Using Henry's law, the concentration of oxygen dissolved in soil water is

$$C = k\,P_t \qquad t = 25°C$$
$$C = (1.28 \times 10^{-3}) \times 0.2034$$
$$= 0.2604 \times 10^{-3} \text{ moles/L}$$

Since 1 mole of O_2 = 2 x 16 = 32 grams, the concentration of oxygen dissolved in grams is

$$C = (0.2604 \times 10^{-3}) \times 32$$
$$= 8.33 \times 10^{-3} \text{ g/L} \quad \text{or } 8.33 \text{ mg/L}$$

The amount calculated above is the maximum concentration of dissolved O^2 at a water temperature of 25°C. The solubility usually decreases as the temperature increases. The amount of CO_2 dissolved in water can be calculated in a similar fashion and amounts to 0.984×10^{-5} moles/L. This is the amount of CO_2 in water of high quality, which is in equilibrium with atmospheric air.

5.3.1 Dissolved CO_2

Carbon dioxide is produced when carbon is burned with O_2. An example is the burning of fuel, such as methane, CH_4:

$$CH_4 + 2O_2 \rightarrow CO_2 + 2H_2O \tag{5.9}$$

In nature, CO_2 is produced by respiration of roots and the aerobic decomposition of organic matter, as discussed earlier. It is a colorless and odorless gas. It is 1.5 times heavier than atmospheric air. Carbon dioxide is considered one of the polluting gases that causes the greenhouse effect and the destruction of the ozone shield. Large amounts of CO_2 can be produced by large scale burning of the tropical rain forests and by the burning of fossil fuels in industry and by automobiles. Supersonic aviation also generates large amounts of CO_2. Another source of considerable amounts of CO_2 is active volcanisms. The latter has received little attention. All these activities and processes contribute to the generation of excessive amounts of CO_2, causing global warming and the destruction of the ozone shield. The amount of CO_2 produced by natural respiration and decomposition processes is usually of no harm, and is in fact a necessary process in the *carbon cycle*. Excess CO_2 in the Earth's atmosphere is usually absorbed by green plants and recycled through photosynthesis into carbohydrates. The oceans with their salt water and high pH are also sinks for CO_2. They are not only capable of absorbing huge amounts of CO_2 and converting it into carbonates and bicarbonates, but the large population of green marine plants, such as seaweed and kelp, absorb CO_2 and function similarly to terrestrial green plants. However, this formidable capacity of the green plants and ocean water to prevent such pollution can be destroyed by excessive and accelerated production of CO_2.

Carbon dioxide forms *carbonic acid*, H_2CO_3, with water, which is a weak acid that gives a weak sour taste to water. Because of this, it is a valuable gas for the manufacture of carbonated water and other beverages, such as Coca-Cola, Pepsi Cola, and other soda pops. Carbonic acid is very unstable, and has never been isolated. Its stability depends on the partial pressure of the CO_2 gas above. When the pressure in a can of soda water is released, *effervescence* takes place. Carbon dioxide is also an important ingredient for certain types of fire extinguishers. Fire extinguishers containing CO_2 are preferred for fighting fires from explosive materials, such as gasoline and aviation fuel. Carbon dioxide is one of the materials that does not support the combustion. Air, containing 2.5% CO_2 is able to extinguish such fires. It is also used in the production of *baking soda*, $NaHCO_3$, and *washing soda*, $Na_2CO_3.10H_2O$. Today baking soda is used in toothpaste, and as water softeners. When frozen, carbon dioxide forms a solid, called *dry ice*. It is often used as a refrigerant in coolers and for cooling of beverages.

As discussed in chapter 4, atmospheric air contains 0.03% CO_2. However, because of respiration and aerobic decomposition of organic matter in soils, the CO_2 content in soil is usually above 0.03%. Therefore, the amount of CO_2 dissolved will be above 1.0×10^{-5} moles/L.

Dissolved carbon dioxide, or CO_2, affects many biological and chemical reactions in soil water. It is used by aquatic plants, such as algae, in photosynthesis. It is a chemically active compound, and interacts with water to form carbonic acid; hence, it affects the pH of soil and soil water. The reaction is usually represented by the following equation:

$$CO_2 + H_2O \leftrightarrow H_2CO_3 \tag{5.10}$$

$$H_2CO_3 \leftrightarrow H^+ + HCO_3^- \tag{5.11}$$

Carbonic acid is a weak acid and will dissociate some of its protons in soil water, as indicated by reaction (5.11). Such a reaction normally increases the acidity of soil water. However, the HCO_3^- is unstable and may dissociate, producing OH^- ions as follows:

$$HCO_3^- \leftrightarrow OH^- + CO_2\uparrow \tag{5.12}$$

The OH^- ions neutralize the H^+ formed by reaction (5.11). Because carbonic acid is capable of producing H^+ and OH^- ions at the same time, it is considered a buffer compound. Therefore, it is capable of stabilizing the acidic conditions of soil and water to a certain extent. This stabilizing effect is especially enhanced when it is present as a bicarbonate of calcium.

Water containing CO_2 is a powerful solvent for limestone and other calcareous materials. Calcium carbonate, which is otherwise insoluble in pure H_2O, becomes soluble in carbonated water. Such a reaction is called earlier *carbonation* and can be illustrated by the reaction below:

$$CO_2 + H_2O + CaCO_3 \leftrightarrow Ca^{2+} + 2HCO_3^- \qquad (5.13)$$

This reaction is the main weathering process by which limestone is decomposed in soil formation.

5.3.2 Dissolved Oxygen

Another important substance dissolved in soil water is oxygen. In nature, oxygen is the most abundant and widely distributed element. Atmospheric air theoretically contains 23% oxygen. In the form of compounds, oxygen is present in rocks and minerals, and makes up a large part of the bodies of plants and animals. It is a colorless and odorless gas, which is slightly more dense than air. Liquid oxygen, however, has a pale blue color, and will boil at -183°C at atmospheric pressure. The element consists of two atoms, hence the formula O_2. In the liquid and solid state, oxygen has *paramagnetic properties*, meaning that it can be attracted by a magnetic field. Chemically, oxygen is the most active element. When oxygen combines with another element, the product formed is called an *oxide*.

Oxygen is needed for the slow oxidation of compounds that generates the energy required by all living organisms for normal functions and maintenance of body temperature. The intake of O_2 by respiration of roots and microorganisms is an example of such a production of energy through burning of tissue carbohydrates. Oxygen is in fact considered the key substance in both soil air and soil water for the existence of all forms of life in soils. Oxygen deficiency in soil air causes many undesirable effects as has been discussed in chapter 4. Oxygen deficiency is detrimental to organisms living in soil water. In lakes and streams, lack of oxygen is fatal to fish and aquatic plants.

The amount of oxygen dissolved in soil water depends on the partial pressure of O_2 and water vapor, as discussed previously.

It is very small; the calculated value of dissolved O_2 is 8.33 mg/L at 1 atm and 25°C. This amount of dissolved oxygen can be depleted very rapidly unless some mechanism for aeration is present. In natural streams and lakes, oxygen content is replenished by aeration through turbulent flows and waterfalls. Artificially, aeration of water is achieved by pumping air in water, or creating fountain sprays, such as in aquariums, hydroponic systems, and sewage treatment plants. Several processes are responsible for the depletion of dissolved organic oxygen. Oxygen can be consumed rapidly in the oxidation process of organic matter as discussed previously. Soil water may contain a lot of organic pollutants, which are washed down from manure, and industrial and domestic wastes during heavy rains. Part of the dissolved organic compounds is sometimes referred to as *dissolved organic carbon* or *DOC*. Microbial decomposition of these organics consumes most of the dissolved oxygen. Moreover, a lack of O_2, rather than the presence of pollutants, may cause aquatic organisms to suffocate in polluted streams, lakes and reservoirs. Pollutants are frequently not the primary source for fish kill, but their presence complicates the effect of other adverse conditions. This is evidenced by the fact that fish and other aquatic organisms thrive in turbulent streams and lakes that are loaded with clay suspensions. Other microorganism-mediated processes depleting the dissolved oxygen content are the *biochemical oxidation* of:

Iron compounds

$$4Fe^{2+} + O_2 + 4H^+ \rightarrow 4Fe^{3+} + 2H_2O \qquad (5.13)$$

Sulfur compounds

$$2SO_4^{2-} + O_2 \rightarrow 2SO_4^{2-} \qquad (5.14)$$

Ammonium

$$2NH_4^+ + 3O_2 \rightarrow 2NO_2^- + 2H_2O + 4H^+ + \text{energy} \qquad (5.15)$$

$$2NO_2^- + O_2 \rightarrow 2NO_3^- + \text{energy} \qquad (5.16)$$

The oxidation of ammonium into nitrate, called *nitrification*, has been discussed previously.

5.3.3 Oxygen Demand

The rate by which oxygen is consumed by the oxidation processes, discussed above, is called *oxygen demand* (OD). Three types of ODs are distinguished:

Biological Oxygen Demand (BOD). This is defined as the amount of oxygen consumed by the microbial decomposition of organic matter during a 5-day incubation period. The test was developed in England, where it was considered that dissolved organic matter not decomposed within 5 days would be transported into the sea.

Chemical Oxygen Demand (COD). This is defined as the amount of oxygen consumed in the chemical oxidation of organic matter by $K_2Cr_2O_7$ in the presence of H_2SO_4. The analysis for determination of C_{org} by the wet oxidation method with $K_2Cr_2O_7$ is today called the *Walkley-Black method*.

Total Oxygen Demand (TOD). This is the amount of oxygen consumed in the catalytic oxidation of carbon. The amount of CO_2 produced in the reaction is measured.

Of these three types of ODs, the BOD is the best known, although the determination of BOD is more difficult than the determination of COD, whereas the 5-day incubation period is subject to many arguments. Nevertheless, many scientists prefer the use of BOD for determining the quality of stream and lake water and the amount of pollution in soils and the environment. Organic wastes are frequently introduced into streams and lakes through runoff and/or leaching. The BOD demand of organic waste decreases the dissolved O_2 content during the decomposition process. The lower the BOD values, the better is the water quality. A BOD value of 1 ppm means that 1 ppm of oxygen was consumed in the decomposition process during a 5-day incubation period. This indicates that only a small amount of organic pollutant was present; hence, the water being analyzed is of high quality. On the other hand, high BOD values (5-20 ppm) in an analysis suggest that the water contains high amounts of organic contaminants, or is water of low quality (Stevenson, 1986). Since the maximum amount of dissolved oxygen is 8.33 mg/L (at 25°C, 1 atm), a value of 8 ppm as the lowest limit of a high BOD value is perhaps closer to reality than 5 ppm (Tan, 1993). Animal waste, runoff from barnyards, and effluent from food processing plants are notorious for their high BOD values. The BOD may run as high as 10 000 ppm in runoff from feed lots (Stevenson, 1986). On the other hand, digested sewage sludge is low in BOD because of microbial oxidation during the digestion process. It is expected that the soil can take care of the amount of dissolved organic substances on its own as long as the level of pollutants can be oxidized by 8.33 mg O_2/L. As soon as this amount of dissolved O^2 is depleted, organic contaminants start to accumulate, decreasing the quality of soil water.

CHAPTER 6

ELECTROCHEMICAL PROPERTIES OF SOLID CONSTITUENTS

As discussed in chapters 2 and 3, the solid constituents of soils consist of a variety of inorganic and organic compounds. Most of the coarse materials, such as sand, silt, and undecomposed organic matter are chemically inert. They are important constituents for building up the soil, and affect many soil properties. Since they are coarse in size, they have low specific surface area and do not exhibit colloidal properties. They may participate in a number of soil reactions and exhibit some adsorption capacities, but they are not really chemically active. However, clay and humus, the smallest soil constituents, have large specific surface areas and exhibit a surface chemistry different from the coarse materials. The surface chemistry of clay and humus is attributed to the presence of electrical charges in their molecules. Due to these charges they are chemically very active and are considered the *seat of soil activity* (Brady, 1990), causing many soil chemical reactions such as cation exchange and complex reactions.

6.1 SOIL CLAYS

Soil clays ordinarily carry electronegative charges, which are the result of one or more of several different reactions. Two major sources for the origin of negative charges are *isomorphous substitution* and *dissociation of exposed hydroxyl groups.*

6.1.1 Isomorphous Substitution

Isomorphous substitution is the substitution of atoms in the crystal structure for other atoms without affecting the crystal structure. It can take place in both the silica tetrahedrons and the aluminum octahedrons of the clay mineral. For example, in the absence of isomorphous substitution, kaolinite is electrically balanced. Assuming that the unit cell formula of kaolinite is $Al_2O.2SiO_2.2H_2O$, the following simple calculation shows that the positive charges carried by the cations are completely neutralized by the negative charges carried by the oxygen atoms:

Al^{3+}	Si^{4+}	H^+	O^{2-}
2x	2x	2x	9x
	18^+		18^+

A replacement of one octahedral Al by Mg by the isomorphic process yields one negative charge unbalanced in the crystal. Since Mg is divalent, it can only contribute two positive charges for the neutralization of the negative charges in the crystal:

Al_{3+}	Mg^{2+}	Si^{4+}	H^{+}	O^{2+}
1x	1x	2x	2x	9x
	17^{+}			18^{-}

A similar substitution can also occur in a Si tetrahedron, where Si can be replaced by Al. This reaction also leaves one negative charge not neutralized. These types of negative charges are called *permanent negative charges*, and are independent of pH. Isomorphous substitution will occur only between atoms of almost equal sizes, and when the difference in valences does not exceed one unit. Permanent charges are of special importance in 2:1 types of clays, e.g., smectites.

6.1.2 Dissociation of Exposed Hydroxyl Groups

Exposed hydroxyl groups are OH groups present on the surface of the Al octahedron sheets. They are prevalent in 1:1 types of clays, sesquioxides, and amorphous clays. These OH groups are in contact with the soil solution and tend to dissociate, releasing thereby their protons as illustrated in the reaction below.

$$\underset{\text{neutral octahedron}}{-Al-OH} \leftrightarrow \underset{\text{neg. charged octahedron}}{-Al-O^{-}} + H^{+} \quad (6.1)$$

This dissociation of the H^{+} leaves one negative charge in the octahedron not neutralized. Such a dissociation reaction is dependent upon pH. The dissociation reaction occurs at high pH, and decreases at low pH. Therefore, the magnitude of the negative charge also increases and decreases accordingly with the change in pH. Because of this, this type of negative charge is called *pH dependent charge* or *variable charge*. It is of importance in the minerals with OH groups present on their surfaces, as indicated above. For example, kaolinite exhibits variable charges. Permanent charges are also present in kaolinite, but to a lesser amounts. The minerals with variable charges are frequently called *variable charge minerals*, and the soils containing these minerals are called *soils with variable charges*.

6.1.3 Protonation of Exposed Hydroxyl Groups

Protonation of exposed OH groups is the addition of H^+ ions to the exposed OH groups of the clay minerals. The H^+ is adsorbed with a relatively weak bond. Because of this addition of H^+, the OH group is oversaturated with protons and the clay surface becomes positively charged, as illustrated by the reaction below.

$$\text{- Al - OH} + H^+ \leftrightarrow \text{- Al -OHH}^+ \qquad (6.2)$$

neutral octahedron — positively charged octahedron

Protonation of exposed OH groups occurs only at low pH, because acid conditions are required for the supply of the extra protons.

6.1.4 Zero Point of Charge (ZPC)

The *ZPC* is the *pH* at which the mineral has no charge, or has equal amounts of negative and positive charges. It has a similar meaning as *isoelectric point*. As discussed above, at high pH values the mineral carries a negative charge, which decreases with a decrease in pH. When the pH is continuously decreased, a point will be reached at which the negative charge equals zero. The pH at which this occurs is called ZPC, as indicated in the definition above. The ZPC is a specific characteristic of the clay mineral, and its value differs from one to another mineral (Table 6.1). When the net charge is zero at

Table 6.1 ZPC Values of Selected Minerals

Mineral	ZPC
Hematite, α-Fe_2O_3	2.1
Corundum, α-Al_2O_3	2.2
Goethite, α-FeOOH	3.2
Gibbsite	4.8
Lepidocrocite	5.4 - 7.3
Maghemite	6.7
Ferrihydrite	8.1
Amorphous $Al(OH)_3$	8.3
Amorphous $Fe(OH)_3$	8.5

Sources: Van Schuylenborgh and Sänger (1949); Van Schuylenborgh and Arens (1950).

ZPC, clay particles in soil water will not repel each other and tend to aggregate forming larger particles. These aggregates precipitate and form the soil structure. In contrast, negatively charged clay particles repel each other, resulting in dispersion. Under such condition, the clay suspension is considered stable. If clays remain dispersed, the soil is puddled and sensitive to water erosion. Puddled soils are also sticky when wet, and become hard and dense upon drying. A compacted soil is undesirable for plant growth. Root growth requires a porous soil for adequate aeration. Such a soil can be formed if aggregation of clay can be enhanced naturally or artificially. Naturally, aggregation is enhanced by the presence of high amounts of Al and Fe, which usually occurs in acid soils. Although aggregation is enhanced, the high amounts of Al and Fe may create toxicity to plants. Artificially, aggregation is increased by liming practices. Calcium and Mg are known to flocculate clay, while at the same time will reduce the toxicity of Al and Fe.

6.1.5 Cation Exchange Capacity

The *cation exchange capacity* is the capacity of clays to adsorb and exchange cations. The negative charges of clays are usually attracting a swarm of cations (positively charged ions). This is Mother Nature's way of maintaining electroneutrality in the soil. A system is then created in the soil composed of particles with a negatively charged layer neutralized by a layer of positively charged ions. Such a system is called in soil chemistry an *electric double layer*. The cations, held electrostatically on the clay surface, can be replaced by other soil cations. These adsorbed cations are, therefore, called *exchangeable cations*, and the process of exchange is referred to as *cation exchange*. The soil particles responsible for adsorption and exchange of cations are called the *exchange complex*. Exchange reactions are instantaneous. To maintain electroneutrality, the reaction is stoichiometric, meaning that the exchange occurs in equivalent amounts, as illustrated by the reaction below:

$$\underset{\text{adsorbed Ca}}{\text{Soil-Ca}} + 2H^+ \leftrightarrow \underset{\text{adsorbed } H^+}{\text{Soil-2H}} + \underset{\text{free Ca ion}}{Ca^{2+}} \qquad (6.3)$$

As shown in reaction (6.3), it needs 2 monovalent ions, e.g., two H^+ to replace one Ca, which is divalent.

The cation exchange capacity (CEC), expressed in milliequivalents (me) per 100g (cmol(+)/kg), differs from soil to soil depending on (1) clay content, (2) types of clays, and (3) organic matter content. The higher the clay content, the larger will be the CEC of the soil. Hence, sandy soils exhibit low CECs. A similar reasoning can also be given for organic matter content. The types of clays may also affect the CEC of soils because different types of clays exhibit different types of CECs as can be adduced from the table below

Soil colloid	**CEC (me/100g)**
Humus (humic acids)	> 150
Vermiculite	150
Smectite	100
Illite	30
Kaolinite	10
Sesquioxides	4

6.1.6 Environmental Importance of Cation Exchange

Cation exchange is of great importance in (1) soil fertility, (2) fertilizers application, (3) nutrient uptake, and (4) environmental quality.

Soil Fertility. Under natural conditions H^+, Ca^{2+}, Mg^{2+}, K^+, and Na^+ are the most common cations in soils. They can replace each other depending on the conditions. When conditions are favorable for the presence of high amounts of protons, H^+ replaces the other cations in the exchange complex. Such an exchange with H^+ ions produces acidic soils, which occur especially in humid regions. The bases released in the soil solution are leached by the percolating waters. Liming such soils is then necessary to replace the adsorbed H^+ by Ca^{2+} and thereby increase soil fertility.

Fertilizer Application. Fertilizers are added to soils to increase soil fertility and improve plant growth. The major nutrients in fertilizers are N, P, K, Fe, Cu, Zn, and Mn. The N in fertilizers can be in cationic (NH_4^+) or anionic form (NO_3^-), whereas P is always anionic in nature ($H_2PO_4^-$, HPO_4^{2-}). The other nutrients are in the form of cations. These cations are released upon dissolution of the fertilizer in soil water. After release, they are either adsorbed or they will replace the original cation on the exchange complex. In this way the fertilizer elements needed for plant growth are stored in the soil, and are less subject to leaching. As such, the adsorption complex gives to the soil a storage and buffering capacity of cations.

Nutrient Uptake. The exchangeable cations serve as storage for large quantities of available nutrients for plant growth. Plant roots obtain the adsorbed cations by cation exchange. The exchanged material used by roots is H^+, which is produced as a by-product of root respiration, as discussed previously. Such an exchange reaction is illustrated in Figure 6.1.

Environmental Quality. A lot of material may be added to soils by agricultural, industrial, and domestic operations. Several of the compounds are hazardous to humans and animals. They may leach with the percolating waters and pollute the groundwater. However, the presence of clays with their cation exchange capacity provides a buffering capacity. Because of the electrical charge and high surface area, clays adsorb a variety of chemical compounds entering the soils as products of microbial reactions as organic waste, gas, heavy metals, and other pollutants. By adsorption to clay surfaces, many toxic

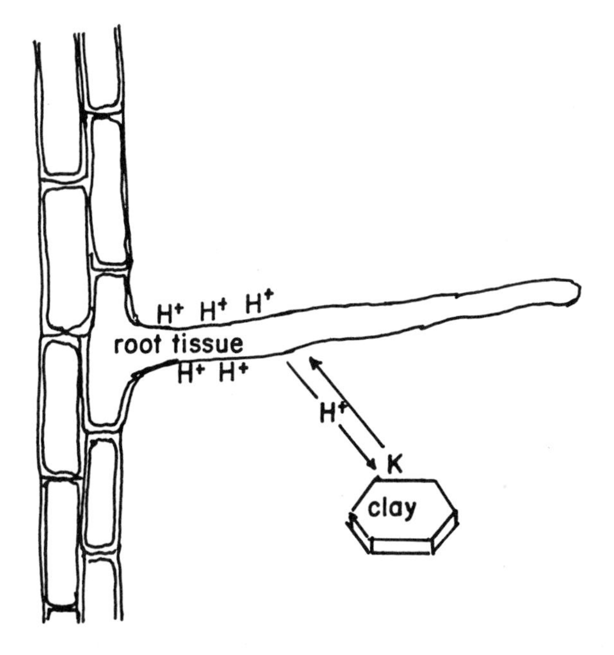

Figure 6.1 Cation exchange reaction between H^+ ions in the root rhizosphere and K adsorbed on the clay surface.

metals are immobilized and/or precipitated into less harmful solid compounds. The clay will intercept a variety of pollutants trickling down the soil with the percolating water. These pollutants will be removed by clay because of cation exchange before they reach the ground water. Consequently, clay acts as a purifying agent in nature and increases the quality of soil and ground water.

6.2 ANION EXCHANGE CAPACITY

The *anion exchange capacity* is the capacity of clay to adsorb and exchange anions. The clay must be positively charged to be able to adsorb negatively charged ions. Positive charges in clays are of importance only in acidic conditions, when the soil pH is below the ZPC of the clay. It can also develop because of broken bonds on the broken edges of the clay mineral. In general, the positive charge, hence the anion exchange capacity of clays, is considerably smaller than the cation exchange capacity. The major anions in soils subject to anion exchange reactions are SiO_4^{4-}, $H_2PO_4^-$, SO_4^{2-}, NO_3^-, and Cl^-. Adsorption of phosphate ions will usually result in phosphate *fixation* and *retention* (Tan, 1993).

6.3 SOIL ORGANIC MATTER

6.3.1 Amino Acids

Amino acids are amphoteric compounds because they contain both carboxyl and amino groups. The carboxyl groups behave acidicly, whereas the amino groups are basic in nature. Therefore, they can be negatively and positively charged depending on the conditions. The pH at which an amino acid exhibits equal amounts of positive and negative charges is called the *isoelectric point* (pH_0). At the isoelectric point, the amino acid is electrically neutral. The neutral ion of amino acid is called a *zwitterion* (zwitter is German for double or pair), and has the following formula:

$$\begin{array}{c} NH_3^+ \\ | \\ H_3C - C - COO^- \\ | \\ R \end{array}$$

Note that the zwitterion carries both positive and negative charges, which neutralize each other. When amino acids are present in soils with a pH > pH_0, the condition is considered "alkaline" for the amino acids, and the excess OH^- ions present in the soil solution react with the NH_3^+ group of the zwitterion. Such a reaction yields a negative charge as can be noticed from the equation below

$$\underset{\text{zwitterion}}{R-\overset{\overset{\displaystyle COO^-}{|}}{\underset{\underset{\displaystyle CH_3}{|}}{C}}-NH_3^+} + OH^- \rightarrow \underset{\text{anionic form}}{R-\overset{\overset{\displaystyle COO^-}{|}}{\underset{\underset{\displaystyle CH_3}{|}}{C}}-NH_2} + H_2O \qquad (6.4)$$

On the other hand, in acid soils (soil pH < pH_0), the system contains large amounts of H^+ ions. The protons will then react with the carboxyl group of the zwitterion and the amino acid is positively charged

$$\underset{\text{zwitterion}}{CH_3-\overset{\overset{\displaystyle NH_3^+}{|}}{\underset{\underset{\displaystyle R}{|}}{C}}-COO^-} + H^+ \rightarrow \underset{\text{cationic form}}{CH_3-\overset{\overset{\displaystyle NH_3^+}{|}}{\underset{\underset{\displaystyle R}{|}}{C}}-COOH} \qquad (6.5)$$

In the anionic form, amino acid reacts with cations, such as metal ions, whereas as a cation it will react with anions or undergoes interactions with clays.

6.3.2 Humic Matter

Humic matter, composed of humic and fulvic acids, are also amphoteric compounds. Although they can be positively and negatively charged, the negative charges are usually of more importance in humic matter than the positive charges. As discussed in chapter 3, the negative charge in humic matter is expressed in terms of *total acidity*, which is defined as the sum of the carboxyl and phenolic-OH groups. In general, these two functional groups control the electrochemical behavior of humic matter. Dissociation of protons from the carboxyl groups starts at pH 3.0, and the humic molecule becomes electronegatively charged (Figure 6.2). At pH < 3.0 the humic molecule exhibits

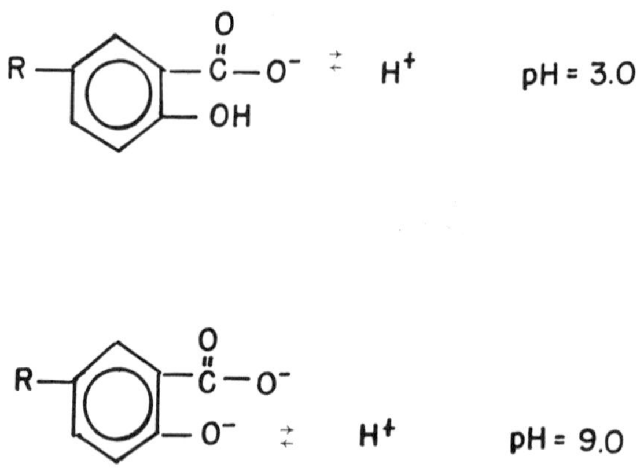

Figure 6.2 Development of negative charges in a humic acid molecule by dissociation of protons from carboxyl (COOH) groups at pH 3.0 and from phenolic-OH groups at pH 9.0.

a small negative charge, but this charge increases with increasing pH. At pH = 9.0, the phenolic-OH group also starts to dissociate its proton, and the humic molecule attains a high negative charge. Since the development of these negative charges is pH dependent, this charge is called *variable charge* or *pH dependent charge*.

Several reactions or interactions can take place because of the presence of these charges. At low pH values, the humic molecule is capable of attracting cations, which leads to cation exchange reactions. The magnitude of the cation exchange capacity (CEC) of humic matter is reflected from the total acidity value. As discussed in chapter 3, the total acidity, hence the CEC, can range from 500 to 1200 me/100g, which is the highest CEC value of all the colloids in soils. When both the carboxyl and phenolic-OH groups are completely dissociated, humic matter is also able to undergo complex reactions or chelation reactions with metal ions or other soil constituents (Figure 6.3). These reactions have been discussed in other chapters of this book as they play an important role in soil fertility, plant nutrition, and in enhancing environmental quality.

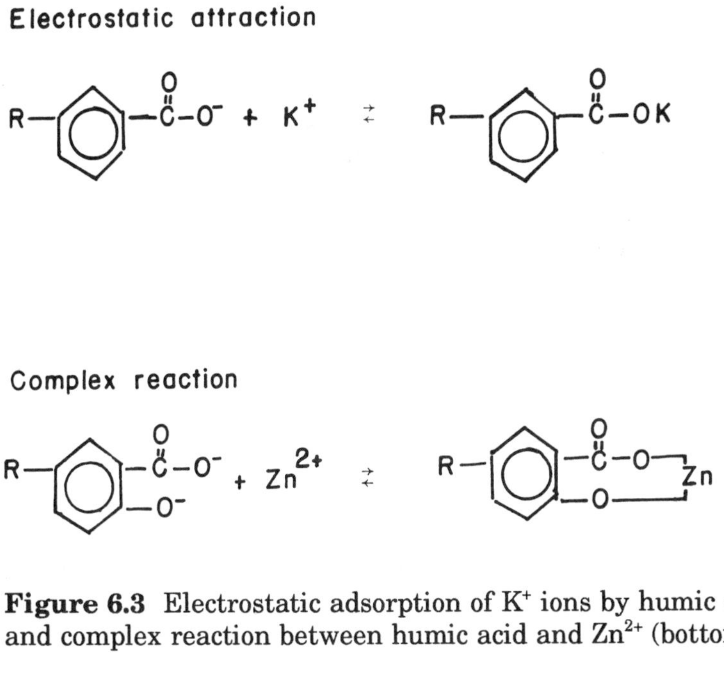

Electrostatic attraction

Complex reaction

Figure 6.3 Electrostatic adsorption of K^+ ions by humic acid (top), and complex reaction between humic acid and Zn^{2+} (bottom).

6.4 SOIL REACTION

Soil reaction is a soil parameter which is also closely controlled by the electrochemical properties of soil colloids. The term is used to indicate the acidity or alkalinity of a soil. The degree of acidity or alkalinity is determined by the hydrogen ion, H^+, concentration in the soil solution. In acidic soils the H^+ concentration is greater than the OH^- concentration, whereas in alkaline soils the H^+ concentration is smaller than the OH^- concentration. In a soil with a neutral reaction, $H^+ = OH^-$. These conditions are usually expressed in pH values, ranging from 0 to 14. The *p* refers to negative logarithm and the *H* means the H^+ ion concentration in grams/L. Thus,

$$pH = -\log (H^+)$$

or

$$pH = \log 1/H^+$$

At a H^+ concentration of 0.001 g/L, the pH = -log 0.001 = -(-3)= 3. At a H^+ concentration of 0.000001 g/L, the pH = -log 0.000001 = -(-6)= 6. Notice that a solution with fewer H^+ ions has numerically larger (higher) pH values.

Acidity and alkalinity reflect both the H^+ and OH^- ion concentrations. The mass action law states that the product of the concentration of H^+ and OH^- ions is always constant. This works out to be

$$(H^+)(OH^-) = 10^{-14}$$

By taking the negative logarithms of both sides, this equation changes into

$$pH + pOH = 14$$

Since the sum of pH and pOH is constant, the concentrations of H^+ and OH^- ions vary inversely. Therefore, only one (pH) needs to be determined to know the other.

Soil acidity or alkalinity is affected by the types of cations adsorbed on colloidal surfaces. The major soil cations adsorbed on colloidal surfaces are Al^{3+}, H^+, Na^+, K^+, Ca^{2+}, and Mg^{2+} ions. An overabundance of adsorbed Al^{3+} and H^+ ions decreases soil pH, whereas a saturation of the exchange sites with the bases Na, K, Ca, and Mg increases soil pH.

6.4.1 Types of Soil Reactions

Based on soil pH values, the following *types of soil reactions* are distinguished:

Soil Reaction	pH	Soil Reaction	pH
Slightly acid	7.0 - 6.0	Slightly alkaline	7.0 - 8.0
Moderately acid	6.0 - 5.0	Moderately alkaline	8.0 - 9.0
Strongly acid	5.0 - 4.0	Strongly alkaline	9.0 - 10.0
Very strongly acid	4.0 - 3.0	Very strongly alkaline	10.0 - 11.0

These terms can be used to identify the degree of acidity in soils. If one says that the soil has a very strongly acidic reaction, it is meant that the soil pH is between 4.0 and 3.0. Similarly when we say that the soil has a slightly alkaline reaction, we are referring to soils in the pH range of 7.0 to 8.0. The use of the terms acidic pH or basic pH should be avoided, since the pH is expressed in numerical values, ranging from low (0) to high (14). Figures are neither acidic nor basic.

Most soils have a pH between 5 to 9. In a humid region, the

surface soil usually exhibits a pH of 5 to 7 because most of the bases are exchanged and leached as can be illustrated by the following reaction:

$$\text{Clay-Ca} + 2H_2O \leftrightarrow \text{Clay-2H} + Ca^{2+} + 2OH^- \quad (6.6)$$

The percolating water provided by the high amount of precipitation in humid regions removes the soluble Ca^{2+} and OH^+, and forces the reaction above to go to the right. The soil is left with clay saturated with H^+ ions. Therefore, due to the leaching of bases, a humid region soil will seldom exhibit a pH > 7.0. The pH can decrease below 3.0 under very special soil conditions, e.g., the presence of S compounds as discussed before. On the other hand, soils in arid regions are characterized by a pH of 7.0 to 9.0 in the surface soil. Here, the adsorbed bases are not leached away, and some of them may even form salts, e.g. $CaCO_3$, Na_2CO_3, and NaCl. These salts provide a reserve of cations that can maintain the saturation of the clay complex. The process can be illustrated as follows:

$$\text{Clay-2H} + CaCO_3 \leftrightarrow \text{Clay-Ca} + H_2O + CO_{2\uparrow} \quad (6.7)$$

Hydrolysis of the carbonate salts contributes toward increasing the soil pH level over the value that would have been expected from a 100% base saturation. The hydrolysis reaction of $CaCO_3$ can be written as follows:

$$CaCO_3 + H_2O \leftrightarrow Ca^{2+} + 2OH^- + CO_2{}^{\uparrow} \quad (6.8)$$

Therefore, because leaching is not important in arid regions, the soil remains saturated with bases, hence the soil pH seldom decreases below 7.0.

6.4.2 Sources and Types of Soil Acidity

A number of compounds contribute to the development of acidic and alkaline reactions in soils. Water is a source for a small amount of H^+ ions. Inorganic and organic acids, produced by the decomposition of soil organic matter, are common soil constituents that also contribute to soil acidity. Respiration of plant roots, hydrolysis of Al, nitrification, oxidation of S, fertilizers, and acid rain are additional sources of H^+ in soils. All these compounds and their reactions contributing to soil acidity have been discussed in previous chapters or will be discussed in the following chapters.

The H^+ ions may be present in soils as adsorbed ions on the surface of the colloidal complex, or as free H^+ ions in the soil solution. The adsorbed H^+ ions are referred to as *potential* or *exchange acidity*, whereas the free H^+ ions are called the *active acidity*. Taken together, the active and potential acidity make up the *total soil acidity*. The system composed of free and exchangeable (adsorbed) H^+ ions is illustrated in Figure 6.4.

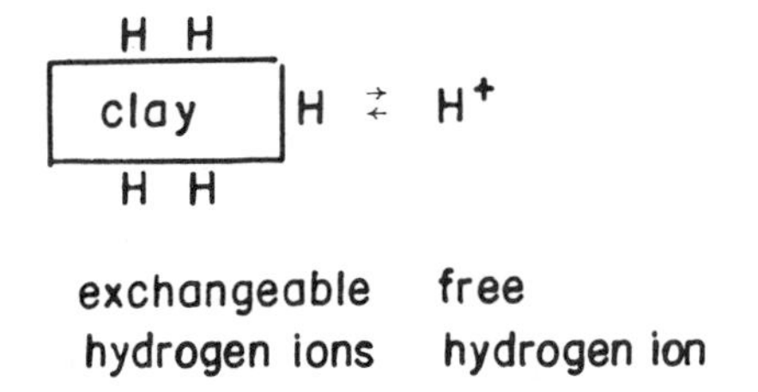

Figure 6.4 Dissociation of exchangeable H^+ ions from clay surfaces.

The free H^+ ion concentration of the soil solution at any particular time is relatively small compared with the reserve H^+ ion concentration. In humid region soils, the removal of bases from the colloidal complex by leaching, especially Ca, occurs constantly through cation exchange. Their place on the exchange sites is taken by H^+ ions. These adsorbed H^+ ions will dissociate free H^+ ions, and the concentration of free H^+ ions is measured and expressed in terms of pH.

The reaction of acid soils can be influenced only when enough lime is added to react with the *total acidity*. The greater the exchange capacity of the soil and the greater the reserve acidity, the more difficult it is to reduce the soil pH. This resistance to change is called *buffer capacity.*

6.4.3 Effect of Soil Reaction on Plant Growth

The soil reaction has a direct and indirect nutritional effect on plant growth. The direct effect is manifested by the toxic effect of H^+ and OH^- ions, whereas the indirect effect is made by controlling availability of plant nutrients.

Most plants grow best in soils with a slightly acid reaction, although some variations may be noticed. For example, alfalfa, clover and cedar require a soil pH closer to 7.0 for maximum growth, whereas pine trees need a soil pH of 5.0. On the other hand, azaleas and rhododendrons do better in a more acidic medium.

In the pH range of 6.0 to 7.0, nearly all plant nutrients are available in optimal amounts. Soils with a pH below 6.0 will likely be deficient in some available nutrients for optimal plant growth. Calcium, Mg, and K are especially absent in acid soils. In strongly to very strongly acidic soils, the microelements Al, Fe, Cu, Zn, and Mn may exist in very high quantities, creating micronutrient toxicity. In strongly alkaline soils Ca, Mg, and K concentrations are very high, whereas the soluble microelement concentrations are very low. For example, Al^{3+} ions, when present, tend to be precipitated in the form of insoluble $Al(OH)_3$. The concentrations of Fe, Mn, Cu, and Zn are decreased by a similar reaction, and become so low that the very strongly basic soils tend to exhibit micronutrient deficiency.

The type of phosphate ion and its concentration in soils are also controlled by the soil reaction. At very strongly acidic conditions, phosphate ion concentration is very low because most of the phosphate is precipitated in the form of insoluble $AlPO_3$ or $FePO_3$, called variscite and strengite, respectively. The major phosphate ion present in soils with an acid reaction is H_2PO_{4-}, and its concentration increases from very low at pH 3.0 to sufficiently high at pH 6.0 to 7.0. Phosphate ion concentration is also low at very strongly basic condition because of precipitation as insoluble tricalcium phosphate, $Ca_3(PO_4)_2$. Tricalcium phosphate is a constituent of animal bones. In slightly to moderately alkaline soils the phosphate ion is present in the form of HPO_4^{2-} and PO_4^{3-}.

CHAPTER 7

SOILS AND CROP PRODUCTION

Soil has been defined previously as the natural portion of the earth's surface that supports plant growth. It is the medium for crop and animal production. Soils, providing good media for an adequate supply of food and fiber, have been one of the reasons for the establishment of large human populations in many parts of the world. In Mesopotamia and Egypt, long considered the cradle of civilization, the fertile soils in the valleys and deltas of the Tigris, Euphrates and Nile rivers were responsible for the creation of flourishing civilizations. Similarly, the Ganges and Indus rivers in India, Bangladesh, and Pakistan, and the Mekong, Yangtze and Hwang Ho rivers in Southeast Asia and China created sites with rich soils where stable and organized human communities could grow food and thrive. The presence of water for irrigation and periodic flooding contributed to the continuous build up of the nutrient supply of the soils for good soil fertility.

As the world's population has expanded and living standards have improved, the demand for food and fiber has increased considerably. Because of recent advances in medical science drastically improving world health, many countries have experienced and are still experiencing an unprecedented population growth. Predictions have been made that by the year

2000 the world population will be 6 to 7 billion, which is 25% higher than it is today (Brady, 1990). This staggering number of people will consume perhaps more food than all other animals combined (Deevey, 1960). The increased demand for food places an increasing load on soil productivity, and several methods to increase soil productivity have been proposed. Brady (1990) suggested three routes to increase food production:

1. Clear and bring new lands into cultivation.
2. Intensify production on lands already under cultivation.
3. Increase the number of croppings per year.

Recent advancements in agricultural technology indicate that three more methods should be added today as possibilities:

4. Use *biotechnology* to create the most high yielding crops.
5. Employ *hydroponics, aeroponics,* or *soilless* agriculture to grow food and fiber without putting pressures on soil resources.
6. Develop *aquaculture*, which utilizes the resources of fresh water bodies, the seas, and oceans.

The first three routes will be discussed below in more detail. *Soilless agriculture* and *aquaculture* will be examined in chapter 8, and *biotechnology in soil science* in chapter 9.

7.1 CLEARING NEW LANDS

This method of increasing food production depends on the quantity and quality of soils. Quantity refers to the available acreages of new soils that can be cultivated. In Europe and the United States most of the soils are already under cultivation, and little is left for further expansion (World Resources, 1987; FAO, 1987; President's Science Advisory Committee, 1967). However, only 25% of the soils are presently being used for crop production in Africa. In South America and Oceania (Australia and New Zealand), 20% and 31% of the soils, respectively, are under cultivation. Most of the unused areas providing a possibility for agricultural expansion are covered by rain forests or savannah-rain forests. In the six Amazonian countries in South America, the total forested area is estimated to be 825 million ha, and an average of 4 million hectares per year are expected to be cleared during the next 6 years. The cultivated area in Brazil alone must be increased by the year 2050 by 70-90 million hectares to support the food requirement of a population increase from an estimated 135 million at present to 250 million in the year 2050 (Fearnside, 1987).

The second point to be considered in clearing new areas for crop production is the quality of soils. Quality refers to the fertility of soils, or the capacity of soils to supply nutrients in adequate amounts and in the proper balance for crop production. The President's Science Advisory Committee report (1967) indicated that many of the soils in the world were low in fertility. Approximately 3.5 billion ha of these infertile soils are entisols. Of this group, 80% are too sandy and too shallow for cultivation. Another 2.9 billion ha are ultisols and oxisols, located mostly in the humid tropics of Africa, South America and Southeast Asia, and are very acidic and low in nutrients. They are highly weathered soils, but their clay mineralogy, composed of 1:1 lattice type of clays (kaolinitic clay) and sesquioxides, permits them to be cultivated even under very humid conditions or under the heavy monsoon rains of the tropics (Arnold and Jones, 1987). Soils with high fertility, such as the mollisols in the United States and Russia, are estimated to be 1.2 billion ha in extent, but 90% of these soils are already under cultivation.

7.1.1 Nutrient Cycling

Nutrient cycling, a natural process that preserves and maintains soil fertility, is examined here in the context of clearing new lands for crop production in the tropical rain forest. The term *nutrient cycling* is used instead of *element cycling* or *mineral cycling*. Element cycling refers to the cycling of elements regardless of their importance as plant food. Mineral cycling is an incorrect term, since minerals are inorganic compounds, such as kaolinite and feldspars, which are not recycled by nature.

In a tropical rain forest, the vegetative cover produces high amounts of organic matter that are very rich in plant nutrients (Follet et al., 1987; Stewart et al., 1987). The organic matter in the form of leaf fall under the canopy of a tropical rain forest in Nigeria is estimated to be annually 7 Mg (tons)/ha. The rate of leaf fall in Nigeria is largest during the dry season in December and January (Ghuman and Lal, 1987). In the nutrient cycling process, this organic residue decomposes, releasing nutrients into the surface soil where they are taken up again by growing plants, in other words recycled (Stevenson, 1986). This recycling process entails the maintenance of a thick forest cover, which preserves the fertility of the surface soil, the soil's A horizon.

A number of factors affect nutrient cycling, e.g., climatic and biotic factors (Jordan, 1985). Important climatic and biotic factors are temperature, soil moisture, and rate of decomposition. Differences in these factors produce differences in nutrient cycling in tropical and temperate region forest. The year-round high temperature in the humid tropics insures a year-round growing season, resulting in high annual nutrient uptake by plants, and high annual return of nutrients to the forest floor. In the temperate region, seasonality in both temperature and precipitation is the reason why production of biomass and decomposition are not as high as in the humid tropics. Decomposition is very rapid in the tropics, and leaf litter is mineralized within approximately 8 months on the average, and little is converted to soil humus (Lavelle, 1987). Humus is usually formed by a decomposition process, called *humification*. The humus accumulated is very beneficial and is composed of a mixture of complex organic compounds, e.g., humic and fulvic acids. As colloids, humus exhibits similar properties as soil clays. Chemically, humus increases the cation exchange and waterholding capacity of soils, and also provides for a large buffer capacity which offsets pH changes. Physically, humus enhances formation of a stable soil structure, which helps to improve poor drainage and control erosion. As indicated above, mineralization dominates over decomposition in the humid tropics resulting in low humus content of the soils.

7.1.2 Plantation Agriculture and Agroforestry

In Africa and South America the increase in crop production

Table 7.1 Plant Nutrient Content in Soil and Vegetation in Tropical Forests (in % of Total Stock)

Region	N	P	K	Ca	Mg
Ivory Coast (Banco)	82.2	50.0	13.3	08.3	15.1
Ghana (Kade)	69.2	08.6	41.6	49.1	49.6
Venezuela (San Carlos de Rio Negro)	62.6	59.3	18.1	38.9	20.2
Panama	00.0	11.6	10.1	84.3	84.3
Puerto Rico	00.0	83.6	08.9	47.1	69.3
Zaire (Yangambi)	89.5	98.0	66.3	33.8	42.0

Sources: Odum and Pigeon (1970); Golley et al.(1975); Herrrera (1979); Bernhard-Reversat et al.(1979); Lavelle (1984).

comes by clearing the tropical rain forests. The soils are usually highly leached and low in plant nutrients. Nevertheless, natural rain forest ecosystems on tropical soils have a large standing biomass. Large amounts of the nutrients are contained in the

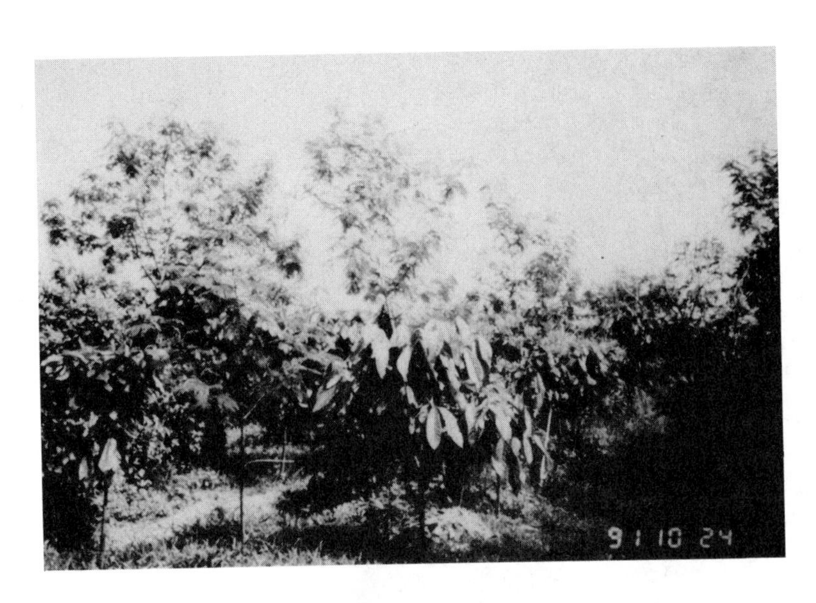

Figure 7.1 Cacao (*Theobroma cacao*) grown in plantation agriculture with *Leucaena glauca* and *Glyricidae* sp. as shade trees (Courtesy: Didiek H. Goenadi, Biotecnnology Research Institute for Estate Crops, Bogor, Indonesia.)

plant biomass (Table 7.1), which will be released upon decomposition of the litter.

A variety of problems develop after deforestation. After deforestation, the surface soil, in which most of the nutrients are recycled, can support crop production for a year or two. Soon, the cultivated crops and leaching processes exhaust the soil's nutrient supply. Crop yields decrease and the land is abandoned, leaving bare soils exposed to the impact of tropical rains, and severe erosion becomes a problem. When the surface soil has been stripped off by accelerated erosion, the exposed subsoil, often rich in iron, hardens and forms an iron pan. This pan formation inhibits further vegetative growth.

The disastrous effect of deforestation as discussed above can

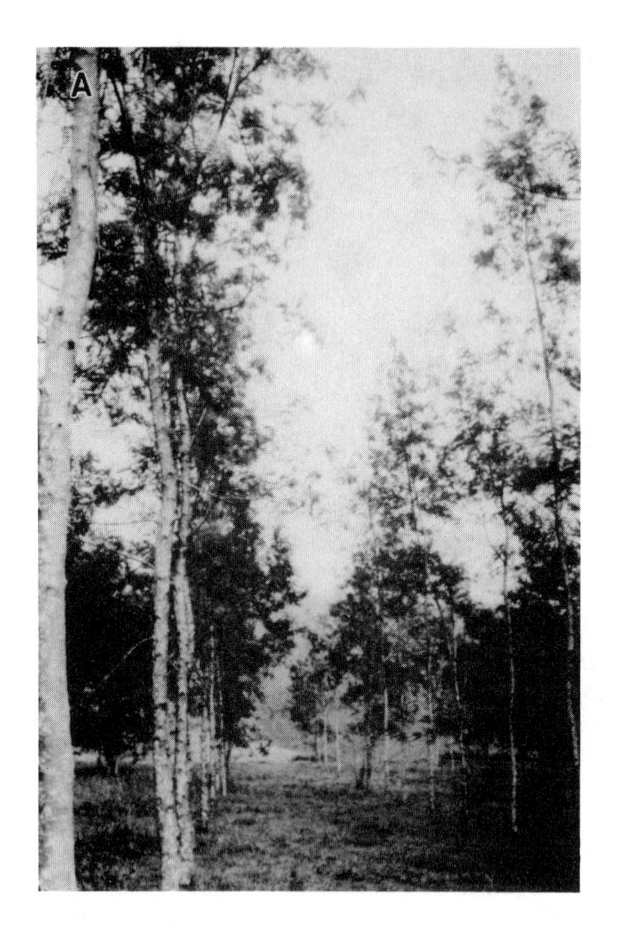

Figure 7.2 (A) Agroforestry of *Leucaena* sp., (B) Closeup of *Leucaena glauca* tree. (Courtesy: Didiek A. Goenadi, Biotechnology Research Institute for Estate Crops, Bogor, Indonesia.)

be avoided, and sustainable economic yields are possible in tropical agriculture by the application of a nutrient cycling system. Such a system has been known in the tropics for decades under the name of *plantation agriculture*, and recently

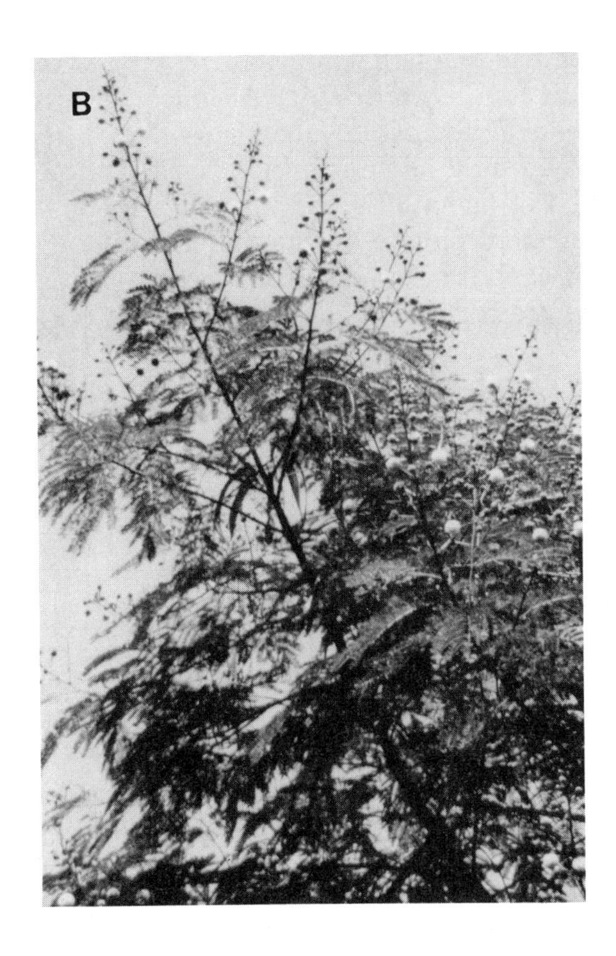

a variation of this is introduced, called *agroforestry*. In *plantation agriculture*, the crops are composed of trees or shrubs (Figure 7.1), and only the fruits or young shoots, such as coffee, cacao, and tea, are harvested. These crops are grown together with nitrogen-fixing legume trees that provide the crop with necessary shade, N_2, and other nutrients. A widely grown legume tree is *Leucaena leucocephala*; another is *Leucaena glauca* (Figure 7.2). When used as mulch, the leaves of these legume trees may add 150 kg/ha of N per year. The roots of these shade trees penetrate deep into the subsoil, and take up nutrients beyond reach of the roots of the coffee, cacao or tea plants. These nutrients are recycled to the surface soil by way of litter- and leaf-fall.

Agroforestry, as defined today, is a system of crop production by growing trees, in association with crops and pastures. The trees are grown in rows, providing the forest system, separated by strips of soils cultivated with food crops. Such a system originates from the indigenous, frequently considered primitive, system called *shifting cultivation*. It was developed by the native people in the tropics to restore soil fertility by nutrient cycling. After the soil has been cultivated for two or three years, it is then abandoned for 5-10 years, allowing hereby the regrowth of the forest and sufficient accumulations of organic matter for recycling purposes. The topsoil is rejuvenated by a combination of effects due to nutrient recycling, accumulation, and conservation. However, large acreages of land are required to produce enough food with shifting cultivation. To minimize the damage to the environment, perhaps 10 to 20 hectares of land per person are required, which is a far bigger acreage than a farmer in the temperate region uses to cultivate.

7.1.3 Environmental Changes

Because of population pressure and poor economic conditions, especially in Africa, South America, and Southeast Asia, large areas containing poor soils have been deforested for food and timber production. Forests have been cut at an alarming rate and frequently insufficient time has been allowed after cultivation to return the cleared areas into forest. This appears to be more harmful to the environment than the benefits it brings of more food for the population. The environmental impact is expected to reach drastic proportions within the foreseeable future. However, such a view is not shared by many scientists in Brazil (Fearnside, 1987). Surveys conducted on deforestation of the Brazilian Amazon using *LANDSAT* satellite images indicated that only 1.55% of the area legally defined as Amazonia had been deforested in 1978. Although, on a regional scale the cleared area has increased from 0.5% to 3.12%, these increases are believed to be not widespread. Most of the increases in deforestation are related to cultivation efforts by large landholders, and transmigration because of improved road access.

Environmental considerations necessitate careful deliberations before clearing rain forest areas, and a suitable balance must be found between the necessity of clearing the tropical rain forest for crop production and the rate or degree of destruction in environmental quality that it brings. The destruction of the tropical rain forest causes permanent changes in the environment. Concern has been expressed in many countries of the world that the extensive slash-and-burn method produces large amounts of CO_2 and other pollutant gasses, contributing to the so-called greenhouse effect. The resulting global warming can bring drastic changes in the earth climate, while cleared areas can turn into desert lands, as has frequently happened in Africa. Deforestation in the Amazon rain forest of Brazil results in a decrease in evapotranspiration, and hence in total cloud formation and cover. Therefore, rainfall also decreases by 0.5-0.7 mm/day, but nevertheless no regional temperature changes have been reported (Henderson-Sellers, 1987). Emission of CO_2 by industry and vehicular transportation, and other factors, related to the distance of the earth from the sun, are perhaps bigger contributors to the greenhouse effect. If global warming is to occur by 0.3° per decade, as predicted, the sea level will rise to such a level so that extensive areas of coastal plains in the world, such as in Bangladesh, will disappear. In upland soils the increase in temperatures may increase the rate of rock and mineral weathering, and organic matter decomposition, accelerating soil degradation.

The increase in CO_2 production by both agricultural and industrial operations may have a pronounced effect on photosynthesis. An increase in CO_2 content in soil air will not only accelerate soil forming processes, as discussed above, but a doubling of the CO_2 content in atmospheric air is believed to increase the yield of C_3 plants, such as soybean, potato, oats, barley, wheat, and rice by 10% to 50% (Wild, 1993). C_4 plants, e.g., corn, sugar cane, and sorghum, appear to be less affected by an increase in CO_2 content in our air. C_3 plants fix CO_2 by the so called *Calvin cycle*, whereas C_4 plants use another process for CO_2 fixation, sometimes also called the *Hatch-Slack cycle*. This cycle was discovered by Hatch and Slack in sugar cane, and enables the plants to store more CO_2 in the chloroplast. It is the reason why C_4 plants do not respond as well as C_3 plants to an increase in CO_2 content. The growth rate of C_4 plants is consequently larger than that of C_3 plants.

The trees and other plants in the rain forest are also the major suppliers of oxygen in the air we breathe. They also purify the air by absorbing excess carbon dioxide produced by our modern industry, and prevent it from accumulating in our atmosphere. With the help of sunlight, green plants produce carbohydrate from carbon dioxide and water. During this process, known as photosynthesis, oxygen is formed and released. When the forest disappears, these processes — so essential to our environment and health — cease.

The destruction of the tropical rain forest also destroys a variety of plants and animals. Such ecosystems are characterized by a highly diverse and interdependent population of plants and animals. The interaction between these plants and animals are so close that the extinction of one species may have direct and indirect effects on other species. For example, the Brazil nut (*B. exelsa*) is pollinated by bees. Any changes that destroy one of these organisms may harmfully affect the other (Mori and Prance, 1987). If the pollinators were to vanish, these nut trees will also disappear. If the trees are destroyed, then the pollinators will become extinct. The seeds have also to be dispersed and birds play an important role in this respect. Even if cleared areas have been allowed to return to forest, original habitats for plant and animal life have been destroyed. Every day and every moment wild animals are vanishing. Plants that are commonplace and animals that are pleasing to the eye are disappearing forever. It will be a global tragedy if most of the animals vanish, except for domestic cats and dogs, and our earth becomes inhabited only by human beings. When the forest disappears, we also lose valuable sources of chemicals, medicine, and fiber. Many of the plants are known to have economic value due to their medicinal properties, and these will be lost forever with the disappearance of the rain forest.

7.2 INTENSIFYING SOIL PRODUCTIVITY

In Europe where population pressures have always been strong, most of the good soils are already being used for food production, and little land remains for agricultural expansion. Approximately 80% of the arable land in Europe is already used for crop production, whereas in North America 60% of all arable land is cultivated (World Resources, 1987; FAO, 1987; President's Advisory Panel on World Food Supply, 1967). In Asia and Russia, 73% and 65%, respectively, of the arable land are in use currently. These figures may be higher today. Therefore, these countries have little opportunity for increasing food production by opening new lands. At the same time, they are already growing as many crops as possible during the year. Thus the third option, increasing cropping intensity, is also infeasible. The only viable option for these countries is to intensify crop production on soils under cultivation. Complicating the situation is the fact that large areas of arable land are constantly being taken out of agricultural use for housing and urban development. In addition, younger generations are leaving the farms for the cities, and more food must be produced by fewer farmers on less land than ever before. Only through the combined efforts of scientists, professionals, and others loyal to agriculture can intensification of crop production be achieved.

7.2.1 Green Revolution

Ironically, the push for intensification of food production in the world was set off by the *green revolution* (Uribe, 1975) in Central America and Southeast Asia. The green revolution, a revolution in agricultural production, was initiated by a team of scientists from the Rockefeller Foundation. Under the leadership of George Harrar, these scientists were sent to Mexico in 1943 to improve and increase corn production. At the onset, it was an attempt to transfer U.S. techniques in crop production to the farmers in Mexico. However, today the green revolution has developed into a global effort in improving food and fiber production.

The innovations that George Harrar's team introduced — genetic improvement of local corn, proper soil management, use of fertilizers and weed, pest and disease control — enabled Mexico to become self-sufficient in this important staple food. The success of the Mexican project led to expansion of the program toward improving wheat production in the Punjab, India, and Mexico (Reitz, 1968). Results of this team effort enabled farmers in India and Mexico to double their wheat production and boost their total tonnage in food production. Norman Borlaug, who played an important role in the wheat improvement program, was later awarded the Nobel Prize in agriculture and food production. The effort in improving world food production was continued in 1961 by the establishment of the International Rice Research Institute (IRRI) at Los Banos, the Philippines, under the combined sponsorship of the Rockefeller and Ford Foundations (Uribe, 1975).

Rice is the major staple food grain in Asia, and attempts to increase local rice yields in Southeast Asia were at first disappointing. The use of fertilizers and proper control of weeds, pests, and diseases caused the local varieties to grow excessively tall, hence caused the plants to lodge or fall over easily. At the IRRI, crossings were made between a tall tropical "indica" variety from Indonesia and the "ponlai" variety from Taiwan. The "ponlai" rice variety was a small "japonica" variety developed for tropical and subtropical conditions. The result of the crossing was a dwarf, stiff-straw, high-yield variety of rice, introduced for the first time under the name *IR8-288-3*, or better known as *IR-8* (Chandler, 1968). This new variety had a grain-straw ratio of 1.2, instead of 0.6 as in the local varieties of rice. It had, therefore, more grain than straw and it matured early and was photoperiod insensitive. Not only could the rice yield be doubled by planting IR-8, but the farmers could also have three crops a year.

Although there is no doubt that food production has been increased considerably, several scientists remain skeptical about the green revolution. Among their major concerns are the social and economic factors indicating that too high a price is paid for the increase in crop yields (Moore and Moore, 1976). The new crops need more fertilizers and pesticides, affordable only to rich farmers and big landowners. More energy-intensive cultivation methods must be applied, which require mechanization. The latter may result in unemployment and increased migration of rural folks to the cities. Another question raised about the green revolution is the decrease in variability in the gene pool. Breeding of high yielding varieties has resulted in genetic uniformity, and cultivation of these new plants as monocultures increases the chances of the development of pests and diseases. The control of these pests and diseases will then be very difficult since breeding new resistant plants would be impossible due to the loss of genes. The latter will be discussed in the next section in relation with the southern corn blight disease in the USA.

Although urban migration has occurred in Southeast Asia, the reason for such a migration can be traced to a multitude of factors, and it is somewhat incorrect to blame it solely on the green revolution. The vulnerability of the high yielding crops to pests and diseases is perhaps also true, but this is a general problem with plant breeding and not necessarily the effect of the green revolution. The rice tungro disease reported during 1970–1971 (Moore and Moore, 1976) did not affect the millions of hectares of rice, but was limited to a few thousand hectares only, and was controlled rather quickly.

It is apparent that the positive effects of the green revolution outweigh their negative effects. The effort started by the IRRI has spread to neighboring countries, especially Indonesia, where a long-standing project from the time of Dutch colonialism, to improve rice yields, is revitalized. Due to the introduction of its own high yielding varieties, Indonesia is currently reported to be not only self-sufficient in rice production, but has become an important rice-exporting country.

7.2.2 Hybrid Corn

In the USA, intensification of crop production preceded the green revolution. It started perhaps in the period of 1812—1877 with the discovery of open-pollinated corn, which became known later as *hybrid corn* (Harpstead, 1975). The practical seed production of hybrid corn and the use of the *double cross* led to the development of the *corn belt* in the Midwest. Today increasing the yield of corn to 10 000—20 000 kg/ha (equivalent to 200 to 300 bushels/acre) by the use of high yielding hybrid corn and proper management of the soil is not an impossible task (Aldrich et al., 1975).

As is the case with intensification of rice production, the efforts in breeding new high yielding corn varieties and their cultivation in monocultures create some concern about the vulnerability of the crops to pests and diseases. As indicated earlier, many scientists were alarmed about a possible loss of beneficial genes that can be used to develop new resistant plants. However, the sudden explosion of the southern corn blight in the USA, destroying in 1970 almost one-fifth of the U.S. crops, has not supported the negative concerns. The corn blight disaster was controlled rather quickly within the year by producing new varieties with plant breeding.

Such intensive production methods, producing high yields, require a large investment of capital. Heavier application of fertilizers than usual, and larger amounts of chemicals for controlling weeds, insects and diseases must be used. This need for such capital expenditures is a major obstacle in Africa, South America and Southeast Asia, where economic conditions present major problems. Some observers also feel that the modern agriculture of the northern hemisphere is too energy–intensive, and that methods requiring less energy input per unit area are preferable, especially in the third world countries. Less intensive methods are less expensive, but more land is then required for farming to increase food production. The consequence of cultivating more land at lower yield levels is that less desirable soils will be used for agriculture. Not only will this result in lower output per unit energy input, but also the danger of destroying the environment will increase.

7.2.3 Use of Fertilizers

Fertilizers are defined as any material applied to soils to increase yield to improve quality and nutritive value of crops. The bulk of fertilizers are artificially produced by chemical companies and the oil industry. These fertilizers contain one or more of the elements essential for plant growth. The elements are carried in forms available to plants. Among the many nutrients required by plants, three elements, N, P, and K, are the major components of inorganic fertilizers. Based on these three major *fertilizer elements*, the artificial fertilizers can be distinguished into (1) nitrogen fertilizers, (2) phosphate fertilizers, and (3) potash (potassium) fertilizers. The three groups of fertilizers are considered single element fertilizers, in contrast to a fourth group called mixed fertilizers. The mixed fertilizers contain two or all three of the major fertilizer elements, and may also have other plant nutrients, such as the micronutrients.

The N, P, or K content, or quality of the fertilizers, is indicated by the *fertilizer grade*. This fertilizer grade is usually expressed in % total N, % available P_2O_5, or % soluble K_2O. The grade of mixed fertilizers is composed of three figures, e.g. 10-10-10, 4-12-12, etc. A 4-12-12 fertilizer mixture contains 4% total N, 12% available P_2O_5, and 12% soluble K_2O. Currently, there is a trend toward expressing fertilizer grades in the elemental percentage for scientific purposes, and in the oxide percentage for fertilizer sales. Some of the common artificial fertilizers and their grades are listed in Table 7.2. The equivalent acidity listed in the table is the amount of lime required to bring the soil pH back to pre-fertilizer application levels. For example, the use of 1 Mg (1000 kg)/ha of ammonium nitrate will decrease the soil pH enough so that 599 kg/ha of limestone is needed to restore the original soil pH. Therefore, the equivalent (or potential) acidity of 1000 kg ammonium nitrate equals 599. Fertilizers that decrease soil pH are called *acid forming fertilizers*. All ammonium fertilizers are acid forming fertilizers. In contrast, nitrate fertilizers, such as $NaNO_3$, are *basic forming fertilizers*. The equivalent acidity of $NaNO_3$ is, therefore, -294.

The importance of artificial fertilizers in crop production dates back to 1842 when J.B. Lawes and J.H. Gilbert invented

Table 7.2 Major Inorganic Fertilizers in Agriculture

Fertilizer	**N*** %	**P_2O_5** %	**K_2O** %	**Equiv. acidity**
Nitrogen fertilizers				kg/ha
Ammonium nitrate, NH_4NO_3	33.5			599
Anhydrous ammonia, NH_3	82.0			1492
Sulphate of ammonia, $(NH_4)_2SO_4$	20.0			1109
Urea, $CO(NH_2)_2$	45.0			756
Phosphorus fertilizers				
Superphosphate		20.0		
Triple superphosphate		48.0		
Potassium fertilizers				
Muriate of potash, KCl			60	
Sulfate of potash, K_2SO_4			50	

*Total N, available P_2O_5, and water soluble K_2O.

the production of superphosphate at the Rothamsted Experiment Station in England (Brady, 1990; Tisdale et al., 1993). However, the growth of the fertilizer industry was propelled to its current dimension after the discovery of the production of ammonia, NH_3, by reacting N_2 gas with H_2 gas, according to the so-called *Haber-Bosch process* (Tisdale et al., 1993). Intensifying crop production requires higher yields per unit area of soil. This increases the demand placed on soils to provide sufficient amounts of nutrients, and fertilizers are applied to remove the limitation of crop production caused by an inadequate supply of plant nutrients in soils. The use of fertilizers worldwide has, therefore, increased considerably since 1950. For example, the yield of wheat has improved steadily from 800 kg/ha in 1950 to 2382 kg/ha in 1987. During the same period corn yield increased from 2272 kg/ha to 7250 kg/ha. Corn yields exceeding 300 bu/a (18142 kg/ha) are not uncommon today by the application of fertilizers in combination with the use of hybrid corn and the proper management practices (Tisdale et al., 1993). However, as the use of inorganic fertilizers increases, the potential hazard for contamination of surface and ground water increases considerably. Therefore, new techniques have to be developed to control the harmful effect on environmental quality. The use of fertilizers has been shown to increase yield and prolong the period of good yield. However, even fertilizers have been known to fail in halting yield decline over a period of years in upland rice fertilization trials in Peru (Jordan, 1985).

7.2.4 Residue- or No-Till Farming

To reduce the hazard in decreasing the quality of the environment by intensification of crop production, a new method is currently introduced to the United States.

With the development of the moldboard plow in 1837, farmers settling in the Great Plains of the United States plowed through the tough root system of prairie grasses. Exposing the black topsoil of the mollisols, rich in organic matter and plant nutrients, they planted corn and wheat. Despite several years of ravaging dust bowls when drought-stricken soil was lifted by storms and carried as far east as the eastern seaboard, America became the breadbasket of the world. During those years, more plows and more heavy machinery of mounting complexity were developed. Notwithstanding the availability of modern equipment, fertilizers and the use of high yielding crops, farmers today appear to be making little economic headway. They are financially strapped and over-burdened by overhead expenses from a task force of monstrous machines needed to plant and harvest corn, wheat, and soybeans. Additionally, farm legislation in 1955 forced them to adopt conservation methods in order to receive crop support payments. This factor, together with a strong desire to reduce the overhead in machinery and to convert from an intensive into a less labor-intensive operation, led farmers to investigate more efficient farming methods. Recently, a new method called *residue farming* by the USDA Soil Conservation Service, popularly known as *no-till farming*, seems to have set hold. This technique has been known for some time, but has not attracted too much attention because of the lack of economic and environmental urgency. However, following recent years of severe economic depression and disastrous farm surpluses, farmers permitted millions of acres of farmlands to lie fallow. This compelled the farmers to adopt better and more efficient farming methods on the lands still under cultivation. One of these methods is residue farming, which is now being applied on more than 70 million acres of U.S. crop lands. This method is spreading as a renewed burst of the green revolution from the coastal plains of the Atlantic seaboard to the rich floodplains of the Mississippi River valleys and on to the great plains in Nebraska and the highlands in Oregon, where corn, soybeans, wheat, and other crops are grown.

In residue farming, the residue or stubble from the previous year's crop is not plowed under. Instead, it is left undisturbed (in place) to hold soil and conserve soil moisture. The plows and machines are retired, and the seeds for the new crop are chiseled in between the stubbles. The seedlings are allowed to sprout through the decomposing vegetative residue, hence, the name residue or no-till farming (Figure 7.3). It is sometimes also referred to as *mulch-till farming*. Weeds are controlled by newly developed biodegradable herbicides. Insects are also controlled with biodegradable insecticides or by adoption of crop rotations to break the insect life cycles. Unconfirmed reports

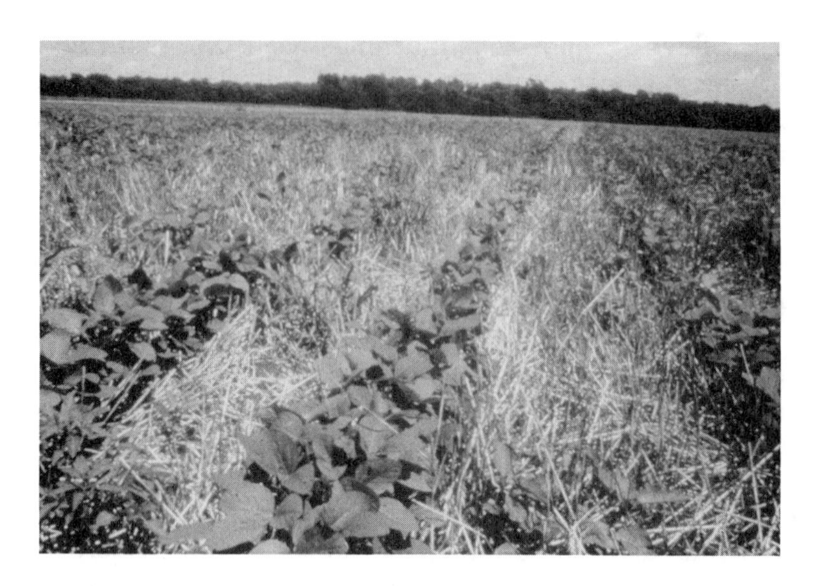

Figure 7.3 Residue farming of soybean (*Glycine max*). (Courtesy: D.L. Armstrong, editor, Potash & Phosphate Institute, Atlanta, GA.)

indicate that the application of residue farming has enabled farmers to decrease their labor input considerably, allowing them to cut expenses of producing crops by 30% to 40%.

7.3 ORGANIC FARMING

This system of farming does not fall in the category of intensifying crop production, but is somewhat related to residue farming. Organic farming is also a system of low external input of crop production, but without using artificially produced agricultural chemicals. It has as a main objective the production of food void of chemical contaminants and relatively safe for human consumption. The use of commercial fertilizers, insecticides, and pesticides is avoided. Artificial fertilizers are replaced by organic manures and compost, whereas soil organic matter and nitrogen content are maintained by growing leguminous green manures. Pests and diseases are controlled by the proper selection of resistant crops, and use of the appropriate agronomic practices, such as crop rotations and *buffer plants*. The latter may kill or expel insects from the main crops. Mixed reports are available on the yield and quality of the crop produced by organic farming. A report from the Council for Agricultural Science and Technology (CAST, 1980) shows a wide range in crop yields as a result of organic farming, from 56% to 107% of the yield of *conventional farming*. The crops, especially fruits and vegetables, are frequently deformed, and display some blemishes or imperfections due to slight pathogenic infection. They are otherwise free of chemical contaminants, and are usually more expensive. Their market value depends on the willingness of the customer to accept a less perfect shape of fruit or vegetable at a higher price.

CHAPTER 8

SOILLESS AGRICULTURE

8.1 HYDROPONICS

Hydroponics, from the Latin words *hydro* (water) and *ponos* (labor), is by definition "growing plants in water." It is also referred to as soilless culture of plants (Jones, 1983), *water culture,* or *nutriculture* (Hoagland and Arnon, 1950). Water culture or hydroponics is a method of growing plants with their roots in a solution containing a balanced proportion of nutrient elements essential for plant growth. In the past, the names *tray agriculture* and *tank farming* were also used for this method. Today water culture has been revised and expanded to include a variety of growth media. These methods now include all methods of growing plants in an artificial medium supplied with nutrient solutions. Although it is frequently assumed that hydroponics is a soilless culture, some of the growth media today often include *artificial soil*, which is made up of a mixture of sand, or vermiculite, and organic compounds such as peat and the like, especially in the aggregate and adsorbed nutrient techniques. All these materials are soil constituents. This method allows intensification of agricultural production without using natural soils or destroying valuable areas of rain forest.

Related to hydroponics is *aeroponics*, which involves growing plants in the air (*aero* = air; Figure 8.1). In hydroponics, plants

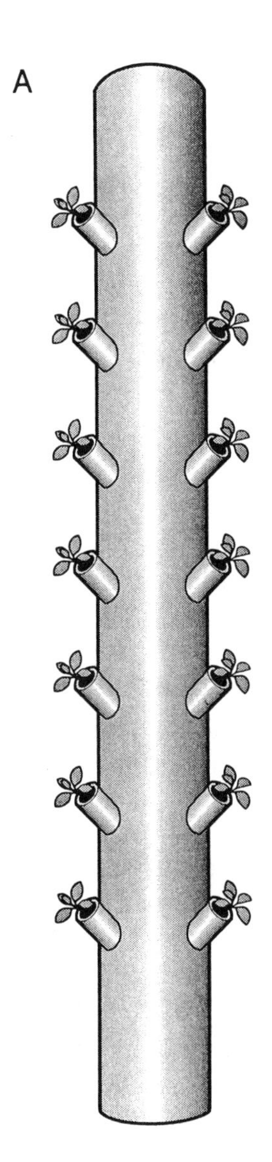

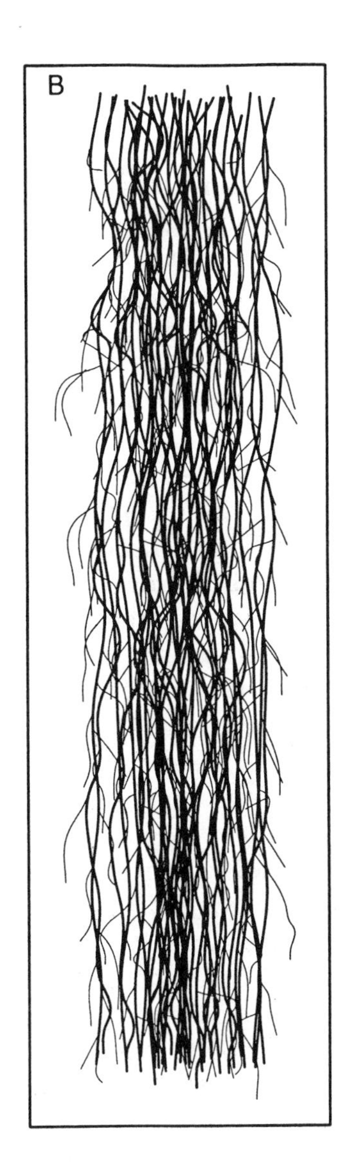

Figure 8.1 (A) Aeroponics, or the culture of plants in the air. The plants are allowed to grow in hollow plastic tubes. (B) Roots of plants, grown in aeroponic cultures, hanging vertically in the tubes. They are sprayed periodically with nutrient solutions. Excess nutrient solutions flow or fall down in the tube and are collected and recycled. Aeroponics are suitable only for growing certain plants, e.g., lettuce. (Drawings by W. G. Reeves, Art Coordinator, University of Georgia.)

are grown in water to which nutrient mixtures have been added. On the other hand, in aeroponics plants are grown in the air, and dilute nutrient solutions are sprayed onto the hanging roots. The idea with aeroponics is to reduce the amount of water and nutrients used in growing plants to the bare minimum for maximum yields. No scientific data are available yet to support this contention. Data on water consumption of tomatoes grown side by side in water and soil culture indicate some differences. The amount of water used to produce 45 kg (100 lbs) of tomatoes was 971 L (257 gallons) in water cultures as opposed to 839 L (222 gallons) in soil (Hoagland and Arnon, 1950). The water requirement of growing plants, as expressed in terms of *transpiration ratio*, is in fact the same for one species of plant, whether it is grown in soil or in water. The transpiration ratio is by definition the units of water needed to produce a unit of dry matter. The transpiration ratio varies from plant species to plant species. It is low for sorghum (126 kg = 277 lbs), but high for alfalfa plants (387 kg = 853 lbs). Rice plants are characterized by a transpiration ratio of 310 kg (682 lbs), which is less than the water requirement of alfalfa. The transpiration ratio is on the average 227 kg (500 lbs) of water for 0.454 kg (1 lb) of dry unit produced.

A number of nutrient solutions have been developed for hydroponic and aeroponic cultures, such as the *Hoagland, Sach's, Knop's, Pfeffer's*, and *Crone's* solutions (Jones, Jr., 1983; Douglas, 1976; Hewitt, 1966; Hoagland and Arnon, 1950). One of the nutrient solutions frequently used is the so-called *Hoagland* solution with a composition as listed in Table 8.1. However, the other types of nutrient solution are equally as effective for water cultures as the Hoagland solution. As correctly indicated by Hoagland and Arnon (1950) there is no one composition superior over an other. Plants will adapt remarkably to different chemical environments, otherwise they would not be growing in all kinds of soils in nature. In the opinion of the authors above, water culture is not superior to

Table 8.1 Composition of a Hoagland and Arnon Nutrient Solution

Compound	Concentration
	moles/L
$NH_4H_2PO_4$	0.001
KNO_3	0.006
$Ca(NO_3)_2$	0.004
$MgSO_4$	0.002
	mg element/L
H_3BO_3	0.5
$MnCl_2.4H_2O$	0.5
$ZnSO_4.4H_2O$	0.05
$CuSO_4.5H_2O$	0.02
$H_2MoO_4.H_2O$	0.05
Fe tartrate	1.37

growing plants in natural soil. The yields are not strikingly different, and growing plants in water cultures does not guarantee the production of food safer for human consumption than that grown in the traditional manner in soil. Regardless of the method used for food production, rigid sanitation measures must be observed to prevent contamination of the products by insecticide and/or other chemical residues and pathogenic infections. Another issue in water culture is plant spacings for maximum yields. Plants can perhaps be more closely spaced together in water cultures than in soil. However, the rules in plant physiology indicate that the density of stand giving the highest yield is determined by the amount of light received by plants, when all other growth factors are optimum.

Although this technique of growing plants in water has been known for centuries, hydroponics has only recently gained its present popularity for growing vegetables and other plants.

Early in the 17th century, Jan Baptista Van Helmont indicated, as a result of his now famous willow tree experiments, that water was the most important nutrient for growing plants (Brady, 1990). The importance of water was contended later by John Woodward, who experimented with growing spearmints in river water, rain water, and muddy water. He argued that the mud, not water, was the substance necessary for increased plant growth. Although others indicated that organic matter or *humus* was consumed by plants instead of mud, the concept of mud as a plant food was supported by Jethro Tull's discovery in the 18th century. Tull noticed that increased plant growth was obtained by tilling the soil, and believed that fine soil particles, produced by cultivation, were taken up by the growing plants. In the beginning of the 19th century, De Saussurre discovered the process known today as *photosynthesis*. This process, that plants absorbed CO_2 from the air and at the same time released O_2 with the help of sunlight, was not well understood at that time. However, this new approach brought a change in the concept in plant nutrition. It was finally realized that plants obtain nutrients from both the air and water.

Hydroponics, used in combination with biotechnology, allows for immense possibilities in intensification of crop production. However, the method is considered more difficult to apply for commercial crop production than the conventional method using soil. Not only does the commercial grower require a thorough knowledge in plant nutrition, but the grower must perfectly design and manage a routine procedure of growing, which involves the diagnosis and testing of plants, rooting media, and nutrient solution. However, hydroponics is perhaps the best alternative for crop production in the desert regions of the world It may one day become the method for growing food and fiber on the moon (Ming and Henninger, 1989). Jones (1983) also indicated that in cases of space and soil limitations, such as in many urban areas, the individual can apply hydroponics to grow food for his family.

A less widely known application of hydroponics is the cultivation of algae, which can be carried out indoors or outdoors in ponds (Figure 8.2). Algae are lower plants that

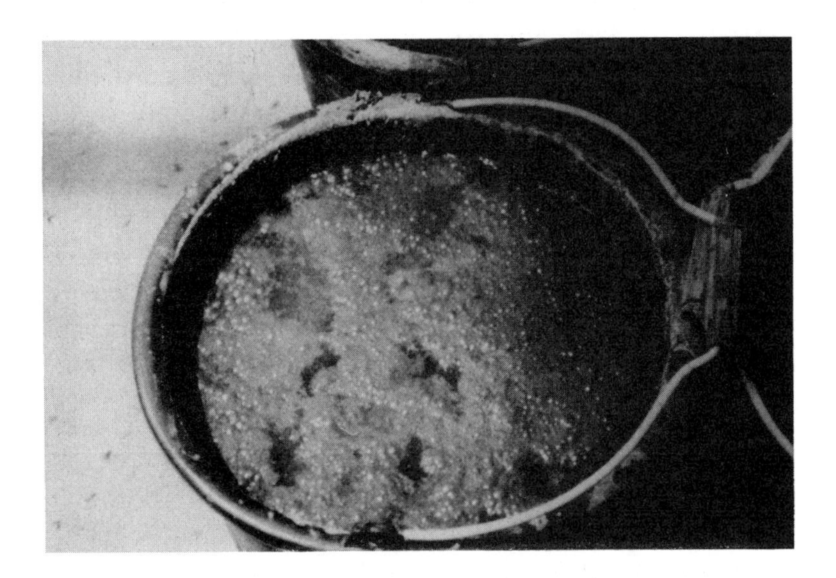

Figure 8.2 Indoor cultivation of algae. (Courtesy: Didiek H. Goenadi, Biotechnology Research Institute for Estate Crops, Bogor, Indonesia.)

contain chlorophyll, enabling them to produce carbohydrates by photosynthesis. Blue-green algae are also known to be capable of fixing nitrogen from the air. Algae are also important as a protein source. Their capacity for protein production far exceeds that of the peanut, pea, or legume plants, and their protein content is believed to be greater than that of beef. Some types of algae are high in vitamin B12, whereas others may contain ß-carotene.

Algae grow best in the tropics and subtropics, areas characterized by high temperatures and abundant sunlight. Today, large scale production of algae in outdoor-ponds is found in California and Israel. In northern Israel, liquid municipal sewage is treated with algae to produce water suitable for irrigation. The algae is periodically harvested and pelletized for use as chicken and fish feed. It was estimated that algae production uses only 2% of the land area required in conventional agriculture to produce an equal amount of organic matter.

In several other countries, algae is an important food source for humans. It is a major component of the diet in Japan, where a variety of seaweed is used for human consumption. In addition, algae is a source for the manufacture of agar and gelatin, ingredients for making desserts and cakes in the United States.

8.2 AQUACULTURE

Aquaculture is by definition the culture and husbandry of aquatic organisms. It encompasses the control and management of aquatic plants and animals in controlled or selected environments for economic or social benefits (Bell and Canterbery, 1976). In a narrow sense it is fish farming, which is considered more of an art than a science. Fish farming has been practiced since ancient times. The cultivation of fish in ponds today originates from the practice of prehistoric people living in coastal regions keeping live fish in baskets submerged in the river or sea (Tiddens, 1990). Fish farming can be traced back to the Egyptians in 2000 B.C., who grew tilapia (*Tilapin nilotica*) and to the ancient Chinese people, who were known for their carp (*Cyprinus carpo*) culture. From these ancient methods, aquaculture has developed into its present modern science in the same way as the development of agriculture. Some consider it a type of agriculture, with the main difference being that aquaculture is aquatic, whereas agriculture is terrestrial in nature. However, its progress to the present level has been much slower than that of agricultural science. In their quest for food, human beings have directed their attention to the cultivation of soils. The oceans and lakes were until recently a mysterious and impenetrable domain.

Several factors have contributed to the current heightened interest in aquaculture. Over-fishing of oceans and lakes by huge fishing vessels, using improved netting techniques that act literally as gigantic vacuum cleaners, has markedly decreased the worldwide catch of wild fish. Salmon, herring, and halibut populations are decreasing at an alarming rate. Discharge of pollutants from coastal towns, maritime shipping, and offshore oil production are compounding the problem. Not only do these contaminants threaten the safety of human consumption of fish, they also play an important role in the decline of reproduction of several species of fish, such as salmon. As one response to these concerns, the United Nations Conference in 1987 formulated the *Law of the Sea*. Many nations in the world sought to protect their fishing rights by claiming a 200-mile zone extending seaward from the coast of each nation as their exclusive property. Consequently, such a law means the end of the freedom of fishing in the high seas (Tiddens, 1990).

In the early days, aquaculture was practiced for the simple production of a cheap source of animal protein. It was conducted at first by growing fish which was hardy, easy to grow and popular as a food source, such as carp, catfish, tilapia, milkfish, and mullets (Bell and Canterbery, 1976). This has expanded in several countries, such as in Japan, into a modern operation to include growing aquatic organisms which command high prices in the market. The "inexpensive" fish is grown and processed into feed for cultivating the higher priced fish and shellfish (Kafuku and Ikenoue, 1983). Aquaculture is a highly specialized operation in Japan, and can be distinguished into *freshwater aquaculture* and *marine aquaculture.*

8.2.1 Freshwater Aquaculture

Freshwater aquaculture in Japan involves the cultivation of highly priced freshwater fish, such as chum salmon (*Oncorhynchus keta*), ayu (*Plecoglossus altivelis*), eel (*Anguilla japonica*), and several species of carp. It has been expanded recently into growing terrapin *(Tryonix sinensis)*, a soft shell turtle considered an expensive delicacy, and freshwater oyster (*Hyriopsis schlegelii*). This type of oyster is grown not for food but for the pearls, which are of high quality and have been compared to the once world-famous, now extinct, Persian Gulf natural pearl (Kafuku and Ikenoue, 1983).

8.2.2 Marine Aquaculture

In Japan, marine aquaculture includes growing valuable sea items, such as green turtle (*Chelonia mydas*), nori (*Porphyra yezoensis*), and wakame (*Undaria pinnatifida*). Kuruma prawn (*Penaeus japonicus*), scallop (*Patinopecten yessoenensis*), oyster (*Crassostrea gigas*), and abalone (*Haliotis(Nordotis) discus*) are also favored sea crops because of the high prices they bring in the marketplace. Nori and wakame are seaweed or algae, and are important foodstuffs in Japan. Wakame is used as an ingredient in soybean paste (miso) soup, whereas nori sheets are employed for making sushi and rice balls. In Southeast Asia, seaweed is an important source for agar production. Japan has intensified its cultivation of pearl oyster (*Pinctada fucata*) in the sea since 1919, when cultured pearls became acclaimed in the London pearl market (Kafuku and Ikenoue, 1983). A high-tech center for the cultured pearl is located at Mikomoto Pearl Island, where oysters are surgically implanted with a small pellet of ground oyster shell that serves as seed for the growth of pearl. The implanted oysters are returned to the bay to grow. Mikomoto pearls are famous for their beauty, and Mikimoto and similar companies have given Japan a monopoly in today's world pearl market.

8.2.3 Aquaculture in the United States

Aquaculture has not flourished in the United States as it has in Japan. In contrast to Japanese people, Americans prefer to consume beef and chicken rather than fish. At present, fishery science in the United States has been largely limited to managing and improving the population of wild fish. Fish hatcheries have been established to produce young fish, such as trout, for restocking streams and lakes. Perhaps the closest concept in the United States to modern aquaculture is an operation called *salmon ranching*. It is usually conducted by large corporations, such as the Weyerhauser Timber Company and British Petroleum Anadromous, Inc. (Tiddens, 1990). Salmon are born in freshwater, but spend most of their adult life in the oceans, hence the salmon is an *anadromous fish*. They may return to their original breeding grounds to spawn and die. In the salmon ranching operation, salmon eggs are hatched artificially, and the young fish are released in the rivers. It is hoped that this process of releasing young fish, called *imprinting,* to the surroundings will encourage the adult fish to return in the future to be harvested.

Another development toward modern aquaculture in the United States is the cultivation of freshwater fish in ponds. This practice started in 1927 when scientists from the Agricultural Experiment Station, University of Alabama, under the leadership of H.S. Swingle, raised blue gills, bass, and other fresh water fish in ponds (Shell, 1975). At first, the fish were grown for sport fishing, but the experiment was later expanded for food production. Swingle and his group demonstrated that fertilizing ponds with N, P, and K increased the growth of algae and other aquatic organisms, which are major food sources for many types of fish. An optimum NPK:fish ratio was developed for optimum fish production. Later, Swingle added channel catfish to his experiments, and his report in 1959 became the basis for much of the U.S. channel catfish industry today. Finally worth mentioning is the intensive shrimp farming in ponds conducted by the Marine Culture Enterprises in Hawaii. Shrimp is also grown artificially in Panama by the Purina Company, as a joint venture between Panamanians and Americans.

CHAPTER 9

BIOTECHNOLOGY IN SOIL SCIENCE AND AGRICULTURE

The advancements in *biotechnology* have created new frontiers, and new vistas of opportunity for increasing and improving food and fiber production. Biotechnology involves the application of organisms or their subcellular components to create new substances or organisms (Persley, 1990; Smith and Lewis, 1991). It can be distinguished into *food biotechnology* and *agricultural biotechnology*. In the author's opinion, there is also room for the division of *Soil Biotechnology*, a science which has yet to be developed. The manufacture of soil organic compounds, e.g., humic acids, and the application of soil-borne organisms in the control of pests and diseases fall in this category. Often soil biotechnology is closely related to agricultural biotechnology, blurring the distinction between the two sciences.

9.1 FOOD BIOTECHNOLOGY

Food biotechnology involves techniques for the production and processing of food. Modern food biotechnology finds its origin in the fermentation of food and beverages, techniques practiced since ancient times. Beer was produced by Sumerians and Babylonians as far back as of 6000 BC, whereas bread making was already known by Egyptians in 4000 BC. Cheese production was also known in ancient times. Although these ancient people can be considered pioneers in biotechnology, it is Louis Pasteur (1857—1876) who is commonly regarded as the founder of modern biotechnology.

Today the techniques in biotechnology are applied to improve the fermentation of beverages and the production of a variety of food products from cereal and soybean, such as bread, soysauce, tofu, and tempeh. Soysauce and tofu were introduced in Europe and the USA from China via Japan. Because of their high protein, low fat, and low cholesterol content, they are important additions to vegetarian diets. In Japan, sophisticated biotechnological operations are used to make these products. Less well known in the United States is *tempeh*, which was developed centuries ago in Indonesia. Tempeh is produced by fermentation of soaked soybean with a fungus, *Rhizopus oligosporus* (Smith and Lewis, 1991). The Netherlands, which has close historical ties with Indonesia, is an active center for tempeh production, using advanced biotechnological methods. In the USA, tempeh enjoys increasing popularity as a healthy vegetarian food with meat-like texture.

9.2 AGRICULTURAL BIOTECHNOLOGY

Agricultural biotechnology is the science of creating new strains of plants and animals, and improving agricultural products and chemicals by *genetic engineering*. The discovery and advent of new recombinant DNA technology opens new possibilities for the development of superior crops and animals. The green revolution, started by George Harrar and his team, is hereby propelled into new areas and dimensions. Breeding programs can be accelerated with greater speed than usual. The application of genetic engineering to plants can confer novel properties in the recipient crops. Crop improvements which were previously not possible in a traditional way are now made possible by the application of recombinant DNA techniques. The shelf life of food and vegetables has been lengthened considerably by the use of biotechnological methods, and several plants have been made more resistant to pest and diseases.

As has been known for years, plants can produce chemical compounds of importance for pesticides as well as for pharmaceutical purposes. *Pyrethrum* is one example of an insecticide produced by chrysanthemums. The production of such a chemical compound is the plant's natural defense mechanism to combat the attack by insects and microorganisms. Another example is the oily aromatic substance in citrus skin which has a toxic effect on many insects. Other plants can produce a proteinase inhibitor to attack an invading pathogen. Such a chemical is *trypsin* inhibitor, which is carried by cowpea seed (Smith and Lewis, 1991). When trypsin inhibitor is introduced into tobacco plants, it appears to increase the resistance of tobacco plants to infestation by the tobacco budworm, *Heliothis virescens*. Such bioinsecticides and other engineered microorganisms are being developed currently with promising results for the biological control of pests and diseases.

9.3 TISSUE CULTURE

Another important aspect of agricultural biotechnology is *plant tissue culture* (Lebaron, 1987). Although it has not received as much publicity as genetic engineering, tissue culture has, nonetheless, enjoyed practical applications in agriculture. Long before the term biotechnology came into existence, tissue culture was used extensively in the propagation of orchids. This method of growing orchids, called in the past *asymbiotic orchid cultures*, was used at first only for the production of orchid plants from seed. This technique accelerates the time for germination and growth of seedlings by at least 10 to 20 times that of plants produced in the conventional way, sowing seeds on well-rooted plants. However, some growers believe that stronger growing plants are usually produced in the conventional way than those from the same seed pod raised asymbiotically in the laboratory. The asymbiotic propagation of orchids from seed succeeded after Lewis Knudson in 1918 made the discovery that orchid seedlings would grow only in a nutrient medium containing an organic compound in the form of sucrose (Sander, 1969). His nutrient formula, known as the *Knudson's formula*, has enjoyed great popularity and was for some time the most used formula for the asymbiotic cultures of orchids. The standard Knudson's formula is composed as follows:

KH_2PO_4	0.25 g
$CaNO_3$	1.00
$(NH_4)_2SO_4$	0.50
$MgSO_4$	0.25
$FePO_4$	0.05
Sucrose	20.00
Agar	17.50
Distilled water	1000 mL

The pH of this nutrient mixture is adjusted to 5.0 before autoclaving. Today a variety of organic additives are used in the nutrient media of orchids. The technique has also been expanded to grow orchids from meristematic tissue or orchids buds. Such a technique allows for the preservation of superior plants by the production of genetically identical plants. It also has an immense potential for mass propagation of plants.

The term tissue culture is considered a misnomer, because when it was introduced, it was restricted mainly to the culture of pieces of plant tissue *in vitro* (Bonga and Durzan, 1982). As indicated above, currently meristematic cells, parenchyma cells, embryos, callus, and/or other plant organs can be used in tissue culture (Kyte, 1983). Hence two groups of tissue culture methods can be distinguished: (1) methods using organized cell masses, such as meristems and embryos, which is frequently referred to as *micropropagation*, and (2) methods using unorganized cell masses, such as callus (see Figure 9.1).

The first attempt to culture plant cells was conducted by Gottlieb Haberlandt. Although his experiment in growing aseptically palisade cells isolated from *Lamium purpureum* and *Pulmonaria mollisima*, was unsuccessful, Haberlandt is regarded today as the *founder* of plant tissue culture. The application of tissue cultures became successful only after the right formula and additives, including growth hormones, were discovered. In the early attempts, it was noticed that many plants cultivated *in vitro* behaved *heterotrophically* rather than *autotrophically*. Plants grown in cultures were unable to manufacture carbohydrates on their own from inorganic nutrients only. The usefulness of cold filtered or autoclaved organic supplements, such as sugar, malt extract, yeast, fruit juices, coconut milk, thiamine, and growth hormones has been examined with mixed results. After numerous attempts, the first successful growth medium was formulated by Murashige and Skoog (1962). This medium, called the *MS medium* after the name of the developers, was for some time a popular medium in tissue cultures. It is used in its original or modified form in the aseptic propagation of plant tissue and a variety of culture media is now available.

Micropropagation enables the multiplication of clones and hence the production of plants of high uniformity and quality. On the other hand, tissue culture using callus or unorganized cell masses is often done to create variations in the regenerated plants, a phenomenon known as *somaclonal* variation. The regenerated plants differ from the parent plants.

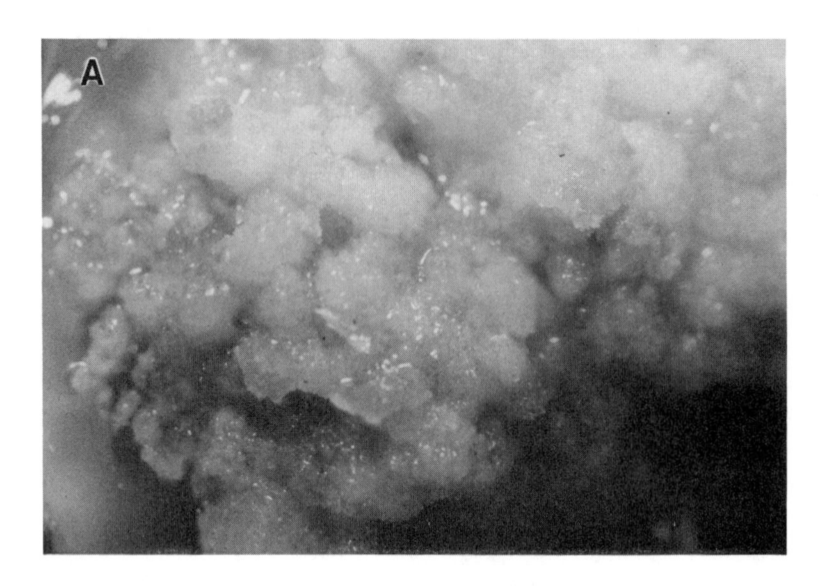

Figure 9.1 (A) Callus culture of slash pine (*Pinus elliottii* Engelm) seen with the light microscope, (B) Scanning electron micrograph of individual callus cells. (Irianto, 1991; Irianto and Tan, 1993.)

In general, tissue culture is practical because it permits mass production of plants. Large numbers of planting stocks can be produced in a very small area at a reasonable cost within a relatively short time. Moreover, this technique is applicable to ornamental plants, horticultural and agronomic crops, as well as commercially important fruit and forest crops (Bajaj, 1989). Tissue culture may provide the answer to the cultivation of plants that are very difficult to propagate by conventional or traditional means. For example, many forest trees valuable for timber in the humid tropics, such as teak (*Tectona grandis* L.),

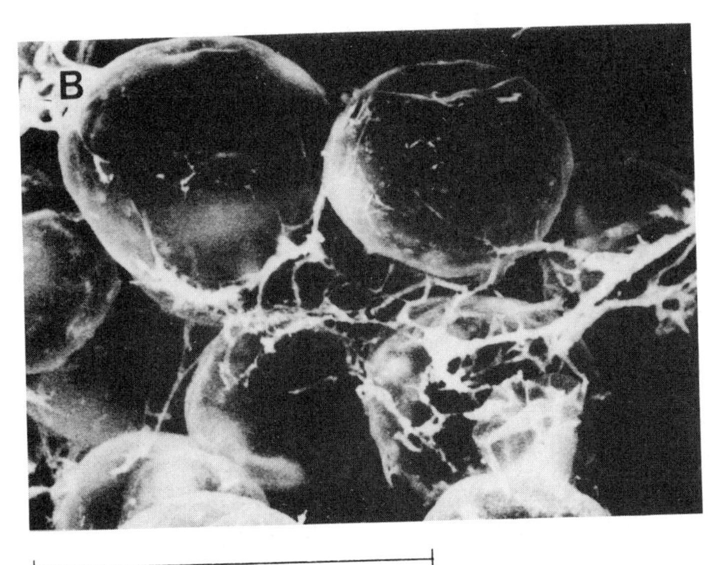

iron wood (*Mesua ferrea* L.), and mahagony (*Swietenia mahagony* Jacq.), grow extremely slowly, and are difficult to propagate by conventional vegetative methods or through seeds (Irianto, 1991). Tissue culture opens new possibilities for a rapid propagation of these trees. This method also enables the mass production of new tree stock for a rapid re-establishment of the tropical rain forest that is disappearing at an alarming rate due to increased demand for food, timber, pulpwood, fuel, fodder, and other forest products, as discussed previously.

CHAPTER 10

SOIL AND POLLUTION

10.1 DEFINITION AND CONCEPT OF WASTE

Waste is defined as useless, unwanted, or discarded material (U.S. Environmental Protection Agency, 1972). It can be distinguished into solid and liquid waste. Liquid waste is often referred to as *effluent*.

Agricultural, industrial, and other operations in our modern society produce large amounts of waste. The soil is traditionally the site for disposal of all these wastes, and people have been discarding waste since prehistoric times. However, there was little concern in the old days about pollution because the human population was not that large and there was plenty of space on earth for the amount of waste produced. However with the population growth and the revolutions in industry and agriculture, huge amounts of waste and a variety of new types of pollutants have been produced. For example, beef cattle in the USA were estimated to produce 92 million and dairy cattle 27 million metric tons/yr of manure (Donahue et al., 1983). Some of these types of wastes are difficult to deal with because of their diffuse or *nonpoint* nature, such as manure deposited at random by livestock, which may be washed into nearby streams (Troeh et al., 1980). Therefore, troubled by the degradation in environmental quality starting in 1970, a number of methods of waste disposal were explored. Today waste is buried in landfills, incinerated, dumped in the sea or used again on farmlands. When material called waste is used again as soil amendment or for any other purpose, it is no longer considered as waste but rather as a valuable resource material. If the demand for waste in energy and crop production increases, production of waste may well become an important process in the future (McCalla et al., 1977).

The major types of waste reaching the soil can be classified as: (a) agricultural waste, (b) industrial waste, (c) municipal waste, and (d) nuclear waste.

10.2 AGRICULTURAL WASTE

Agricultural wastes include the many forms of fertilizers, pesticides, plant residues, animal waste, and forest residues. Many of them are very beneficial when returned to the soil, such as plant residues and cattle and barnyard manure. However, the improper handling and disposal of them may cause pollution.

10.2.1 Fertilizers

The use of inorganic fertilizers, though essential to increasing crop production, can also prove to be hazardous to the environment. Of much concern is, for example, nitrate (NO_3^-) fertilizers or fertilizers that can be converted into nitrates. Ammonium (NH_4^+) fertilizers, for example, when used in well-drained soils may be converted into nitrates. This conversion of NH_4^+ occurs in two steps and is conducted by two types of bacteria: *Nitrosomonas* sp., responsible for the conversion of NH_4^+ into nitrite (NO_2^-), and *Nitrobacter* sp., responsible for the conversion of nitrite into nitrate (NO_3^-). The biochemical reactions, called *nitrification*, have been discussed in chapters 2 and 3.

Nitrates are taken up by plants, but high nitrate contents in plants are considered unhealthy, especially when the crops are used for the manufacture of baby food. When not taken up by plants, concern is expressed for contamination of ground water by nitrate ions. Nitrate ions, being negatively charged, are not adsorbed by the also negatively charged clay colloids, and hence are subject to leaching. By EPA standards, water containing >10% NO_3-N is unfit as a source for drinking water. In addition to these hazards, the nitrification process produces protons (see reaction 2.4) which may increase soil acidity. Because of this and because the nitrate is in the form of nitric acid (HNO_3), ammonium carrying fertilizers are frequently called *acid forming fertilizers*.

Another fertilizer element considered to be a hazard in soils and the environment is phosphorus. Phosphorus is a plant nutrient and is required for plant growth. However, by the excessive use of phosphate fertilizers, large amounts of the phosphate may leach into streams and lakes. An over-enrichment of lake water with phosphate and nitrate ions causes excessive growth of unwanted aquatic plants, a process called *eutrophication*.

10.2.2 Pesticides

Pesticides, another group of necessary agricultural chemicals in crop production, are used for the control of pests and diseases in crops. They include insecticides, fungicides, nematocides, rodenticides, and herbicides. Most of them are aromatic compounds, and chemical structures for some of the most widely used pesticides are shown in Figure 10.1. Their potential as a pollutant depends on their biodegradability and toxicity to animals and people. Pesticides that can persist in soils for a long time affect the food chain by a process called *biological magnification*, meaning accumulation and subsequent concentration in the food chain. They may also cause severe damage to non-target animals. Persistence of pesticides is often expressed in terms of *half-life*. The half-life of a pesticide is defined as the length of time required for one-half of a given amount of the pesticide to disappear or decompose to other compounds. The possibility arises that the decomposition products can be equally or even more harmful than the original compound. DDT, a chlorinated hydrocarbon widely used during and after World War II as an insecticide, is banned today

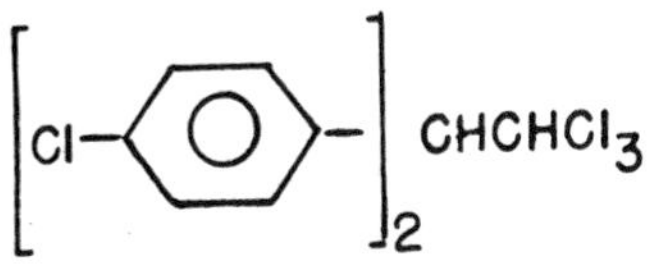

DDT, Dichlorodiphenyl-trichloroethane

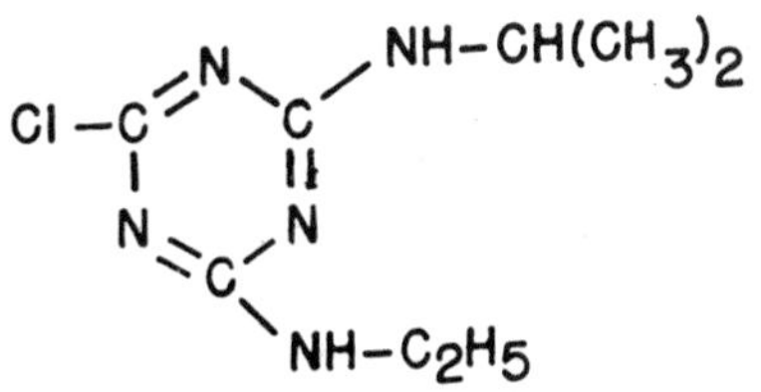

Atrazine

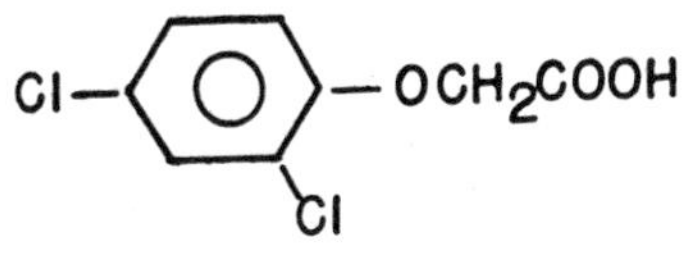

2,4-D

Figure 10.1 Chemical structure of DDT, triazine (atrazine), and 2,4-D.

because of its persistence in soils and its toxicity to animals and humans. The principal degradation product of DDT, called DDE, is also persistent, and has been implicated for the development of thin eggshells in birds. Aldrin, another common pesticide at the time of DDT use, yields a decomposition product called dieldrin. Dieldrin is reported to be more toxic than aldrin. Triazines and 2,4-D, used as herbicides, are more biodegradable and less toxic than DDT. Therefore, they are less likely to accumulate in the food chain than DDT.

10.2.3 Crop Residue

Crop residues are generally very beneficial for soils and will cause no serious pollution when disposed off in a proper manner. They are the main source of food and energy for soil microorganisms. Used as mulch, they control loss of water by evaporation from soils, and protect the soil at the same time against erosion. They contain plant nutrients which will be released upon decomposition. The nutrient content is, however, very variable and depends on the type of plant material (Table 10.1). Generally the C/N ratio of plant residues varies from 80:1 in wheat straw to 20:1 in legume material. During the microbial decomposition process the C/N ratio is reduced to the narrowest ratio at which C and N can exist together in soils, i.e., around 10:1. However, because of continuous turnover of plant residue, this narrowest ratio is seldom reached in soils under vegetation (McCalla et al., 1977).

Differences in plant species may affect the quality of crop residues. Generally crop residues from legume plants are higher in N than those from nonlegume plants. Therefore, used as soil amendment or used as cattle feed, these crop residues can have different results. At one time, during 1970—1980, cattle fed with fescue grass acquired underdeveloped hind legs, a disease called *fescue foot disease*. The exact cause is still unknown, but

Table 10.1 Nutrient Composition of Leaves of Selected Crop

Crop	N	P	K	Ca	Mg	Fe	Cu	Zn	Mn	B
	---------------%--------------					-----------mg/kg-----------				
Wheat	2.80	0.36	2.26	0.61	0.58	155	28	45	108	23
Corn	2.97	0.30	2.39	0.41	0.16	132	12	21	117	17
Peanuts	4.59	0.25	2.03	1.24	0.37	198	23	27	170	28
Soybeans	5.55	0.34	2.41	0.88	0.37	190	11	41	143	39
Potatoes	3.25	0.20	7.50	0.43	0.20	165	19	65	160	28
Sugar beets	3.76	0.38	4.01	0.78	0.68	126	26	40	086	53
Cotton	3.29	0.37	2.07	2.48	0.49	132	10	24	241	25
Alfalfa	4.63	0.48	2.76	2.38	0.66	140	21	46	065	56
Coastal bermuda	2.55	0.25	1.67	0.33	0.15	103	09	21	082	08
Tall fescue	2.78	0.33	3.01	0.43	0.32	098	08	20	135	08

Sources: author's unpublished data; Anderson et al (1971); McCalla et al.(1977); Donahue et al.(1983); and Jones et al.(1991).

the disease is believed to be caused by a fungus living in fescue, poisoning the cattle. The fungus produces alkaloids toxic to cattle. When cattle are raised on bermuda grass, they become excited. This disease is called *bermuda grass stagger*. The cows will recover if fed with grain-feed or rye grass (R. Wilkinson, USDA-ARS, personal communications).

10.2.4 Animal Waste

Animal wastes from agricultural operations include manure from cattle, swine, chickens, horses, sheep, and other types of animals. They vary considerably in chemical composition (Table

Table 10.2 Wet-Mass Percentages of Nutrient Elements in Animal Waste

Source	N	P	K	Ca	Mg	S	Fe
Dairy cattle	0.53	0.35	0.41	0.28	0.11	0.05	0.004
Beef cattle	0.65	0.15	0.30	0.12	0.10	0.09	0.004
Horse	0.70	0.10	0.58	0.79	0.14	0.07	0.010
Poultry	1.50	0.77	0.89	0.30	0.88	0.00	0.100
Sheep	1.28	0.19	0.93	0.59	0.19	0.09	0.020
Swine	0.58	0.15	0.42	0.57	0.08	0.14	0.020

Sources: Loehr (1974); Peterson et al. (1971); Tan et al.(1975), Brady (1990).

10.2), due to the type and amount of feed used and also the methods of collection, storage, and handling. For example, Donahue et al.(1983) reported figures for N content which were ten times higher than those listed in Table 10.2. This difference is caused perhaps by differences in analyses and calculations. The data presented by Donahue et al.(1983) were apparently percentages on a dry-mass basis.

As can be noticed from Table 10.2, poultry litter is the highest in N, P and Mg contents. When poultry litter is used as a fertilizer on fescue grass, the imbalanced K/N ratio in poultry litter was believed at one time to cause a disease in grazing cattle called *fescue foot disease*. As indicated previously, poisoning of cattle by the fungus living in fescue grass is considered a more likely reason for this disease.

In general, the plant nutrient content in all types of manure is lower than that in commercial fertilizers. But, manure is usually applied in large quantities, which then amounts to the addition of considerable quantities of nutrients. The data in Table 10.2 indicate that one metric ton of fresh (wet) dairy manure can supply approximately 5 kg N, 3.5 kg P, and 4.1 kg K, 2.8 kg Ca, and 1.1 kg Mg.

Most of the nutrients in manure are not easily available to plants. Their release depends on the rate of decomposition or mineralization. As such, they compare to the reaction of slow-release fertilizers. Crops are reported to seldom recover more than 2% of the soil nitrogen from humus (McCalla et al, 1977). This low availability is attributed to nitrogen's presence as organo-complexes,i.e., nitrogen is present as microbial protein and as complexes with humic acids or lignin-like substances.

Biologically, animal manures contain a large number of saprophytic, disease carrying, and parasitic microorganisms, which need to be taken into consideration in the disposal of manure. Chicken manure is known to contain *Salmonella sp.*, whereas swine manure may contain *Mycobacterium tuberculosis* (Azevedo and Stout, 1974). Feedlot waste was reported to contain 10^{10} organisms per gram, of which 10^{9}/g are various types of anaerobic organisms. They may also contain large amounts of *enterobacteria*, which is a health hazard if unsterilized waste is refed to animals (Hrubant et al, 1972).

10.2.5 Compost

Large piles of organic matter can be composted. Composting is a process resulting from controlled biological decomposition of organic residue into partially humified material. It seldom occurs naturally in soils, since large accumulation of vegetative residue in nature occurs where excessive amounts of water is present or where temperatures are low during most of the year. These conditions are not ideal for a composting process, which needs temperatures of 55°C (131°F). The materials for composting vary considerably, from materials high in N to materials low in N but high in C. For example, manure and sewage sludge are high in N, but dead leaves, grass clippings, straw, saw dust and wood chips or shavings are low in N but high in C. Materials very rich in carbon (sawdust) are preferably combined with nitrogenous materials, such as stable manure, poultry litter, or sewage sludge in a 4:1 ratio. During incubation the temperature of the mixture rises and levels off at 60-65°C (140—150°F) when the composting process is completed.

10.2.6 Forest Waste

Forest waste is composed of leaves and twigs remaining from the harvest of forest trees. It also includes inferior and nonharvestable trees. The amount of waste from the harvest of forest trees, commonly known as *slash*, was estimated in the USA to be 23 million metric tons per year (Donahue et al., 1983). Due to problems in collecting and processing it for further use, little effort has been made to recycle this type of waste. In Africa, Southeast Asia, and South America, slash is removed by burning, as discussed in chapter 7.

In general, forest waste has many properties in common with crop residues. As is the case with crop residue, forest waste also contains significant amounts of organic matter and plant nutrients. Therefore, it is a very valuable material for amending physical and chemical soil conditions. The nutrient content appears to not be affected by differences in tree species. Only small differences were noticed in C and N content between hardwood and softwood trees (Table 10.3). The nutrient content depends more on whether the forest waste is composed predominantly of leaves, twigs, branches, or bark. Lutz and Chandler (1947) reported that among hardwood trees, leaves had the highest nutrient content followed by stems (Table 10.4). The bark of hardwood is generally lower in C, but higher in N content than bark of softwood trees.

Another type of waste related to the forest is the residue from the forest industry in the form of wood chips, bark and

Table 10.3 Differences in C and N Contents Between Softwood and Hardwood Trees

Source	WOOD		BARK	
	C	N	C	N
	------%------		------%------	
Softwood*	48.5	0.10	50.4	0.14
Hardwood**	47.1	0.09	45.3	0.24

* Average of 19 tree species, including cedar, cypress, hemlock, fir, spruce, and pine.
** Average of 9 tree species, including oak, hickory, red gum, chestnut and black walnut. Sources: Allison (1965) and McCalla et al.(1977).

sawdust. Totalling almost 63 million metric tons annually (Donahue et al., 1983), this type of waste finds extensive application in industry, nurseries, and as soil amendment. Sawdust is used commercially for the production of pressed wood utilized in the furniture and housing industry. Bark has been applied extensively as mulching material and potting mixtures in nurseries. Both bark and wood chips are valued for landscaping purposes. However, the use of sawdust and bark in soils to improve physical and chemical soil conditions has received mixed reactions. Depending on the type of wood, both sawdust and bark have been noted to exhibit a harmful effect on the germination and growth of pea seedlings (Allison, 1965), and caution was expressed in the use of this type of waste in crop production (McCalla et al., 1977).

10.3 INDUSTRIAL WASTE

A variety of industrial waste products is currently causing

Table 10.4 Percentages of Major Nutrient Elements in the Ash Content of Selected Trees

Source	P	K	Ca	Mg	Fe	Si
			%			
Ash, *Fraxinus excelsion*						
Leaves	9.9	15.5	28.1	4.9	0.8	1.2
Stem	3.0	10.9	44.3	3.5	1.3	1.0
Bark	1.7	06.9	57.3	1.4	0.8	0.7
Aspen, *Populus tremula*						
Leaves	3.8	15.3	35.4	2.4	1.4	3.5
Stem	1.9	09.8	50.8	2.3	0.7	1.3
Bark	1.4	06.4	52.0	4.3	2.1	1.0
Beech, *Fagus sylvatica*						
Leaves	3.4	18.1	31.6	4.4	1.6	4.9
Stem	1.2	12.0	43.0	2.7	1.6	4.7
Bark	0.9	04.2	59.5	2.2	0.5	1.7
English Oak, *Quercus robur*						
Leaves	5.4	18.6	33.6	1.7	2.2	2.4
Stem	1.6	08.1	54.4	2.2	1.1	1.1
Bark	1.3	02.4	62.8	1.2	0.7	0.4

Sources: Lutz and Chandler (1947), and McCalla et al.(1977).

concerns regarding proper disposal. This waste can be in the gas, liquid and solid form. The most important gases are CO_2, CO, NO, NO_2, and SO_2. They are produced by the combustion of fossil fuels in industry and automobiles, and they pose a hazard to the environment. Liquid waste, called effluent, and solid waste are produced by food processing plants. Much of this solid waste is organic in nature and has properties almost similar to crop residue. For example, soybean, peanut, cotton seed, and sugar cane pulp have great recycling potential. Other forms of solid waste are also produced by other industrial operations. They can be introduced in the soil or in the atmosphere as industrial sludge or as dust or very fine particulates, such as elemental sulfur, S. This constituent is linked to the formation of acid rain, which will be discussed in a following section.

10.3.1 Carbon Monoxide

Carbon monoxide, CO, is the result of incomplete oxidation of fossil fuel. Most of it (approximately 80%) is produced by the combustion of oil by automobiles. During rush hours in large cosmopolitan cities, the CO content in the air can reach levels of 50 to 100 mg/L (Manahan, 1975). High levels of carbon monoxide are also frequently detected in the craters of volcanos.

In contrast to CO_2, carbon monoxide does not dissolve in water. This type of gas is hazardous to animals and humans because it reacts with hemoglobin to form CO-hemoglobin. This *carboxyhemoglobin* is unable to carry O_2, causing respiratory failures. It is an odorless and tasteless gas and gives no warning of its presence. Therefore, the hazard of CO poisoning by CO from faulty home heaters, exhaust from automobiles, and in volcano's craters is very great. However, in contact with soil, CO gas is either rapidly adsorbed or oxidized into CO_2 by certain types of microorganisms. Manahan (1975) stated that OH radicals in the atmosphere are also capable of converting CO into CO_2. In the atmosphere, CO is usually oxidized and converted into CO_2 by reaction with O_2, O_3, N_2O, or NO_2 gas. It burns readily with oxygen forming carbondioxide according to the following reaction:

$$2CO + O_2 \rightarrow 2CO_2 + \text{energy} \qquad (10.1)$$

This reaction indicates that CO can be used as a fuel source.

10.3.2 Carbon Dioxide

Carbon dioxide, or CO_2, is produced naturally by the decomposition of organic matter and respiration of plant roots and microorganisms. The chemical properties and environmental aspects of this gas have been discussed in chapter 5. In natural conditions, the CO_2 content of atmospheric air is very small and by volume it constitutes only 0.031% of our air. Because of this low level, some scientists are not concerned about pollution of atmospheric air by CO_2. They believe that the low amounts are insufficient to affect photochemical reactions. Absorption of infrared radiation is not energetic enough to induce chemical reactions (Moore and Moore, 1976; Manahan, 1975). Moreover, photosynthesis by terrestrial green plants may be able to absorb excess CO_2 from the air. Another sink for CO_2 is the seawater of the oceans. These bodies of salt water exhibit high pH values and are able to absorb large amounts of CO_2 as indicated in chapter 5. The huge amounts of seaweed and kelp, which are green plants, also contribute tremendously in absorbing the CO_2 for use in photosynthesis.

Under normal condition, the presence of CO_2 has a buffering effect on the pH of rain water. Carbon dioxide dissolves in rain water to produce carbonic acid, which gives to the water some acidity, stabilizing at a pH of 5.6-6.0 (see reactions 5.9 and 5.10).

Many environmentalists reported substantial increases in the CO_2 content of the atmosphere due to the industrial revolution and the burning of fossil fuel in automobiles. Large-scale burning of tropical rain forests to clear the land for crop production has also introduced large amounts of CO_2 into our atmosphere. The increase in CO_2 content in the Earth's atmosphere is believed to create a *greenhouse effect* on earth. Such an increase in temperature may increase the rate of weathering of soil minerals and decomposition of organic matter, whereas doubling the CO_2 concentration of the air may increase the yield of C_3 plants, such as soybeans, by 10 to 50% (Wild, 1993). C_4 plants, e.g. corn and sugar cane, are less affected by an increase in CO_2 content. C_3 plants fix CO_2 according to the *Calvin cycle.* These are mostly temperate region grasses and trees. On the other hand, C_4 plants fix CO_2 with a different process that enables the plants to store larger amounts of CO_2 in the chloroplast, which is the reason why they do not respond as well to an increase in CO_2 as C_3 plants. The growth rate of C_4 plants are consequently greater than that of C_3 plants.

10.3.3 Nitrogen Oxides

Nitrogen, N_2, nitrous oxides, N_2O, nitric oxide, NO, and NO_2 gas are common constituents of atmospheric air. The mixture of NO and NO_2 is usually referred to as NO_x (Manahan, 1975; Brady, 1990). Nitrogen gas is part of the *nitrogen cycle*, whereas the nitrogen oxide gases are the products of oxidation of N_2 gas. Nitrogen is the most abundant constituent of atmospheric air. Its concentration in normal atmospheric air is approximately 78%. In contrast, the nitrogen oxide gases are present only in very small amounts. For example, under normal conditions the concentration of N_2O in atmospheric air is 0.25 mg/L. However, due to the industrial revolution the concentration of nitrogen oxide gases in atmospheric air has increased 10 times or more. It is estimated that production of nitrogen oxide gas in 1975 amounts to 13 million tons per year (Moore and Moore, 1976; Manahan, 1975), and has increased since then. The resulting increase in nitrogen oxide content in the atmosphere has created much concern over harmful effects to the environment because of the formation of so-called *acid rain*, global warming, and destruction of the ozone shield. These environmental issues will be the topics of separate sections below.

In atmospheric air, nitrogen oxide gases are mostly produced by oxidation by lightning. They can also be introduced by emissions from Earth because of combustion of fossil fuel in the industry and automobiles. Supersonic air transport is also suspected to contribute to releasing large amounts of nitrogen oxide into the atmosphere. The three types of nitrogen oxide gases (nitrous oxide, nitric oxide, and dinitrogen oxide) will be discussed in more detail below and their production, emission, and implications in environmental quality will be examined.

Nitrous Oxide, N_2O, is a colorless gas with a mild pleasant odor. It tastes sweet and was used in the past as an anesthetic by dentists. It is sometimes referred to as *laughing gas*. Under high temperatures, N_2O decomposes to N_2 and O_2 gases according to the reaction

$$2N_2O \rightarrow 2N_2 + O_2 + \text{energy} \tag{10.2}$$

Because the decomposition reaction yields oxygen, N_2O gas is frequently used today as a fuel source in atomic absorption spectroscopy.

This gas is a *greenhouse gas*, and may also be detrimental to the ozone shield in our atmosphere. The gas is formed naturally by microbiological processes in soils. Denitrification of NO_3^- yields N_2O. Agricultural operations, biomass burning, and combustion of fuel in power stations and automobiles are considered important *anthropogenic* sources of N_2O gas. It is estimated that about 1/3 of the total emissions of N_2O is of anthropogenic origin (Granli and Bφckman, 1993). Other sources are wastewater treatment plants and medical and industrial use of N_2O. Because of these, the concentration of N_2O gas has increased by about 0.25% annually, which is hardly of concern at all. However, several scientists believe that such an increase in N_2O emission may bring about a 5% increase/year in the greenhouse effect (Granli and Bϕckman, 1993).

Nitric Oxide, NO, is a colorless gas and is insoluble in water. It is also a pollutant gas produced by burning fossil fuels in power plants, industry, and automobiles. Although it can also release its oxygen, it is not used as a fuel source as N_2O gas. NO acts more often as an oxidizing or reducing agent. The reduction reaction may convert NO into NO_2 gas according to the reaction:

$$2NO + O_2 \rightarrow 2NO_2 \qquad (10.3)$$

Such a reaction can occur spontaneously in the air and the NO_2 formed is a polluting gas contributing to the development of acid rain.

Nitrogen Dioxide, NO_2, is a red gas, and can rapidly form *dimers*, called dinitrogen tetroxide, N_2O_4. Nitrogen dioxide usually occurs in equilibrium with its dimer

$$2NO_2 \leftrightarrow N_2O_4 \qquad (10.4)$$

Nitrogen dioxide is a colorless gas, but it is a condensable gas, and will dissolve in water to form nitric and nitrous acids. For these reason, it is considered a polluting gas contributing to acid rain, which will be discussed in section 10.7.2.

10.3.4 Sulfur and Sulfur Oxide

Sulfur occurs in soils in organic form, e.g., humus, and in inorganic form, e.g., in the minerals gypsum, $CaSO_4$, and pyrite, Fe_2S. As discussed in chapter 5, pure elemental S is produced in the craters of active volcanos, and a large amount of S is also emitted into the air by these volcanos in the form of small particulate matter. Sulfur oxide, also called sulfur dioxide, SO_2, is the product of oxidation by natural sources or by the combustion of coal and oil in power plants and other industries. It is a colorless gas and soluble in water. It condenses rapidly into a liquid. This liquid boils at -10°C. Liquid SO_2 must be really dry when stored in steel tanks for shipping. A trace of moisture will convert it into sulfuric and sulfurous acid, which is very corrosive to the steel tankers. Because of its easy conversion into these acids, it is a polluting gas contributing to acid rain. Large amounts of sulfur oxides are also produced by ore smelting in factories.

This S, and its oxides produced by industry are frequently referred to as *anthropogenic sulfur* in contrast to the natural sulfur emitted by active volcanos. Like N_2, sulfur is an essential plant nutrient, and is necessary for the production of proteins, vitamins, and hormones.

The S content of soils varies considerably from 0.002% in highly weathered soils in the humid regions to 5% in the alkaline soils of arid regions (Stevenson, 1986). The element and its oxide are part of the *global sulfur cycle* (Manahan, 1975; Stevenson, 1986). Currently, a lot of concern has been expressed over the S and its oxides released in the atmosphere by industry. Sulfur can also enter the air by biological processes in the form of H_2S. The amount of SO_2 released in the atmosphere by industry is estimated to amount to 65 million tons per year (Manahan, 1975), and approximately 200 kg S per ha are deposited in soils from the air in highly industrialized areas of Europe, the eastern part of North America, and parts of east Asia. The amount of sulfur gases introduced in the air by industry is now perhaps one-half as much as from natural sources (Stevenson, 1986).

These sulfur gases are particularly harmful to the environment, plant growth and human health. Exposure to high levels of SO_2 gas may cause leaf necrosis in plants. The harmful effect increases when the stomata in the leaves are fully open. Some plants require acid soils for optimum growth, such as azaleas, rhododendrons, tea, and pine trees. The soils are usually acidified by applying S as discussed in a previous section.

Oxidation of sulfur and sulfur dioxide in the air and their subsequent reaction with raindrops form sulfuric acid and contribute toward the formation of acid rain. Sulfuric acid dissolves in rainwater and dissociates its proton, H^+, decreasing in this way the pH of rainwater. The reactions and effect of acid rain on environmental quality will be discussed in a separate section below.

Both the salts of this acid and the SO_2 gas have been associated with the formation of turbid haze, fog, and smog, which at one time was dangerously covering many industrial towns in the Midwest, California, and England. Not only is this kind of air pollution corrosive, but it also causes eye irritation and respiratory difficulties in humans. The seriousness of the effect depends on the time of exposure. Prolonged exposures to smog containing sulfuric acid may damage lung tissue.

A number of methods have been used to remove S and SO_2 from coal. The sulfur in coal is usually present as pyrite, Fe_2S, and as organic sulfur. Upon burning the coal, the pyrite minerals are oxidized and sulfur dioxide is produced. To prevent the formation of SO_2, pyrite minerals can be removed physically, e.g. by magnetic separation. Another method is to reduce the amount of SO_2 released in air after burning the coal by using extremely tall smokestacks and a series of *scrubbers*. Some of the scrubbers are dry, whereas others are wetted with water. In the *wet-limestone scrubbing* process, powdered limestone is injected into the oven or boiler along with powdered coal and the S or SO_2 is removed according to the following reactions:

$$\underset{\text{limestone}}{CaCO_3} \rightarrow \underset{\text{burnt lime}}{CaO} + CO_2\uparrow \qquad (10.1)$$

$$CaO + SO_2 \rightarrow \underset{\text{calcium sulfite}}{CaSO_3} \qquad (10.2)$$

$$CaSO_3 + SO_2 + \tfrac{1}{2}O_2 \rightarrow \underset{\text{calcium sulfate}}{CaSO_4} \qquad (10.3)$$

Calcium sulfate can be removed easily and is a valuable liming material.

Magnesium hydroxide can also be used in the same way as $CaCO_3$, and the SO_2 can be removed by catalytic oxidation. By any method, removing the S and SO_2 to keep SO_2 emissions at relatively low levels appears to be a costly process.

10.4 WASTE FROM FOOD PROCESSING PLANTS

Waste from the food processing industry can be in the form of solid waste or liquid waste (effluent).

10.4.1 Solid Waste

Solid waste from food processing plants varies considerably depending on the types of food processed ranging from plant products to animal products. Nevertheless these types of waste are invariably organic in nature, and are related in chemical composition with agricultural waste products.

Most of the solid waste can be recycled by using them as organic soil amendment or as compost. However, their nutrient content, especially their high N and P content, makes their disposal in soils uneconomical. Instead, most of them, such as soybean, peanut, cottonseed, sugar cane, and sugar beet pulp are processed today for animal feed. Solid waste from the chicken, meat, and fish industries are especially high in protein, hence in N content. They are excellent sources for recycling into fish feed and cat and dog food. Bones from the meat industry contain large amounts P in the form of $Ca_3(PO_4)_2$. They are processed into bone-meal, an excellent source of P fertilizer.

10.4.2 Liquid Waste (Effluent)

The *effluent* produced from the food processing industry is generally rich in inorganic nutrients, such as N, P, and K, as well as in dissolved organic compounds. They create a pollution hazard when disposed of improperly in streams and lakes. The excessive enrichment of stream and lake water with the above plant nutrients causes *eutrophication*, as discussed previously. The dissolved organic compounds reduce the oxygen content of soil, stream, and lake waters, because of an increase in the so called *oxygen demand*. The definition and concept of oxygen demand has been discussed in chapter 5. *The Biological Oxygen Demand*, or *BOD*, values in the effluent of food processing plants can, depending on dilution, run as high as 10 000 ppm. Runoff entering streams and lakes is a hazard to environmental quality if the BOD exceeds 20 ppm. High levels of organic pollutants causes microorganisms, responsible for the oxidation processes, to consume all the dissolved oxygen. The oxygen deficiency created in the effluent creates an anaerobic condition, which is highly undesirable.

10.5 MUNICIPAL WASTE

Municipal waste is distinguished by McCalla et al. (1977) into *municipal refuse* and *sewage sludge*.

10.5.1 Municipal Refuse

Municipal refuse, also called *municipal garbage*, is composed of discarded material by people in the home, and in industry. It is composed of paper, plastic, food, and plants. An average composition of municipal refuge is given in Table 10.5. Paper

Table 10.5 Average Composition of Municipal Refuse

Component	%
Paper	58.8
Food residue	09.2
Garden refuse	10.1
Metals	07.5
Glass, ceramics, and ash	08.5
Miscellaneous (plastic, rags, etc.)	05.9

Source: McCalla et al (1977).

makes up the largest amount of this refuse, whereas plastic comprises only very little and is considered a miscellaneous item. With the increasing use of plastics recently, they are an increasingly important component of refuse today and their percentage of total refuse is expected to become as high as paper. Toxic household and agricultural chemicals, fertilizers, solvents, and medicines are additional components of importance in today's refuse. The latter creates serious disposal problems.

Municipal garbage can be recycled by *composting*, by burning, or it can be disposed of in *landfills*. Burning is the least desirable method because of air pollution and because a large amount of the garbage is noncombustible. Composting has attracted increasing attention recently. For the purpose of composting, the organic components are of value and have to be separated carefully from glass, metals and other inorganic components. Composting non-toxic organic waste is currently receiving increasing attention. It relieves the municipalities of some of the heavy volume of garbage, and the compost is a very valuable product as a soil amendment in agricultural and horticultural operations. The process of composting has been discussed in a previous chapter.

10.5.2 Environmental Problems in Disposal of Municipal Refuse

Most municipal garbage is still discarded in *sanitary landfills*. Because of the many environmental problems created by sanitary landfills strict rules have been set up by the Environmental Protection Agency (Donahue et al., 1983). One of the problems in landfills is the generation of gases, such as methane, CH_4, gas. As discussed before, this gas is produced by the anaerobic decomposition of organic matter (See chapter 4). It is a flammable gas that can cause explosion, hence is a potential hazard to public safety. Improving aeration in landfills to create aerobic conditions may perhaps decrease formation of methane gas. Some municipalities have taken advantage of this problem by using the garbage for the commercial production of methane, as indicated earlier.

10.5.3 Sewage Sludge

Sewage sludge is the product of wastewater treatment plants. The materials processed in the treatment plants are domestic and industrial wastes. They are usually a liquid mixture, composed of solid and dissolved organic and inorganic material. The water is separated from the solid part, and undergoes a number of treatments before it is declared environmentally safe for discharge in streams and lakes. The solid part is composed of organic matter mixed with some inorganic compounds. It is biologically unstable, and is stabilized by a series of aerobic and anaerobic digestion processes. This solid waste product is usually referred to as *sewage sludge* (McCalla et al., 1977; King, 1986). Depending on the sources, sewage sludge varies in macro- and micronutrient content. The average macronutrient composition of municipal sewage sludge is given in Table 10.6. The data indicates that the N content of municipal, textile, and fermentation sludge is generally high. On the other hand, sludge from wood-processing plants are lower in N, but higher in K and Ca than the other three sludges. Sludge cake from England is also low in N, though its N content is slightly higher than that in wood processing sludge.

Table 10.6 Average Macronutrient Content of Sewage Sludges from the Southern United States and England

Origin	N	P	K	Ca	Mg
			%		
Municipal sludge (USA)	3.0	1.8	0.2	1.5	0.2
Textile sludge (USA)	4.1	1.1	0.2	0.5	0.2
Fermentation sludge (USA)	4.1	0.4	0.1	4.5	0.1
Wood processing sludge (USA)	0.8	0.1	1.9	3.3	0.2
Sludge cake (England)	1.2	0.6	0.3	0.0	0.0

Sources: King et al (1986); Wild (1993).

Heavy Metals in Sewage Sludge. Of great public concern is the heavy metal content in sewage sludge. A metal is defined as a substance that has (1) large electrical and heat conductivity, (2) has a *metallic luster*, (3) is malleable, and (4) is ductile (can be drawn into wires). Eighty of the elements in the periodic system are considered metals. They can be distinguished into *alkali metals* (Li, Na, K, Rb, and Cs), *alkali-earth metals* (Be, Mg, Ca, Sr, Ba and Ra), and *transition metals* (Al, Fe, Mn, Cu, Co, and Cu). However, a definition of *heavy metal* is not available in pure chemistry, but Wild (1993) indicated that *heavy metals* are by definition metals with a density of >5—6 g/cm^3. In the literature, the term is generally used very loosely, since it includes other metals that are not officially considered heavy metals. Often the term refers to the elements Al, As, Cd, Co, Cr, Cu, Fe, Hg, Mn, Ni, Pb, and Zn. Some of them are required in trace amounts for plants, animals and humans, whereas others are hazardous to human health. Present at even minute concentrations, these heavy metals tend to accumulate in biological systems. In passing through the food chain associated with plant and animal life, their concentrations may increase to harmful levels in the top members of the food chain, e.g., fish, eagles, and humans.

The heavy metal content in sewage sludge varies considerably depending on the contribution of industry (Table 10.7). In general, municipal sludge is very high in Al, Fe, Zn, Cr, and Cu content. The Pb, Ni and Cd content are on the average relatively small, whereas Hg is hardly detected in sewage sludge. Cadmium, Pb, Hg, and Ni are not considered plant nutrients, but these metals can potentially be taken up by plants together with Fe, Cu, Mn and Zn. Aluminum is officially not recognized as a plant nutrient, but plants develop necrotic spots when grown in Al deficient media. Much concern has been expressed about the harmful effects of Pb, Cd, and Hg to animals and humans.

Table 10.7 Average Metal Compositon of Sewage Sludge in the Southern United States and United Kingdom

Origin	Al	Fe	Mn	Cu	Zn	Pb	Ni	Cd	Cr	Hg
				mg/kg						
Southern United States:										
Municipal sludge	7280	2370	150	565	2220	520	100	28	1040	5
Textile sludge				390	864	129	63	4	2490	
Fermentation sludge				81	255	29	18	2	117	
Wood proc. sludge				53	122	42	119	2	81	
England and Wales:										
Sludge				800	3000	700	80		250	

Sources: Tan et al (1971); King and Giordano (1986); Stevenson (1986); Wild (1993).

Lead, Pb, is a soft metal with a dull gray color and low tensile strength. It is the heaviest of the metals, except for gold and mercury. The element is used for covering electric cables, and insulation in x-ray instruments and has been used in the past for the layering of water pipes. It is used as a paint pigment in the form of lead carbonate, $Pb_3(OH)_2(CO_3)_2$, which is called *white lead*. Because of its high toxicity, its use in paint is now replaced by ilmenite. The organometal chelate of lead, called *lead tetraethyl*, $Pb(C_2H_5)_4$, has been used as an *anti-knock* additive in gasoline (to prevent knock in automobile engines). Its use as an anti-knock additive has now been replaced by other less toxic compounds. The oxides of lead, e.g., lead monoxide, also called *litharge*, and *red lead*, Pb_3O_4, are used in making lead crystals and lead glass. Red lead is also used in red paint for protecting iron against corrosion. These applications have been discontinued because of the hazard of Pb toxicity.

Lead, Pb, is physiologically not a nutrient and its accumulation in soil may, therefore, cause pollution. This metal is implicated in causing liver damage. However, no adverse effect has been reported by the intake of Pb below the required threshold values.

Cadmium. Another element considered a liability to the environment (Lagerwerff, 1972) is cadmium, Cd. Cadmium, a silvery metal resembling Zn, is a rare metal and is present in soils and minerals in very low concentrations. The mineral source of Cd is *greenockite*, CdS, a mineral related to *sphalerite*, ZnS. The Cd concentration of phosphate fertilizers, another likely source of Cd in soils, is approximately 7 μg/g. The Cd content is slightly higher in sewage sludge, but still substantially lower compared to Al and Fe contents.

The element is used in electroplating iron and steel and for the production of a number of alloys. Cadmium-plated iron has a better appearance and is more resistant to corrosion than galvanized iron. Galvanized iron is coated (plated) with zinc. Cadmium is also used for making standard cells for measuring electrical potentials, whereas Cd rods find application in nuclear reactors to control chain reactions or absorb neutrons.

Cadmium is also not required as a nutrient, but can replace Zn in plant and animal nutrition, and may cause renal and testicular damage in the latter. Cigarette smoking is one reason for a high daily intake of Cd. The application of Cd in industry as a stabilizing agent in the production of polyvinyl plastics, its use in electroplating of metals, and in the production of batteries and pigments have alarmed environmentalists worried about its harmful accumulation in soils, though very few human health problems have been noted because of Cd toxicity. The only case of Cd fatality was reported in 1950 in Japan, due to the consumption of rice containing high amounts of Cd. The paddy fields had been irrigated with water polluted by materials high in Cd from a neighboring zinc mine (Wild, 1993). Zinc smelters are notorious for the environmental damage they cause by emitting large amounts of ZnO and CdO fumes.

In view of the fact that the Cd content in sewage sludge is relatively low, overconcern for the pollution hazards of Cd and Hg, when sludge is applied in soils for crop production, is perhaps somewhat overstated. Cadmium and Hg are indeed very toxic to humans and animals, and their content in soils may build up with repeated application of sewage sludge over time. However, a build-up of Cd to dangerous levels may take a long time and only with very large amounts of sewage sludge application. It must be realized that huge amounts of materials are required to accumulate minute concentrations of the hazardous metal in soil. For example, Rainey (1967) points out that 5000 tons of material must be dissolved to reach a concentration of 1 ppb (part per billion) of a polluting metal in Lake Michigan (4871 km^3). With sewage sludge, Stevenson (1986) reported that an annual application of 20 metric tons/ha of digested sludge for 20 years would result in an increase of 8 mg/kg of Co, 180 mg/kg of Cu, 270 mg/kg of Pb, and 890 mg/kg of Zn. No data on Cd were presented, but since the Cd content was, for example, 35 times smaller than the Cu content, theoretically only 5 mg Cd/kg is expected to accumulate in soils with the above treatment of sludge in 20 years.

Therefore, of greater concern should be the Al content, which tops all the other metal concentrations in sewage sludge. Large amounts of Al are also toxic to plants, humans, and animals. Large amounts of Al intake have been implicated to damage brain cells in humans. The presence of 50 mg Al/kg has been noted to create Al toxicity in plants. Much of the Al taken up is, however, retained in the roots, especially in the root epidermis in the form of organic chelates (Tan and Binger, 1986). It should also be realized that the metals in sludge are bound strongly to the organic matter by complex and chelation reaction. They will be released gradually as free ions as the sludge decomposes over a period of years. Even then, the presence of fulvic and humic acids in soils may regulate the metal concentrations in the soil solution to the extent that toxicity is suppressed (Tan and Binger, 1986). Its entry into the food chain can, therefore, be kept to a minimum.

Mercury, Hg, is a third element that has created a lot of concern among environmentalists. It is the only metal which is in a liquid state at room temperature. Because of its presence in the liquid state and its silvery luster, the metal is often called *quicksilver*. It exhibits a high boiling point and a uniform expansion and contraction. Therefore, mercury is an excellent substance for making thermometers, barometers and the like. All metals, except Fe and Pt, will dissolve in Hg, including gold. Mercury vapor emits light, hence Pb is also used in mercury vapor and fluorescence lamps. Mercury is also useful in the production of explosives, detonators, and percussion caps. In the form of HgS, it is used as a paint pigment, called *vermillion*.

Mercury and all mercury compounds are toxic in large amounts. However, in small amounts they are used in medicines. Ointments for treating infection of open wounds contain Hg, such as *mercury-chrome*. The critical amount of Hg in the form of $HgCl_2$ for Hg poisoning is approximately 0.3 g. The Hg^{2+} is reported to destroy the kidney. Hg poisoning is often cured by consuming milk and/or egg whites. These substances inactivate the Hg ions by forming organo-Hg chelates, which precipitate in the stomach.

As indicated above, the amount of Hg detected in sewage sludge of the southern United States is so small that it would take tons of sewage sludge to accumulate significant amounts of Hg in soils. Theoretically, if it takes 20 years for 5 mg Cd to accumulate per kg of soils with an annual application of 20 metric tons of sewage, it will take 100 years (5 times longer) to accumulate an equivalent amount of Hg. As indicated in Table 10.7, the Hg concentration is 1/5 or less than that of Cd in sewage sludge of the Southern United States. As indicated earlier, Al, Fe, and Zn top all the other elements in concentration. An oversupply of soluble Al, Fe, and Zn ions is also harmful to plants, since they are needed only as micronutrients.

10.6 DETOXIFICATION OF WASTE

As indicated in chapter 6, soil has the ability to resist changes in soil reaction, called *buffer capacity*, which is related to its cation exchange capacity. It appears that the soil's capacity to resist changes is not limited to buffering soil pH only. The soil also has the ability to adsorb, neutralize and detoxify a number of organic wastes, which, if released in streams and lakes, would pollute the environment. This unique detoxifying capacity is attributed to many soil characteristics. Soil water acts as a solvent, whereas the electrically charged surfaces of clay and humic matter provide for binding sites. Humic acid, especially, is known to able to chelate large amounts of heavy metals in solution, reducing in this way the concentration and hence chemical activity of the metal ions. The presence of static electricity in clay minerals can produce an electrical discharge, which has been reported to be strong enough to destroy carbon compounds which are not too complex in molecular structure. Enzymes produced by microorganisms are also contributing toward decomposing many organic wastes. The term *biodegradable compounds* is used today to refer to materials that can be destroyed by such an enzymatic decomposition, such as plastics and pesticides. The enzymes produced by microorganisms are used to attack natural organic matter in soils with the purpose of obtaining food and energy. Such an enzymatic decomposition depends on the complexity of the molecular structure of the organic material. When a foreign substance is introduced into the soil, the enzyme will be able to attack it if the chemical nature of the foreign substance does not differ too much from that of the natural compound normally broken down by the enzyme. In some cases, the soil appears to need some time to accomplish the detoxifying effect. This happens, especially, with compounds that have not previously been introduced into soils. The delay in detoxification reactions is attributed to the length of time the microorganisms need to increase their number sufficiently to produce enough enzymes.

10.7 ENVIRONMENTAL IMPACT OF AGRICULTURAL AND INDUSTRIAL WASTE

10.7.1 Greenhouse Effect

The greenhouse effect is a phenomenon that causes the Earth's temperature to increase. Carbon dioxide and the other so-called *greenhouse gases*, CH_4, N_2O, and chlorofluorocarbons, emitted from the Earth's surface, move to the upper atmosphere, where they are heated by the sunlight. Energy from the sun's radiation is absorbed by these gases and emitted to the surface of the earth, resulting in an increase in temperature of the Earth's surface. The effect is similar to the warming effect attributed to the glass windows in *Florida rooms* or greenhouses. The warming of the interior of a car after standing in the sun is also a form of the greenhouse effect. In this case, the metal roof of the automobile is heated by the sun and becomes very hot. The heat absorbed increases the temperature of the interior of the car. Therefore, the greenhouse effect is not the result of blocking the sun's rays; rather the increase in temperature of the air on the Earth's surface is attributed to the invisible hot shield of CO_2 cloud. This increase in temperature may not only have a disastrous effect on the polar ice caps, but also many areas may be converted to desert lands. Climatic and vegetational zones may shift to northern latitudes.

The resulting global warming attributed to the greenhouse effect has been disputed recently. Several scientists indicate that the greenhouse effect does not affect uniformly the whole Earth, but that it affects only certain parts of the earth where the production of the pollutant gases is most intense, such as in regions where large industrial centers are located. It is contended that the increase in temperature is not long lasting, so that the long term effect of global warming is negligibly small. Nevertheless, global warming and acid rain have become environmental issues of world proportion. However, the fact that it has polarized the nations of the Northern and Southern Hemispheres is not exactly right. A misconception exists that large-scale burning of the rain forest occurred only in the "South" producing the CO_2. Most of the industrialized nations are indeed located in the Northern Hemisphere, but not all of the rain forest is in the Southern Hemisphere. A large part of the tropical rain forest is on the north site of the equator and is also cleared for crop production. It is an issue to be solved by both the nations that cleared the forest and those that are highly industrialized, and "finger-pointing" will not solve the problem.

10.7.2 Acid Rain

The term *acid rain* was first used in the 19th century for the rain in the industrialized region of northwest England that contained acidic compounds (Wild, 1993). Acid rain is in fact a natural phenomenon occurring during any thunderstorm accompanied by heavy lightning or by volcanic eruptions. However, it is the *accelerated pollution* of the air with nitrogen-

and sulfur-containing gases, emitted by industry, power stations, planes, and automobiles that produces acid rain which has alarmed many people because of the increasing potential hazard for environmental degradation.

Acid rain is caused by the presence of sulfuric acid and nitric and nitrous acid in the rain drops. It is better called *acid precipitation*, because these acids can also be present in snow, ice, sleet, moisture in fog and smog, and in other types of precipitation. The nitric and nitrous acids are formed by the reaction of NO_2 gas with moisture in the atmosphere. In the atmosphere, the NO_x gas is converted into NO_2 gas as illustrated by the following reactions:

$$2N_2O + O_2 \rightarrow 4NO \qquad (10.4)$$

$$2NO + O_2 \rightarrow 2NO_2 \qquad (10.5)$$

The NO_2 gas formed dissolves in rain drops forming nitric and nitrous acids:

$$2NO_2 + H_2O \rightarrow \underset{\text{nitrous acid and nitric acid}}{HNO_2 + HNO_3} \qquad (10.6)$$

Nitric and nitrous acids dissolve in rainwater and dissociate their protons, H^+. Because of this, the pH of rain water or water in fog decreases to 2.0 or lower.

Emission of S particulates in the air is another reason for the development of acid rain. The oxidation of S and formation of sulfuric acid are illustrated by the following reactions:

$$S + O_2 \rightarrow SO_2 \qquad (10.7)$$

$$2SO_2 + O_2 \rightarrow 2SO_3 \qquad (10.8)$$

$$2SO_2 + 2H_2O \rightarrow \underset{\text{sulfuric acid}}{2H_2SO_4} \qquad (10.9)$$

Acid rain has become of increasing concern today in Europe and North America because of *die-back* of forest trees, a harmful process also known as *forest decline*. In Germany, Czechoslovakia, and Poland the die-back of the silver fir (*Abies alba*) forest is reported to be caused by acid rain. Reports have also indicated that the increased acidity of lake water in the Adirondack Mountains of the United States, because of acid rain, has contributed to *fish kill*. The disappearance of brown trout (*Salmo trutta*) in mountain lakes of Scandinavia is another example of the harmful effect of acidification of lake water by acid rain.

Two opposing theories are found in the literature explaining the damage to aquatic life by acidification of lake water. One group of scientists believe that fish kill is not caused by the increased acidity itself, but by increased Al concentration in lake water. The latter is produced by the accelerated weathering of rocks and minerals by acidic water. Survival and growth of the fry of brown trout have been noted to decrease in laboratory conditions at concentrations of 250 μg Al/L or lower (Wild, 1993). In contrast, the other theory indicates that fish are sensitive to water pH and will be harmfully affected by a water pH <4.5 (Brady, 1990).

Acid rain is also corrosive to metals. The salts of these acids have been implicated in the formation of turbid haze, smog, and fog covering much of the industrial towns in the Midwest and California.

Today, the problem seems to be a global environmental issue.

Acid rain and global warming have created a confrontation between the people in the Northern Hemisphere and those in the Southern Hemisphere, especially in the tropics. As discussed previously, the industries are located mostly in the North, whereas the tropics in the south are mostly inhabited by people from developing nations who cut the rain forests for making a living. As noted before, the industrial nations blame the South for global warming attributed to emission of polluting gases by large-scale burning of the rain forests. In turn, the South accuses the North of being the primary producers of pollutant gases responsible for acid rain.

The effect of acid rain is of a less serious nature in soils. Soils exhibit a cation exchange capacity (CEC) that provide them with a buffering capacity to adsorb the excess proton from acid rain. However, a prolonged impact by acid rain can saturate this buffer capacity in soils. From this point on, further addition of acid rain will increase soil acidity. Sandy soils are especially critical in this matter, since these soils are weakly buffered by nature, because of their low cation exchange capacity. Two methods have been suggested to control the effect of acid rain on soil acidity, (1) cleaning emissions in industry and motor vehicles and (2) liming soils and lakes. Combining the two methods is perhaps a better alternative.

10.7.3 Destruction of the Ozone Shield

Destruction of ozone in the stratosphere is another environmental issue resulting from accelerated emission of pollutant gases. It is due more to the effects of industrial- and especially transportation-related air pollution than those of an agricultural pollution of the air. Supersonic air transport is suspected to contribute to the destruction of ozone, because of CO_2 and H_2O emission from combustion of hydrocarbon fuel.

Ozone is a form of oxygen with the formula O_3. It is a blue gas with a characteristic smell and its name is derived from the

Greek term *ozein*, which means *to smell*. It is usually formed in air by a photolytic reaction, or the passage of electric sparks or arcs. It is a stronger oxidizing agent than ordinary oxygen, O_2, and it is capable of oxidizing organic substances in the atmosphere.

Ozone is a normal constituent of the stratosphere and is present as an invisible cloud at approximately 15 miles (24 km) above the Earth, called the *ozone layer*, shielding the Earth against harmful radiation from the sun. Under normal conditions, ozone is being destroyed and at the same time being reformed, maintaining in this way a photochemical equilibrium in the stratosphere. The destruction of ozone in nature takes place by the reaction of O_3 with hydroxyl, OH, groups derived from water vapor in the stratosphere. The process can be represented as follows (Moore and Moore, 1976):

$$O + H_2O \rightarrow 2OH \tag{10.10}$$

$$OH + O_3 \rightarrow HOO + O_2 \tag{10.11}$$

The biogeochemical importance of the ozone layer results from its capacity to absorb ultraviolet radiation at wavelengths between 360 to 240 nm. Such an absorption introduces a photochemical reaction, which decomposes the ozone molecule into ordinary oxygen as follows:

$$O_3 + hv \leftrightarrow O_2 + O \tag{10.12}$$

In natural conditions such a reaction is an equilibrium reaction, meaning that O_2 can react with O to form ozone again. In the reaction above, hv is the energy of UV radiation, which is used for the decomposition of ozone. In this way UV radiation from the sun is blocked from reaching the earth surface. Ultraviolet radiation is destructive for many organic compounds, and if this ultraviolet light is permitted to reach the earth, life in its present form could not exist. Increased levels of UV radiation are linked to increased incidence of human skin cancer.

Since ozone reacts rapidly with organic compounds, the introduction of such compounds in the air damages the photochemical equilibrium of importance in formation and decomposition of ozone. Reaction (10.12) is then skewed toward the decomposition of ozone. Combustion of fossil fuel and oxidation of organic compounds on earth yield H_2O and CO_2. Since H_2O can dissociate its OH ion (see reaction 10.10), the effect of H_2O is to accelerate the destruction of ozone. Other gases responsible for decomposing ozone, are N_2O, NO, CH_3, CH_4, and gases from organic synthetics, such as $CFCl_3$ (freon) and CFCs (chlorofluorocarbons) used as refrigerants and aerosols. The decomposition of ozone by these gases can be illustrated by the following reactions:

$$\underset{\text{from freon}}{Cl} + O_3 \rightarrow ClO + O_2 \qquad (10.13)$$

$$ClO + O \rightarrow Cl + O_2 \qquad (10.14)$$

As can be noticed the ClO produced in the decomposition of ozone again yields Cl. In this way, the destruction reaction can be perpetuated until all ozone is converted into O and O_2. It must be emphasized that the examples of the destruction of ozone above are simplified for an easy comprehension of the problem. In nature, the reaction of ozone with Cl, creating the *ozone hole* above Antarctica, is very complex.

On the Earth's surface, incomplete oxidation products of hydrocarbons from automobiles can react with NO_2 to form peroxyacetyl nitrate, the so-called *PAN*. When present in smog at concentrations >0.3 ppm, PAN and ozone are severe irritants to humans.

The soil is a natural source of these pollutant gases. Respiration of roots and microorganisms produces CO_2. Aerobic decomposition of organic matter produces H_2O and CO_2, whereas anaerobic decomposition of organic matter yields CH_4. However, the natural production of these pollutant gases is small compared to that from combustion of fossil fuel and the large-scale burning of the rain forests.

REFERENCES AND ADDITIONAL READINGS

Ahmad, F., and K. H. Tan. 1986. Effect of lime and organic matter on soybean seedlings grown in aluminum toxic soil. Soil Sci. Soc. Am. J. 50: 656- 661.

Aiken, G. R., D. M. McKnight, R. L. Wershaw, and P. MacCarthy (eds). 1985. *Humic Substances in Soil, Sediments, and Water*. Wiley Intersc., New York, NY.

Alexander, M. 1965. Nitrification. pp. 307-343. In: *Soil Nitrogen*, W. V. Bartholomew and F. E. Clark (eds). Agronomy series No.10, Am. Soc. Agronomy, Inc., Publ., Madison, WI.

Aldrich, S. R., W. O. Scott, and E. R. Long. 1975. *Modern Corn Production*. A & L Publications, Champaign, IL.

Allison, F. E. 1965. Decomposition of wood and bark sawdusts in soil, nitrogen requirements, and effects on plants. USDA-ARS Techn. Bull. 1332.

Allison, F. E., and J. H. Doetsch. 1951. Nitrogen gas production by the reaction of nitrites with amino acids in slightly acidic media. Soil Sci. Soc. Am. Proc. 15: 163-166.

Amano, Y. 1981. Phosphorus status of some Andosols in Japan. Japan Agric. Res. Quat. (JARQ), 15: 14-21.

Anderson, O. E., H. F. Perkins, R. L. Carter, and J. B. Jones. 1971. Plant Nutrient Survey of Selected Plants and Soils of Georgia. University of Georgia, College Agric. Expt. Stns.

Research Report 102, Athens, GA.

Arnold, R. W., and C. A. Jones. 1987. Soils and climate effects upon crop productivity and nutrient use. pp. 9-17. In: *Soil Fertility and Organic Matter as Critical Components of Production Systems*, R.F. Follett (chair). Soil Sci. Soc. Am., Inc., and Am. Soc. Agronomy, Inc., Publ., Madison, WI.

Azevedo, J., and P. R. Stout. 1974. Farm Animal Manures: An Overview of their Role in the Agricultural Environment. Univ. California, Calif. Agric. Expt. Stn., Extension Service Manual 44.

Bajaj, Y. P. S. (ed). 1989. *Biotechnology in Agriculture and Forestry. Trees II.* Vol. 5. Springer-Verlag, Berlin, Heidelberg, New York, NY.

Baver, L. D. 1963. The effect of organic matter on soil structure. Pontificiae Academiae Scientiravm Scripta Varia, 32: 383-413.

Bernhard-Reversat, F., C. Huttel, and G. Lemee. 1979. Structure et fonctionnement des écosystèmes de la forêt pluvieuse sempervirente de la Côte d'Ivoire. UNESCO-Paris, Rech. Res. Nat. 14: 605-625.

Birkeland, P. W. 1974. *Pedology, Weathering and Geomorphological Research.* Oxford University Press. London.

Bonga, J. M., and D. J. Durzan. 1982. *Tissue Culture in Forestry.* Martinus Nijhoff, Boston, MA.

Bell, F. W., and E. R. Canterbery. 1976. *Aquaculture for the Developing Countries.* Ballinger Publishing Co., Cambridge, MA.

Brady, N. C. 1984. *The Nature and Properties of Soils.* 9th edition. Macmillan Publ. Co., New York, NY.

Brady, N. C. 1990. *The Nature and Properties of Soils.* 10th edition. MacMillanPubl. Co., New York, NY.

Bremner, J. M. 1965. Organic nitrogen in soils. pp. 93-149. In: *Soil Nitrogen*, W. V. Bartholomew and F. E. Clark (eds.). Agronomy series 10. Am. Soc. Agronomy, Inc., Publ., Madison, WI.

Brewer, R., and J. R. Sleeman. 1988. *Soil Structure and Fabric.* C.S.I.R.O., Div. Soils, Adelaide, Australia.

Broadbent, F. E., and F. E. Clark. 1965. Denitrification. pp. 344-359. In: *Soil Nitrogen*, W. V. Bartholomew and F. E. Clark (eds). Agronomy series 10. Am. Soc. Agronomy, Inc., Publ., Madison, WI.

Buol, S. W., F. D. Hole, and R. J. McCracken. 1973. *Soil Genesis and Classification.* The Iowa State University Press, Ames, IA.

Cannon, W. A., and E. E. Free. 1925. Physiological features of roots, with especial references to the relation of roots to aeration of the soil. Carnegie Inst. Publ. 368. Washington, DC.

CAST. 1980. Organic Farming and Technology. Council for Agricultural Science and Technology. Ames, IA.

Chandler, Jr., R. F. 1968. Dwarf rice - A giant in tropical Asia. pp. 252-255. In: *Science for Better Living*, USDA, The Yearbook of Agriculture. USDA, U.S. Govern. Printing Office, Washington, DC.

Chang, H. T., and W. E. Loomis. 1945. Effect of carbon dioxide on absorption of water and nutrients by roots. Plant Phys., 20: 221-232.

Clarke, J. W. 1924. The data of geochemistry. U.S. Geol. Survey Bull. 770.

Conn, E. E., and P. K. Stumpf. 1967. *Outlines of Biochemistry.* 2nd Edition. Wiley & Sons, Inc., New York, NY.

De Coninck, F. 1980. Major mechanisms in formation of spodic horizons. Geoderma 24: 101-128.

Deevey, Jr., E. S. 1960. The human population. Scientific American, 203: 195-204.

Dobereiner, J., and J. M. Day. 1975. Nitrogen fixation in the rhizosphere of tropical grass. pp. 39-56. In: *Nitrogen Fixation by Free-living Micro- Organisms*, W. D. P. Stewart (ed). Intern. Biol. Programme 6. Cambridge University Press, New York, NY.

Donahue, R. L., R. W. Miller, J. C. Shickluna. 1983. *Soils. An Introduction to Soils and Plant Growth*. Prentice-Hall, Inc., Englewood Cliffs, NJ.

Douchaufour, P. 1976. *Atlas Écologique des Sols du Monde*. Masson, Paris, New York, Barcelona, Milan.

Douglas, J. S. 1976. *Advanced Guide to Hydroponics*. Drake Publ., Inc., New York, NY.

Dudal, R. 1976. Inventory of the major soils of the world with special reference to mineral stress hazards. pp. 3-14. In: *Plant Adaptation to Mineral Stress in Problem Soils*, M. J. Wright (ed). Proc. Workshop Cornell University, Ithaca, NY.

FAO-Food and Agriculture Organization. 1982. FAO Production Yearbook, Vol.36, U.N.-F.A.O., Rome.

Food and Agriculture Organization. 1987. Agriculture: Toward 2000. U.N.-F.A.O., Rome.

Fearnside, P. M. 1987. Causes of deforestation in the Brazilian Amazon. pp. 37- 61. In: *The Geophysiology of Amazonia. Vegetation and Climate Interactions*, R. E. Dickenson (ed). Wiley & Sons, New York, NY.

Flaig, W. 1971. Organic compounds in soils. Soil Sci., 111: 19-33.

Flaig, W. 1975. An introductory review on humic substances: Aspects of research on their genesis, their physical and chemical properties, and their effect on organisms. pp. 19-42. In: *Humic Substances. Their Structure and Function in the Biosphere*, D. Povoledo and H. L. Golterman (eds). Centre Agri. Publ. and Documentation, Wageningen, The Netherlands.

Follett, R. F., S. C. Gupta, and P. G. Hunt. 1987. Conservation practices. Relation to the management of plant nutrients for crop production. pp.19-51. In: *Soil Fertility and Organic Matter as Critical Components of Production Systems*, R. F. Follett (chair). Soil Sci. Soc. Am., Inc., and Am. Soc. Agronomy, Inc., Publ., Madison, WI.

Foth, H. D., 1990. *Fundamentals of Soil Science*. 8th edition.

Wiley & Sons, New York, NY.
Frear, G. L., and J. Johnston. 1929. The solubility of calcium carbonate (calcite) in certain acqueous solutions at 25°. Amer. Chem. Soc. J., 51: 2082-2093.
Garrels, R. M., and C. L. Christ. 1965. *Solutions, Minerals and Equilibria*. Harper and Row, New York, NY.
Ghuman, B. S., and R. Lal. 1987. Effects of deforestation on soil properties and microclimate of a high rainforest in South Nigeria. pp. 225-244. In: *The Geophysiology of Amazonia. Vegetation and Climate Interactions*, R. E. Dickinson (ed). Wiley & Sons, New York, NY.
Gill, W. R., and R. D. Miller. 1956. A method for study of the influence of mechanical impedance and aeration on the growth of seedling roots. Soil Sci. Soc. Amer. Proc. 20: 154-157.
Gingrich, J. R., and M. B. Russell. 1956. Effect of soil moisture tension and oxygen concentration on the growth of corn roots. Agronomy J. 48: 517-520.
Goenadi, D. H., and K. H. Tan. 1991. The weathering of para-crystalline clays into kaolinite in Andosols and Ultisols in Indonesia. Indonesian J. Trop. Agric., 2: 56-65.
Golley, F. B., J. T. McGinnis, R. G. Clements, G. I. Child, and M. J. Duever. 1975. *Mineral Cycling in a Tropical Moist Forest Ecosystem*. University of Georgia Press, Athens, GA.
Gortner, R. A. 1949. *Outlines of Biochemistry*. (Third edition, edited by R. A. Gortner, Jr., and W. A. Gortner). Wiley & Sons, Inc., New York, NY.
Granli, T., and O. C. Bϕckman. 1993. Nitrous Oxide (N_2O) from agriculture. Bull. Norsk Hydro Research Centre, Porsgrunn, Norway.
Harley, J. L. 1969. *The Biology of Mycorrhiza*. 2nd edition. Leonard Hill, London.
Harpstead, D. D. 1975. Man-molded cereal-hybrid corn's story. pp. 213-224. In: *That We May Eat*. The Yearbook of Agriculture. USDA., U.S. Govern. Printing Office, Washing-

ton, DC.

Havelka, U. D., M. G. Boyle, and R. W. F. Hardy. 1982. Biological nitrogen fixation. pp. 365-422. In: *Nitrogen in Agricultural Soils*, F. J. Stevenson (ed). Am. Soc. Agronomy, Madison, WI.

Henderson-Sellers, A. 1987. Effects of change in land use on climate in the humid tropics. pp. 463-496. In: *The Geophysiology of Amazonia. Vegetation and Climate Interactions*. R. E. Dickinson (ed). Wiley & Sons, New York, NY.

Herrera, R. A. 1979. Nutrient distribution and cycling in an Amazon Caatinga forest on Spodosols in southern Venezuela. Thesis, University of Reading, England.

Hewitt, E. J. 1966. Sand and water culture methods used in the study of plant nutrition. Techn. Comm. No. 22 (revised). Commonwealth Agric. Bureaux, Maidstone, Kent, England.

Hoagland, D. R., and D. I. Arnon. 1950. The water-culture method for growing plants without soil. University of California, Agric. Expt. Stn. Cir. 347. Berkeley, CA.

Hrubrant, G. R., R. V. Daugherty, and R. A. Rhodes. 1972. Entero-bacteria in feedlot waste and runoff. Appl. Microbiol., 24: 378-383.

Hu Han and Shao Qiquan. 1981. Advances in plant cell and tissue culture in China. Advances in Agronomy, 34: 1-13.

Hunt, C. B. 1972. *Geology of Soils. Their Evolution, Classification, and Uses*. Freeman and Co., San Francisco, CA.

Hunter, C., and E. M. Rich. 1925. The effect of artificial aeration of the soil on *Impatiens balsamina* L. New Phytol., 24: 257-271.

Hurlbut, Jr., C. S., and C. Klein. 1977. *Manual of Mineralogy* (after James D. Dana). Wiley & Sons, New York, NY.

Hutchinson, G.E. 1944. Nitrogen in the biochemistry of the atmosphere. Am. Scientist, 32: 178-195.

Inoue, K., and P. M. Huang. 1984. Influence of citric acid on the

natural formation of imogolite. Nature (London), 308: 58-60.
Irianto, B. 1991. Effect of humic acid on tissue culture of slash pine (*Pinus elliottii* Engelm.). M.S. Thesis, University of Georgia, Athens, GA.
Irianto, B., and K. H. Tan. 1993. Effect of humic acid on callus culture of slash pine (*Pinus elliottii* Engelm). J. Plant Nutrition, 16: 1109-1118.
Jackson, T. A. 1975. Humic matter in natural waters and sediments. Soil Sci., 119: 56-64.
Jenny, H. 1941. *Factors of Soil Formation*. McGraw-Hill, New York, NY.
Jensen, H. L. 1965. Nonsymbiotic nitrogen fixation. pp. 436-480. In: *Soil Nitrogen*. W. V. Bartholomew and F. E. Clark (eds). Agronomy series 10. Am. Soc. Agronomy, Inc., Publ., Madison, WI.
Jones, J. B., Jr. 1983. *A Guide for the Hydroponic and Soilless Culture Grower*. Timber Press, Portland, Oregon.
Jones, J. B., Jr., B. Wolf, and H.A. Mills. 1991. *Plant Analysis Handbook*. Micro-Macro Publ., Inc., Athens, GA.
Jones, R. A. 1983. Potential of acid resistant and fungicide resistant *Rhizobium japonicum* strains for improvement of nitrogen fixation in soybeans. Ph.D. dissertation, University of Georgia, Athens, GA.
Jordan, C. F. 1985. *Nutrient Cycling in Tropical Forest Ecosystems*. Wiley & Sons, New York, NY.
Kafuku, T., and H. Ikenoue (eds). 1983. *Modern Methods of Aquaculture in Japan*. Kodansha Ltd., Tokyo, and Elsevier Sci. Publ., Co., Amsterdam.
Kardos, L. T., W. E. Sopper, and E. A. Myers. 1968. A living filter for sewage. pp. 197-201. In: *Science for Better Living*. The Yearbook of Agriculture, USDA, U.S. Govern. Printing Office, Washington, DC.
Keller, W. D. 1954. Bonding energies of some silicate minerals. Am. Mineral., 39: 783-793.
Kellogg, C. E. 1941. Climate and soil. pp. 265-291. In: *Climate*

and Man. The Yearbook of Agriculture, USDA, U.S. Govern. Printing Office, Washington, DC.

King, L. D. (ed). 1986. Agriculture use of municipal and industrial sludges in the Southern United States. South. Coop. Series Bull. 314. North Carolina State University, Raleigh, NC.

King, L. D., and P. M. Giordano. 1986. Effect of sludges on heavy metals in soils and crops. pp. 21-29. In: *Agricultural Use of Municipal and Industrial Sludges in the Southern United States*, L. D. King (ed). South. Coop. Series Bull. 314, North Carolina State University, Raleigh, NC.

King, L. D., R. W. Taylor, and J. W. Shuford. 1986. Macronutrients in municipal and industrial sludges and crop response to sludge applications. pp. 11-19. In: *Agricultural Use of Municipal and Industrial Sludges in the Southern United States*, L. D. King (ed). South. Coop. Series Bull. 314, North Carolina State University, Raleigh, NC.

Kononova, M. M. 1975. Humus of virgin and cultivated soils. pp.475-526. In: *Soil Components*, Vol. 1, *Organic Components*, J. E. Gieseking (ed). Springer-Verlag, Berlin.

Krauskopf, K. B. 1956. Dissolution and precipitation of silica at low temperatures. Geochim. Cosmochim. Acta, 10: 1-26.

Kubiena, W.L. 1938. *Micropedology*. Collegiate Press, Inc., Ames, IA.

Kyte, L. 1983. *Plants from Test Tube. An Introduction to Micropropagation*. Timber Press, Portland, OR.

Ladd, J. N., and R. B. Jackson. 1982. Biochemistry of ammonification. pp. 173-228. In: *Nitrogen in Agricultural Soils*, F. J. Stevenson (ed). Am. Soc. Agronomy, Madison, WI.

Lagerwerff, J. V. 1972. Lead, mercury, and cadmium as environmental contaminants. pp. 593-636. In: *Micronutrients in Agriculture*, J. J. Mortvedt, P. M. Giordano, and W. L. Lindsay (eds). Soil Sci. Soc. Am., Madison, WI.

LaRue, T. A., and T. G. Patterson. 1981. How much nitrogen do legumes fix ? Advances in Agronomy, 34: 15-38.

Lavelle, P. 1984. The soil system in the humid tropics. Biol. Int., 9: 2-17.

Lavelle, P. 1987. Biological processes and productivity of soils in the humid tropics. pp. 175-214. In: *The Geophysiology of Amazonia. Vegetation and Climate Interactions*, R. E. Dickinson (ed). Wiley & Sons, New York, NY.

Lawton, K. 1945. The influence of soil aeration on the growth and absorption of nutrients by corn plants. Soil Sci. Soc. Am. Proc., 10: 263- 268.

LeBaron, H. M. (ed). 1987. *Biotechnology in Agricultural Chemistry*. ACS Symposium Series 334. American Chemical Society, Washington, DC.

Lindsay, W. L., M. Peech, and J. S. Clark. 1959. Solubility criteria for the existence of variscite in soils. Soil Sci. Soc. Am. Proc., 23: 357-360.

Lobartini, J. C., K. H. Tan, J. A. Rema, A. R. Gingle, C. Pape, and D. S. Himmelsbach. 1992. The geochemical nature and agricultural importance of commercial humic matter. The Science of the Total Environment, 113: 1-15.

Loehr, R. C. 1974. *Agricultural Waste Management: Problems, Processes and Approaches*. Academic Press, New York, NY.

Lutz, H. J., and R. F. Chandler. 1947. The organic matter of forest soils. pp.140-197. In: *Forest Soils*, R. F. Chandler (ed). Wiley & Sons, New York, NY.

Mackenzie, R. C. 1975. The classification of soil silicates and oxides. pp. 1-25. In: *Soil Components*, Vol. 2, *Inorganic Components*, J. E. Gieseking (ed). Springer-Verlag, New York, NY.

Manahan, S. E. 1975. *Environmental Chemistry*. Willard Grant Press, Boston, MA.

Marx, D. H. 1969. The influence of ectotrophic mycorrhizal fungi on the resistance of pine roots to root pathogenic fungi and soil bacteria. Phytopathology, 59: 153-163.

Marx, D. H., and S. V. Krupa. 1978. Mycorrhizae. A. Ectomycorrhizae. pp. 373-400. In: *Interactions between Nonpathogenic Soil Micro-organisms and Plants*, V. R. Dommerques and S.V. Krupa (eds). Elsevier Sci. Publ. Co., Amsterdam.

Mason, B. 1958. *Principles of Geochemistry*. Wiley & Sons, New York, NY.

McCalla, T. M., J. R. Peterson, and C. Lue-Hing. 1977. Properties of agricultural and municipal wastes. pp. 11-43. In: *Soils for Management of Organic Wastes and Waste Waters*, L. F. Elliot and F. J. Stevenson (eds). Soil Sci. Soc. Am., Am. Soc. Agronomy and Crop Sci. Soc. Am., Madison, WI.

Meek, B. D., T. J. Donavan, and L. E. Graham. 1980. Summertime flooding effects on alfalfa mortality, soil oxygen concentration, and matric potential in a silty clay loam soil. Soil Sci. Soc. Am. J., 44: 433-435.

Millot, G. 1964. *Geologie des Argiles: Alterations, Sedimentologie, Geochimie*. Masson, Paris.

Ming, D. W., and D. L. Henninger (eds). 1989. *Lunar Base Agriculture: Soils for Plant Growth*. Am. Soc. Agronomy, Inc., Crop Sci. Soc. Am., Inc., and Soil Sci. Soc. Am., Inc., Madison, WI.

Mohr, E. C. J., and F. A. Van Baren. 1960. *Tropical Soils*. Les Editions A. Manteau, S.A., Bruxelles.

Mohr, E. C. J., F. A. Van Baren, and J. Van Schuylenborgh. 1972. *Tropical Soils*. Mouton-Ichtiar Baru-Van Hoeve, The Hague.

Moore, J. W., and E. A. Moore. 1976. *Environmental Chemistry*. Academic Press. New York, NY.

Mori, S. A., and G. T. Prance. 1987. Species diversity, phenology, plant-animal interactions, and their correlation with climate, as illustrated by the Brazil nut family (Lecythidaceae). pp. 69-101. In: *The Geophysiology of Amazonia. Vegetation and Climate Interactions*, R. E. Dickenson (ed). Wiley & Sons, New York, NY.

Murashige, T., and F. Skoog. 1962. A revised medium for rapid growth and bioassays with tobacco tissue cultures. Physiol. Plant., 15: 473-497.

Nutman, P. S. 1965. Symbiotic nitrogen fixation. pp. 360-383. In: *Soil Nitrogen*. W. V. Bartholomew and F. E. Clark (eds). Agronomy Series 10. Am. Soc. Agronomy, Inc.,Publ., Madison, WI.

Odum, H. T., and R. F. Pigeon. 1970. *A Tropical Study of Irradiation and Ecology at El Verde*. U.S. Atomic Energy Commission, Washington, DC.

Ollier, C. D. 1975. *Weathering*. Longman Group Ltd., London.

Orlov, D. S. 1985. *Humus Acids in Soils*. English translation, K. H. Tan (ed). USDA and NSF Publ., Amerind Publ. Co., New Delhi.

Paul, E. A., and F. E. Clark. 1989. *Soil Microbiology and Biochemistry*. Academic Press, Inc., San Diego, CA.

Persley, G. J. 1990. *Agricultural Biotechnology. Opportunities for International Development*. C.A.B. International, Wallingford, Oxon, UK.

Peterson, J. R., T. M. McCalla, and G. E. Smith. 1971. Human and animal wastes as fertilizers. pp. 557-596. In: *Fertilizer Technology and Use*, R. A. Olson (ed-in-chief). Soil Sci. Soc. Am., Inc., Madison, WI.

President's Science Advisory Committee Panel on World Food Supply. 1967. *The world food problem*. Volumes I-III. The White House, Washington, DC.

Rainey, R. H. 1967. Natural displacement of pollution from the Great Lakes. Science 155: 1242-1243.

Raman, K. V., and M. L. Jackson. 1964. Vermiculite surface morphology. Clays Clay Miner., 12: 423-429.

Reitz, L. P. 1968. Short wheats stand tall. pp. 236-239. In: *Science for Better Living*. The Yearbook of Agriculture. USDA, U.S. Govern. Printing Office, Washington, DC.

Rovira, A. D., and C. B. Davey. 1974. Biology of the rhizosphere. In: *The Plant Root and its Environment*, E.W. Carson (ed).

University Press of Virginia, Charlottesville, VA.

Ryther, J. H., and J. E. Bardach. 1968. The Status and Potential of Aquaculture. Clearinghouse for Federal Scientific and Technical Information, P.B. 177. Springfield, VA.

Sander, D. 1969. *Orchids and their Cultivation*. Blandford Press, London.

Schnitzer, M., and S. U. Khan. 1972. *Humic Substances in the Environment*. Marcel Dekker, Inc., New York, NY.

Shell, E. W. 1975. A fish story pans out and world is better fed. pp. 149-156. In: *That We May Eat*. The Yearbook of Agriculture. USDA, House document No. 94-4. U.S. Govern. Printing Office, Washington, D.C.

Singer, A. 1979. Clay mineral formation. pp. 76-82. In: *The Encyclopedia of Soil Science*, Part 1, R. W. Fairbridge and C. W. Finkl, Jr. (eds). Dowden, Hutchinson and Ross, Stroudsburg, PA.

Smith, J., and C. Lewis. 1991. *Biotechnology in the Food and Agro Industries*. Special Report No. 234. The Economist Intelligence Unit, London.

Soil Survey Staff. 1951. *Soil Survey Manual*. USDA Agric. Handbook No. 18. U.S. Govern. Printing Office, Washington, DC.

Soil Survey Staff. 1975. *Soil Taxonomy. A Basic System of Soil Classification for Making and Interpreting Soil Surveys*. USDA Agric. Handbook No. 436. U.S. Govern. Printing Office, Washington, D.C.

Soil Survey Staff. 1990. *Keys to Soil Taxonomy*. AID, USDA, Soil Management Support Services, Monograph No. 19. Virginia Polytech. and State University, Blacksburg, VA.

Soil Survey Staff. 1992. *Keys to Soil Taxonomy*. AID, USDA, SCS, SMSS Techn. Monograph No. 19, fifth edition. Pocahontas Press, Inc., Blacksburg, VA.

Stevenson, F. J. 1967. Organic acids in soils. pp. 119-146. In: *Soil Biochemistry*, Vol. 1, A. D. McLaren and G. W. Peterson (eds). Marcel Dekker, Inc., New York, NY.

Stevenson, F. J. 1982. *Humus. Chemistry, Genesis, Composition, Reaction*. Wiley Intersci., New York, NY.

Stevenson, F. J. 1986. *Cycles of Soil Carbon, Nitrogen, Phosphorus, Sulfur, Micronutrients*. Wiley Intersci., New York, NY.

Stewart, J. W. B., R. F. Follett, and C. V. Cole. 1987. Integration of organic matter and soil fertility concepts into management decisions. pp. 1-8. In: *Soil Fertility and Organic Matter as Critical Components of Production Systems*, R. Follett (chair). Soil Sci. Soc. Am., Inc., and Am. Soc. Agronomy, Inc., Publ., Madison, WI.

Sticher, H., and R. Bach. 1966. Fundamentals in the chemical weathering of silicates. Soils Fertilizers (Harpenden), 29: 321-325.

Stoops, G., and H. Eswaran (eds). 1986. *Soil Micromorphology*. Van Nostrand Reinhold Co., New York, NY.

Tan, K. H. 1965. The Andosols in Indonesia. Soil Sci., 99: 375-378.

Tan, K. H. 1982. *Principles of Soil Chemistry*. Marcel Dekker, Inc., New York, NY.

Tan, K. H. 1984. *Andosols*. Van Nostrand Reinhold Co., New York, NY.

Tan, K. H. 1986. Degradation of soil minerals by organic acids. pp. 1-27. In: *Interactions of Soil Minerals with Natural Organics and Microbes*, P. M. Huang and M. Schnitzer (eds). Soil Sci. Soc. Am. Special Publ. No.17. Soil Sci. Soc. Am., Inc., Madison, WI.

Tan, K. H. 1993. *Principles of Soil Chemistry*. Second Edition. Marcel Dekker, Inc., New York, NY.

Tan, K. H., and A. Binger. 1986. Effect of humic acid on aluminum toxicity in corn plants. Soil Sci., 14: 20-25.

Tan, K. H., L. D. King, and H. D. Morris. 1971. Complex reactions of zinc with organic matter extracted from sewage sludge. Soil Sci. Soc. Am. Proc., 35: 748-751.

Tan, K. H., and R. A. McCreery. 1975. Humic acid complex

formation and intermicellar adsorption by bentonite. pp. 629-641. In: *Proc. Intern. Clay Conf.*, S. W. Bailey (ed). Mexico City, Mexico. Applied Publ. Ltd., Wilmette, IL.

Tan, K. H., V. G. Mudgal, and R. A. Leonard. 1975. Adsorption of poultry litter extracts by soil and clay. Env. Sci. & Techn., 9: 132-135.

Taylor, S. A., and G. L. Ashcroft. 1972. *Physical Edaphology.* Freeman and Co., San Francisco, CA.

Theng, B. K. G. (ed). 1980. *Soils with Variable Charge.* New Zealand Soil Sci. Soc., Soil Bureau, D.S.I.R., Lower Hutt, New Zealand.

Thorp, J., and G. D. Smith. 1949. Higher categories of soil classification. Soil Sci., 67: 117-126.

Tiddens, A. 1990. *Aquaculture in America. The Role of Science, Government, and the Entrepreneur.* Westview Press, Boulder, CO.

Tisdale, S. L., and W. L. Nelson. 1975. *Soil Fertility and Fertilizers.* MacMillan Publ. Co., Inc., New York, NY.

Tisdale, S. L., W. L. Nelson, J. D. Beaton, J. L. Havlin. 1993. *Soil Fertility and Fertilizers.* Macmillan Publ. Co., New York, NY.

Troeh, F. R., J. A. Hobbs, and R. L. Donahue. 1980. *Soil and Water Conservation for Productivity and Environmental Protection.* Prentice-Hall, Inc., Englewood Cliffs, NJ.

Uribe, I. 1975. George Harrar sets off the green revolution. pp. 312-322. In: *That We May Eat.* The Yearbook of Agriculture. USDA, U.S. Govern. Printing Office, Washington, DC.

U.S. Environmental Protection Agency. 1972. Glossary of solid waste management. Publ. GP-1972-3. National Center for Resource Recovery, Inc., Washington, DC.

Van Schuylenborgh, J., and P. L. Arens. 1950. The electrokinetic behaviour of freshly prepared Y- and α-FeOOH. Rec. Trav. Chim. Pays-Bas, 69: 1557-1565.

Van Schuylenborgh, J., and A. M. H. Sanger. 1949. The electrokinetic behaviour of iron- and aluminium-hydroxides and

oxides. Rec. Trav. Chim. Pays-Bas, 68: 999-1010.
Wiegand, C. L., and E. R. Lemon. 1958. A field study of some plant-soil relations in aeration. Soil Sci. Soc. Am. Proc., 22: 216-221.
Wild, A. 1993. *Soils and the Environment*. Cambridge University Press, New York, NY.
World Resources. 1987. A report of the International Institute for Environment and Development, and World Resources Institute, Washington, D.C.
Yoshinaga, N., and S. Aomine. 1962. Imogolite in some Ando soils. Soil Sci. Plant Nutr., 8: 6-13.

APPENDIX A

Atomic Weights of the Major Elements in Soils

Element	Symbol	Atomic number	Atomic weight
Aluminum	Al	13	027.0
Antimony	Sb	51	121.8
Argon	Ar	18	039.9
Arsenic	As	33	074.9
Barium	Ba	56	137.3
Beryllium	Be	04	009.0
Bismuth	Bi	83	209.0
Boron	B	05	010.8
Bromine	Br	35	079.9
Calcium	Ca	20	040.1
Carbon	C	06	012.0
Cesium	Cs	55	132.9
Chlorine	Cl	17	035.5
Chromium	Cr	24	052.0
Cobalt	Co	27	058.9
Copper	Cu	29	063.5
Fluorine	F	09	019.0
Gallium	Ga	31	069.7
Germanium	Ge	32	072.6
Gold	Au	79	197.0
Helium	He	02	004.0
Hydrogen	H	01	001.0
Iodine	I	53	126.9
Iridium	Ir	77	192.2
Iron	Fe	26	055.9
Krypton	Kr	36	083.8

Element	Symbol	Atomic number	Atomic weight
Lanthanum	La	57	138.9
Lead	Pb	82	207.2
Lithium	Li	03	006.9
Magnesium	Mg	12	024.2
Manganese	Mn	25	054.9
Mercury	Hg	80	200.6
Molybdenum	Mo	02	095.9
Nickel	Ni	28	058.7
Nitrogen	N	07	014.0
Oxygen	O	08	016.0
Phosphorus	P	15	031.0
Platinum	Pt	78	195.1
Potassium	K	19	039.1
Radon	Rn	86	222.0
Radium	Ra	88	226.1
Rhodium	Rh	45	102.9
Rubidium	Rb	37	085.5
Selenium	Se	34	079.0
Silicon	Si	14	028.1
Silver	Ag	47	107.9
Sodium	Na	11	023.0
Strontium	Sr	38	087.6
Sulfur	S	16	032.1
Tantalum	Ta	03	180.9
Tellurium	Te	52	127.6
Thallium	Tl	81	204.4
Thorium	Th	90	232.1
Tin	Sn	50	118.7
Titanium	Ti	22	047.9
Tungsten	W	74	183.9
Uranium	U	92	238.0
Vanadium	V	23	050.9
Xenon	Xe	54	131.3

Element	Symbol	Atomic number	Atomic weight
Yttrium	Y	39	088.9
Zinc	Zn	30	065.4
Zirconium	Zr	40	091.2

APPENDIX B

International System of Units (SI)

Basic unit	Symbol
Ampere (electrical current)	A
Candela (luminous intensity)	cd
Kelvin (thermodynamic temperature)	K
Kilogram (mass)	kg
Meter (length)	m
Mole (amount of substance)	mol
Second (time)	s

Factors for Converting U.S. Units into SI Units

U.S. unit	SI unit	To obtain SI unit multiply U.S. unit by
Acre	Hectare, ha	0.405
Acre	Square meter, m^2	4.05×10^3

U.S. unit	SI unit	To obtain SI unit multiply U.S. unit by
Ångstrom	Nanometer, nm	10^{-1}
Atmosphere	Megapascal, MPa	0.101
Bar	Megapascal, MPa	10^{-1}
Calorie	Joule, J	4.19
Cubic foot	Liter, L	28.3
Cubic inch	Cubic meter, m^3	1.64×10^{-5}
Curie	Becquerel, Bq	3.7×10^{10}
Degrees, °C (+273, temperature)	Degrees, K	1
Degrees, °F (-32,temperature)	Degrees, °C	0.556
Dyne	Newton, N	10^{-5}
Erg	Joule, J	10^{-7}
Foot	Meter, m	0.305
Gallon	Liter, L	3.78
Gallon per acre	Liter per ha	9.35
Inch	Centimeter, cm	2.54
Micron	micrometer, µm	1
Mile	Kilometer, km	1.61
Mile per hour	Meter per second	0.477
Millimho per cm	decisiemens per m, dS m^{-1}	1
Ounce (weight)	Gram, g	28.4
Ounce (fluid)	Liter, L	2.96×10^{-2}
Pint	Liter, L	0.473
Pound	Gram, g	454
Pound per acre	Kilogram per ha	1.12
Pound per cubic foot	Kilogram per m^3	16.02
Pound per square foot	Pascal, Pa	47.9
Pound per square inch	Pascal, Pa	6.9×10^3
Quart	Liter, L	0.946
Square foot	Square meter, m^2	9.29×10^{-2}
Square inch	Square cm, cm^2	6.45

U.S. unit	SI unit	To obtain SI unit multiply U.S. unit by
Square mile	Square kilometer, km^2	2.59
Ton (2000 lbs)	Kilogram, kg	907
Ton per acre	Megagram per ha	2.24

APPENDIX C

U.S. Weights and Measures

LAND MEASURE

1 foot	12 inches
1 yard	3 feet
1 mile	5280 feet
1 mile	1760 yards
1 square foot	144 square inches
1 square yard	9 square foot
1 square mile	640 acres
1 acre	4840 square yards
1 acre	43 560 square feet

AVOIRDUPOIS WEIGHT

(Used in weighing all articles except drugs, gold, silver and precious stones)

1 pound, lb	16 ounces
1 hundredweight (cwt)	100 lbs
1 ton	20 cwt
1 ton	2000 lbs
1 long ton	2240 lbs

TROY WEIGHT (Used in weighing gold, silver and precious stones)

1 pound, lb	12 ounces

DRY MEASURE

1 quart	2 pints
1 bushel	32 quarts

LIQUID MEASURE

1 quart	2 pints
1 gallon	4 quarts
1 barrel	31.5 gallons

FLUID MEASURE

1 fluid dram	60 minims
1 fluid ounce	8 fluid drams
1 pint	16 fluid ounce
1 gallon	8 pints

GRAIN WEIGHTS PER BUSHEL

Barley	48 lbs
Beans	60 lbs
Bran	20 lbs
Buckwheat	42-52 lbs
Clover seed	60 lbs
Corn (in the ear husked)	70 lbs
Corn (shelled)	56 lbs
Corn meal	48 lbs
Flax seed	56 lbs
Malt	30-38 lbs
Millet seed	50 lbs
Oats	32 lbs
Peas	60 lbs
Rye	56 lbs
Wheat	60 lbs

INDEX